MEN'S HEALTH TODAY 2003

PLAYBOOK FOR LIFE: Finish First at the Gym, Score in the Bedroom, Win at Work, and Beat Everything from Heartburn to Heart Disease

Edited by Deanna Portz, Men'sHealth. Books

RODALE

© 2003 by Rodale Inc.

Back-Cover Photographs by Blake Little (top), Mitch Mandel/Rodale Images (center), and Beth Bischoff (bottom)
Spine Photograph by Todd France

Interior Photographs
Pages v (top left) and 1 by Svend Lindbaek; pages v (bottom left) and 53 by Diego Uchitel; pages v (top right) and 101 by Colin Cooke; pages v (bottom right) and 137 by Sally Ullman; pages vi (top left) and 185 by Blake Little; pages vi (bottom left) and 219 by Stefan Nyvang; pages vi (right) and 257 by Peter Berson; pages 3, 4, 55 (left), 56, 139, and 140 by Wendy Hope; pages 12, 13, 15, 16, 17, 18, 32, 33, 37, 38, 39, 40, 41, and 259 (center) by Beth Bischoff; pages 34, 35, and 36 by Todd France; page 55 (center) by Toby Seger; page 55 (bottom) by Fernando Sanchez; page 103 (left) by Christopher Lake; page 103 (center) by Brett Panelli; pages 103 (right) and 104 by Kathleen Dooher; pages 187 (left) and 188 by Matthew Lipton; page 187 (center) by Mike Bednar; page 187 (right) by Lloyd Grotjan; pages 221 (left and right) and 222 by Michelle Pedone; page 221 (center) by Kurt Wilson; page 259 (left) by Scott Robinson; pages 259 (right) and 260 by Annie Etheridge

Illustrations
Page 20 by Paul Mirto; pages 152 and 154 by Jennifer Gibas

Printed in the United States of America
Rodale Inc. makes every effort to use acid-free ∞, recycled paper ♻.

ISBN 1-57954-678-1 hardcover

2 4 6 8 10 9 7 5 3   hardcover

Visit us on the Web at www.menshealthbooks.com, or call us toll-free at (800) 848-4735.

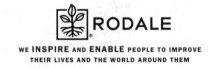

RODALE

WE **INSPIRE** AND **ENABLE** PEOPLE TO IMPROVE
THEIR LIVES AND THE WORLD AROUND THEM

Men's Health Today 2003 Staff

EDITOR: Deanna Portz

CONTRIBUTING WRITERS: Rick Ansorge; Steve Calechman; Adam Campbell; Michael Crowley; Shannon Davis; Debora Dellapena; Ann Marie Dodd; Shelley Drozd; Tracy Erb; Leigh Farr; Kimberly Flynn; Desi Gallegos; Rebecca Gardyn; Gil Gaul; Brian Good; Melissa Gotthardt; Bill Gottlieb; Jennifer Haigh; Kristin Harmel; Brooke Herman; John Hyduk; Karen Jacob; Lauren Janis; Lisa Jones; Chris Kilham; Joe Kita; Alex Koch; Chris Lawson; Jeff Lindenmuth; Matt Marion; Bill Minutaglio; Holly McCord; Katrin McDonald; Christopher McDougall; Colin McEnroe; Sam Neuman; Peggy Noonan; Hugh O'Neill; Laura Ongaro; TN Ooltewah; Francine Parnes; Carol Potera; Steven Raphael; Jessica Rozler; Richard Rhys; Lou Schuler; Nicole Serr; Larry Shadday; Ted Spiker; Laurence Roy Stains; Jeff Stevenson; Bill Stieg; Alix Strauss; Bill Stump; Duane Swiercyznski; Andrew Taber; Neal Thompson; Amy Jo Van Bodegraven; Sara Vigneri; Jonathan Wander; Elizabeth M. Ward, R.D.; Donovan Webster; Kara Wetzel; Mike Zimmerman; Tom Zoellner

ART DIRECTOR AND INTERIOR DESIGNER: Charles Beasley

COVER DESIGNER: Joanna Williams

EDITORIAL RESEARCHER: Bernadette Sukley

LAYOUT DESIGNER: Keith Biery

PRODUCT SPECIALIST: Brenda Miller

Rodale *Men's Health* Books

SENIOR VICE PRESIDENT, MANAGING DIRECTOR: Tom Beusse

U.S. PUBLISHER: Mary Ann Bekkedahl

EXECUTIVE EDITOR: Jeremy Katz

SENIOR EDITOR: Leah Flickinger

ASSOCIATE EDITOR: Kathryn C. LeSage

ASSOCIATE CUSTOMER MARKETING MANAGER: Matt Neumaier

CONTENT ASSEMBLY MANAGER: Robert V. Anderson Jr.

OFFICE MANAGER: Alice Debus

ASSISTANT OFFICE MANAGER: Marianne Moor

ADMINISTRATIVE ASSISTANT: Pamela Brinar

Contents

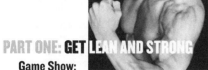

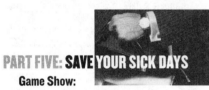
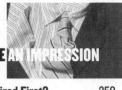

Introduction

Be a Winner

The man who said "Winning isn't everything" may have been content to come in second, but we don't know many guys who are. Whether you're playing a round of golf, picking up a beautiful woman, or pitching an idea at the office, you want to take home the trophy.

It's from that inborn instinct to be better than the next guy that we compiled this book. We jammed hundreds of the latest health and fitness tips, strategies, and life-saving advice into these 296 pages so that your mind and body can easily handle whatever curveballs are thrown your way. Because when it comes right down to it, the *Men's Health* philosophy is simply this: We want you to win at life.

To do that, of course, you must be *alive*. That's why we put together the 46-page bonus section, Beat the Men Killers. We tell you how to ward off the Reaper with blood tests your doctor may not even know about. We warn you about a life-threatening condition that may be suffocating you in your sleep. Plus, we share surprising symptoms you should never ignore.

Sure, we don't want you to die on our watch, but that's only the half of it. We're not content that you merely *survive*. We want you to *thrive*—to be successful at everything you do in life, be it at work, at play, or in the bedroom. Consider *Men's Health Today 2003* your playbook to do just that. Want to land a great job? Be the top candidate with the pointers on page 261. Looking for the love of your life? We'll show you how to win her over. Ashamed to go shirtless at the beach? Lose weight and build a body you can bare with our 8-week program.

That's just the starting lineup. Here are some of the other game plans in our playbook.

- **Cut your training time in half.** Get in and out of the gym fast with six 15-minute workouts starting on page 32.
- **Score big in the bedroom.** Get what *you* want in bed and make *her* beg for more with our 75 steamy sex secrets.
- **Stay on top of your game.** Keep your edge when you're exhausted, with tips from a transplant surgeon who operates for 12 hours at a stretch.
- **Stay off the DL.** Whether headaches or heartburn are slowing you down, feel better fast with the best over-the-counter drugs for the job.

Let *Men's Health Today 2003* make you into a champion at life. We think it's a real winner. We hope you'll agree.

—**Deanna Portz, Editor**

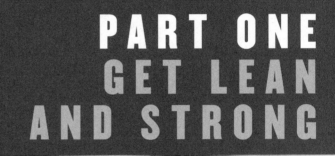

PART ONE
GET LEAN
AND STRONG

GAME SHOW

Who Will Lose 20 Pounds First?

Will one of these guys get rid of his gut? Or will you?

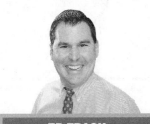

ED FRACK
Age: 39 Height: 5'8"
Waist: 35" Weight: 205

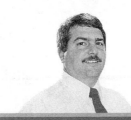

JIM MILLER
Age: 37 Height: 5'7"
Waist: 38" Weight: 226

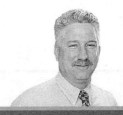

GARY YENCHO
Age: 43 Height: 5'11"
Waist: 40" Weight: 220

HOW HE GOT HIS GUT

• Hectic work schedule and family life make it impossible to exercise and eat well; can't resist doughnuts, chips, candy, beer, sofas.

HOW HE PLANS TO LOSE IT

• No change in diet, but lots of calorie-burning exercise; bicycle to and from work (50 miles per week); swim at least once a week during lunch hour. Promises not to wear a Speedo.

HIS BIGGEST RISK FACTOR

• Dunkin' Donuts is on his way to work. The beer store is on the way home.

ED'S PREDICTION

• "The other two tubs don't have a chance. While they're nibbling carrot sticks, I'll eat what I want and still lose weight."

HOW HE GOT HIS GUT

• Zero exercise and lots of fast food, soda, and 10 P.M. dinners; considers chocolate ice cream one of the four major food groups.

HOW HE PLANS TO LOSE IT

• 2,300 calories per day (60 percent carbohydrates, 25 percent fat, 15 percent protein) spread over four meals (7 A.M. breakfast, 11 A.M. lunch, 3 P.M. snack, 7 P.M. dinner); 75 percent of total daily calories eaten by 3 P.M.

HIS BIGGEST RISK FACTOR

• Staying on the diet while traveling on business. How can you resist the Frank & Stein at Pittsburgh International?

JIM'S PREDICTION

• "Frack is going to drop dead of a heart attack before he drops 20 pounds on his plan. If I can stick to this diet while I'm on the road, I'll be in new pants before all of them."

HOW HE GOT HIS GUT

• No exercise; poor eating schedule (nothing all day, then major feed at night); weakness for meat and pasta; can't resist second and third helpings.

HOW HE PLANS TO LOSE IT

• Jenny Craig's prepackaged meals totaling 1,700 to 2,000 calories per day (60 percent carbs, 20 percent fat, 20 percent protein), walking (20 minutes, four times a week), and private weekly consultation with a program advisor.

HIS BIGGEST RISK FACTOR

• Stigma of going through a program that's named after a woman, for cripes' sake; taste and cost of food (about $80 per week); not having enough to eat.

GARY'S PREDICTION

• "There's no way I can lose. This is a proven program. All I have to do is eat what they give me."

And the Big Loser Is . . .
Jim Miller

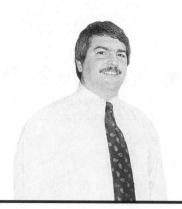

WHY HE ATE THE OTHER GUYS FOR LUNCH

Miller, a former high school lightweight wrestler, dropped 20 pounds in 6 weeks on his front-loaded diet (see below). There are a number of reasons this plan worked so well for Miller, according to Cindy Moore, R.D., director of nutrition therapy at the Cleveland Clinic Foundation and spokesperson for the American Dietetic Association. Those reasons amount to good advice for lots of men.

A simple plan yields the best results. It didn't require Miller to juggle new things in his already busy life. The focus was on making just two behavioral changes: rearranging his meal schedule and eating less.

Do it yourself. Since Miller travels, a program that required prepackaged meals wouldn't have worked for him.

THE FRONT-LOADED DIET

Jim Miller found his meal plan in a past issue of *Men's Health* magazine; it was developed by Nancy Clark, R.D., author of *Nancy Clark's Sports Nutrition Guidebook*. Here's how it would work for a 200-pound guy.

Start the day with a big breakfast: 500 to 600 calories.

Eat lunch 4 hours later: 700 to 800 calories.

Four hours after that—snack time: 400 to 500 calories.

Have dinner 4 hours after the snack: Your last 600 to 700 calories. (For a specific meal plan, go to www.menshealth.com.)

Why It Works

You front-load your calories during the day and end up with 4 food-free hours before bedtime. Add that to 8 hours of sleep, and you're fasting for 12 hours. You'll wake up hungry and eat a huge breakfast, which will help you eat moderately the rest of the day. An empty stomach at night is a flat stomach in the morning.

IF YOU WANT TO LOSE, JUST ASK

1."Is this a diet plan I can follow for the rest of my life, or is it something I'll probably abandon after a few weeks or months?" Although fad diets are often effective in the short term, they're not realistic lifetime eating plans.

2."Does this weight-loss plan incorporate activities I like to do and foods I enjoy eating?" If it doesn't, you're setting yourself up for frustration.

3."Does my dietitian approve of this regimen?" What? You don't have one? If your belly has been growing for years, then you need professional help. Visit the American Dietetic Association Web site (www.eatright.org) or call (800) 366-1655 for a referral. Charges for an initial consultation range from $60 to $100. A bargain.

Replace old habits with healthier ones. Miller taught himself how to eat smaller portions more frequently throughout the day; that kept his appetite in check. And that's a habit that can stick.

For maximum weight loss, add exercise. Moore predicts that Miller will soon plateau and be unable to drop any more weight by simply eating this way. The answer: exercise. It'll increase his activity level and raise his metabolism, so he'll be melting pounds all day long. If he does that, he won't just have won a game show; he will have changed his life.

WHY FRACK FAILED

After an early lead, he stalled at 8 pounds. Here's what you can learn from him.

Don't fall for the common guy belief that if you keep the furnace hot, you can throw in any fuel you want. Exercise without calorie reduction is only half of the equation.

Make sure you have a backup plan. Frack lost his early lead when a week of rain, an unexpected pool closing, and a sale on Pabst derailed his exercise program. The key is to leave yourself no excuses.

Never increase your exercise level more than 10 percent per week. To go from sedentary guy to superathlete in such a short time can result in injury and even death.

WHY YENCHO ALMOST WON BUT IS IN TROUBLE NOW

Yencho lost 15 pounds with Jenny Craig's help, steadily shaving 2 to 3 per week. He liked the food, the convenience, the motivation, and the effects (renewed energy, plus 8 total inches off his hips, waist, and chest). And since his consultations were always private, he never felt like the only bull at the cow trough. But according to Moore, his challenge is just beginning.

When the commercial weight-loss program ends, so do the benefits. For the past month and a half, Yencho hasn't had to think about food. Every week, he met with his advisor, stepped on the scale, picked up his meals, then simply followed the program. He was a robot with a digestive system.

"He's been in an artificial environment," says Moore. As a result, he's in danger of falling back into his old eating habits and regaining the weight.

Make the change part of your life. A common weakness of some weight-loss programs is that the individuals acting as counselors often do not have proper nutrition training. For long-lasting effects, you need to teach yourself how to read product labels, assess portion sizes, and prepare healthful food. In that respect, Yencho is now starting all over again.

AMOUNT OF MUSCLE THE AVERAGE SEDENTARY GUY LOSES EACH YEAR: 1 POUND

FAT HE GAINS EACH YEAR: 1.1 POUNDS

MUST READS

Bust Your Gut

It's simple: If you try this program, you will lose weight

By Lou Schuler

Friend, we need to talk about that gut of yours. We know you're not proud of it. You may crack jokes about how you're aiming for a gold medal in the splash-diving competition at Athens in 2004. But other than the impressive column of water you spew with each cannonball, you know that belly isn't doing you any good. You don't like looking at it in the mirror, women are turned off by it, children ask if you have a baby in there. You have more trouble sleeping than you used to, your lower back hurts, and exercise makes your knees ache.

But the problem is actually worse than that. Much worse.

You see, the fat around your belly is different from fat elsewhere in your body. It's metabolically active tissue that actually functions like a separate organ, releasing substances into the rest of your body that, in excess, can increase your risk of disease.

That's right: Your own belly could be poisoning you.

GUT-CHECK TIME

The notion that abdominal obesity is the most dangerous kind isn't new. Back in the 1940s, the French physician Jean Vague observed that some obese patients had normal blood chemistry, while some moderately overweight patients showed serious abnormalities that predisposed them to heart disease or diabetes. Almost always, the latter patients carried their fat around the middle. And almost always, they were men.

Multiple studies since then have shown that abdominal fat—the cause of the classic apple-shaped body—is more than nature's way of telling you that you'll never become a soap opera star, news anchor, rock legend, or *Men's Health* magazine cover model. It's a sign that your body chemistry is seriously out of whack. There are a number of substances your bloated belly secretes to your heart, liver, and other vital organs. Among them:

Free fatty acids. Released directly to the liver, they impair your ability to break down insulin, which over time can lead to diabetes.

Cortisone. High levels of this hormone are associated with diabetes and heart disease.

PAI-I. This blood-clotting agent increases your risk of heart attacks and strokes.

CRP. This protein inflames blood vessels, making them more susceptible to artery-clogging plaque.

All these chemicals floating around spell big trouble for big-bellied guys. In a study at the University of Alabama at Birmingham, researchers took 137 men of all ages and sizes and used seven different measurements to determine their risks of cardiovascular disease. The single best sign of multiple risks for heart disease? No, it wasn't the guys' family histories or their cholesterol profiles. It was the amount of abdominal fat they carried.

By the way, heart disease and diabetes are only two of the ways belly fat can ruin your health. If you count them all up, you'll find at least 39 different conditions associated with abdominal obesity (40, if you include looking lousy with your shirt off).

THIS WAY OUT

When we set out to create the *Men's Health* Belly-Off Program, the book from which this article is adapted, our mission was simple. We weren't looking for fancy dieting gimmicks. We weren't looking for amazing weight-loss theories. We weren't looking to invent electronic gizmos or miracle pills. We just wanted to create a simple, instinctive, and satisfying eating-and-exercise plan that would attack the fat around any man's middle.

You and your gut will be the judges of how well we did, but if you ask us, we think we hit it out of the park. The diet portion of the Belly-Off Program not only attacks belly fat specifically but also lets you eat regular food while you're at it. And our 8-week workout plan relies on the radical notion that you should do the kind of exercise you like to do.

So keep reading. Following our plan may kill your chances in the Olympic cannonball competition. But your odds of a gold-medal body will skyrocket.

THE FOOD PLAN

Diets generally fail for one of two reasons: Either they're too restrictive about the kind of food you put in your belly, or they too frequently leave you feeling as if you haven't put any food in your belly. In either case, it's usually not long before you have chocolate cruller crumbs on the corners of your mouth.

You won't be sabotaged by either of those problems with the Belly-Off Program Diet, which was created for us by the trainer and nutritionist Thomas Incledon, Ph.D., R.D. Incledon built our program around three simple weight-loss principles.

I. If you want to shrink your gut, get enough protein in your diet. In this case, about 25 percent of calories. Why? For starters, protein makes you feel full and helps you build muscle (which increases metabolism, thereby making it easier to lose weight). Just as important, high-protein diets have been shown to be the best way of attacking belly fat. Consider a 1999 study published in the *International Journal of Obesity*. Danish researchers put 65 people on either a 12 percent protein diet or a 25 percent protein diet. The low-protein dieters lost an average of 11 pounds, which isn't bad. But the high-protein subjects lost an average of 20 pounds—including twice as much abdominal fat as the low-protein group.

2. Get enough fat. About 30 percent of your calories. First, fat helps you feel fuller longer between meals, slowing your appetite. Second, it provides essential fatty acids needed for optimal health. Above all, fat makes you feel you're eating real food, not starving in the land of plenty. Deprivation? Hey, man, you don't need no stinkin' deprivation.

3. If you get enough protein and fat, your total calorie intake should take care of itself. Because you feel full, you won't binge on a can of Pringles and blow your calorie count for the day. The remaining 45 percent of calories in our plan come from carbohydrates—enough to give your palate a full range of tastes and your body a combination of fast- and slow-burning fuel.

HOW TO USE THE DIET

The meals shown here are "templates" that you can vary any number of ways to please your tastebuds and avoid eating the same old thing every day. Follow them and you'll get between 2,400 and 2,800 calories per day. That should provide plenty of calories for all but the most severely obese while allowing most guys to lose fat around their middles at a steady pace. (Don't worry about hitting the numbers on the nose every time. If you exceed your fat quota during lunch, for instance, just cut back a little during dinner.)

Breakfast

- Whole grain cereal or oatmeal (1¼ cups)
- Fat-free milk (2 cups)
- Almonds or other nuts (4 tablespoons)
- Raisins (2 tablespoons)

Total: 591 calories, 29 grams (g) protein, 78 g carbohydrates, 18 g fat

Lunch

- Sandwich made with whole grain bread (2 slices)
- Lunchmeat or canned tuna (5 ounces)
- Reduced-fat cheese (1 slice)
- Lettuce and tomato (2 leaves/2 slices)

- Mayonnaise (1 tablespoon)
- Carrot (1)
- Orange juice (1 cup)

Total: 666 calories, 41 g protein, 71 g carbohydrates, 25 g fat

Dinner

- Meat (pork, chicken or turkey breast, lean beef, seafood) (5 ounces)
- Salad (1 cup)
- Dressing (2 tablespoons)
- Dark green vegetable (broccoli, asparagus, green beans, peas) (1 cup)
- Starch (bread, potato, pasta, rice) (1 slice or 1 cup)
- Fruit (¾ cup)

Total: 379–953 calories, 23–53 g protein, 33–109 g carbohydrates, 12–43 g fat

Floater Meal (Eat this as one meal or split into two snacks.)

- Whole grain bread (2 slices)
- Peanut butter (2 tablespoons)
- Fat-free milk (2 cups)
- Apple (1 medium)

Total: 629 calories, 31 g protein, 83 g carbohydrates, 20 g fat

THE EXERCISE PLAN

Can diet alone help you lose belly fat? Probably. In a 2000 study in the *Annals of Internal Medicine,* a group who only dieted dropped just as much weight (16½ pounds) and just as much belly fat (about 2 pounds) as the group who simply exercised.

That said, the combination of diet and exercise is still the best ticket to permanent gut reduction. The diet-only group in the above study lost less total fat and more muscle than the exercise-only group. What's more, another, very scary study in the journal *Obesity Research* looked at people who had lost 14 pounds on a 28-day crash diet. Five years later, they had regained all the weight, with a twist: All the new weight was fat, whereas they'd originally lost a combination of fat and muscle. And their health had deteriorated in multiple ways, including increased insulin resistance and higher LDL cholesterol.

So what's the best kind of exercise for losing your gut? The short answer is any kind that you'll actually do. But intriguing new research suggests that for many guys, particularly big guys with big bellies, weight lifting may be the best way to lose weight.

In a study published in the journal *Preventive Medicine,* researchers separated a group of people by overall build—thinner or thicker—then put them on a 12-week weight-training program. Slender guys didn't get much benefit from weight lifting, but the guys who were big to begin with gained about 3½ pounds of muscle. The implication: Bigger guys benefit most from weight training.

(If you prefer to exercise on a bike or a running trail—hey, you'll get no argument from us. Go to www.menshealth.com for "The Weights-Hater's Guide to Exercise," an 8-week beginner's guide to aerobic exercise.)

But if you're a weights guy, this is the plan for you. The goal of the program, designed by Canadian strength-and-conditioning coach Craig Ballantyne, C.S.C.S., is to increase energy expenditure while building muscle. Successful gut reduction through weight training combines these two elements. You need to burn calories to lose weight now, and you need to build muscle to increase metabolism and prevent future weight gain.

HOW TO USE THIS PROGRAM

Every week, do three workouts; each should use different exercises and different systems of sets and repetitions. Working three different ways each week ensures that your body takes longer to get used to the workouts and works harder to make adaptations. Hard work elevates metabolism, making you burn more calories between workouts.

Weight. If you've never lifted before, trial and error can determine the amount of weight you'll lift in each exercise. Try to increase the amount by about 10 percent each week.

Cardiovascular work. This program relies on what Ballantyne calls the new cardio. Rather than long, slow, steady aerobic exercise, it calls for you to go hard for short periods, then easy for a minute or two. Do the cardiovascular workout one to three times a week.

Results. While muscle growth occurs after only one training session, it probably won't be visible for about 4 weeks. Fat loss, on the other hand, will be apparent much sooner. As soon as you start expending more calories than you take in, you'll start burning stored fat for energy. With the diet changes and this exercise program, you could lose a pound or two of fat each week for 8 weeks.

THE MONDAY WORKOUT

- Do 10 repetitions of each exercise in a circuit—that is, do one set of every exercise before repeating any of them.
- Start with a warmup circuit, using one-half to two-thirds of the weight you'll use in your actual work circuits.
- Then do one, two, or three circuits, depending on your experience, fitness level, and time allotted. If you're a total beginner, aim for one circuit the first week or two, and gradually build up to three circuits.

SQUAT

(1) Stand holding a barbell across your upper back. Set your feet shoulder-width apart, toes pointed forward, lower back in its naturally arched position, and eyes focused straight ahead. (2) Push your hips backward, as if you were sitting in a chair, and bend your knees until your thighs are slightly below parallel to the floor. Stand back up to the starting position.

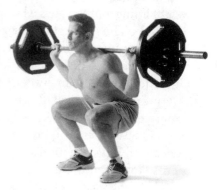

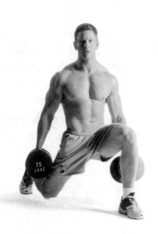

45-DEGREE TRAVELING LUNGE WITH DUMBBELLS

(1) Hold a pair of dumbbells at your sides. With your left leg, take a large diagonal step forward, and drop until your left thigh is parallel to the floor. (2) Stand, bringing your right foot next to your left, and repeat with your right leg. Lunge five times with each leg, then turn and lunge back to your starting position.

BARBELL BENCH PRESS

(1) Lie on your back on a flat bench and grab a barbell with an overhand grip, your hands about shoulder-width apart (or as wide as they would be if you were doing a pushup). Hold the bar over your chin at arm's length. (2) Slowly lower the bar to your chest. Pause, then push the bar back up until your arms are straight and the bar is over your chin again.

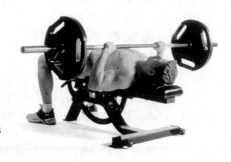

WIDE-GRIP SEATED ROW

(1) Attach a straight bar to a low cable and sit so your feet are braced against the footrest and your knees are slightly bent. Grab the bar with a wide overhand grip, and sit upright so your torso is perpendicular to the floor and your lower back is in its natural alignment. (2) Pull the bar to your lower abdomen. Slowly return the bar to the starting position.

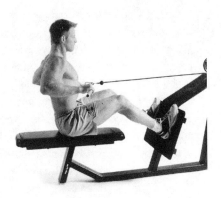

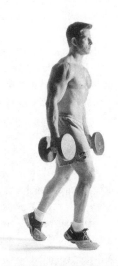

FARMER'S WALK ON TOES, WITH DUMBBELLS

(1) Grab a pair of dumbbells and hold them at your sides. (2) Rise on your toes and walk forward 10 steps with each leg, staying on your toes the entire time. Turn and walk back 10 steps with each leg.

SWISS-BALL CRUNCH

(1) Lie on your back on a Swiss ball, with both feet on the floor, just wider than shoulder-width apart. Your head should be slightly lower than your chest. Place your hands behind your ears and point your elbows out. (2) Curl your rib cage toward your pelvis while keeping your head and neck still. Hold, then return to the starting position.

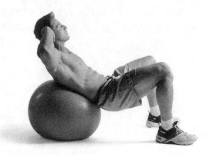

GET MOTIVATED

If you're looking for the reason why American men are fatter than ever, these stats might be enlightening: Fewer than one in five guys exercises long enough or consistently enough to produce any health-enhancing effects. Not that they don't know better—97 percent say they understand the benefits of exercise. Problem is, 50 percent of exercisers bail out within 6 months of starting an exercise program. After 21 months, the dropout rate reaches an astounding 75 percent.

Jim Annesi, Ph.D., an exercise psychologist with the YMCA of Metropolitan Atlanta, has done groundbreaking research on exercise adherence and identified three reasons people turn into quitters: lack of self-management skills (you always find an excuse not to work out); lack of social support (nobody is around to keep you pumped up); and physical discomfort (basically, you just think exercise sucks).

How can you beat those problems? Adopt these survival tactics.

Tell your brain to shut its pie hole. When your brain tells you not to exercise ("The boss is on the warpath, and I'm too stressed to work out"), force a more rational, positive thought into your head: "Exercise will help me relieve stress. I'll feel worse if I don't exercise this week." For every negative thought your brain generates, we bet you can counter with three positive ones. Use 'em.

Mark off the days. After you complete a workout, mark down on your calendar what you did that day. If you perform a cardiovascular exercise, such as running, for 20 minutes, jot down "C-20." If you complete your weight-lifting program, write "WL." This gives you written proof of your accomplishments, which studies have shown is strong motivation and reinforcement.

Give yourself a reward. After an especially good workout, treat yourself to a whirlpool. After a week of consistent exercise, go out to dinner with a friend. After a month, buy yourself a CD boxed set. Or come up with your own plan. A longterm study of slightly overweight men showed that self-chosen rewards helped them reach their exercise goals.

Join a group or work out with friends. A review of 113 studies published in the *Journal of Sport and Exercise Psychology* showed you're more likely to make a lifetime commitment to exercise if you have some kind of social support.

Distract yourself from the pain. Psychologists call this "disassociation." You call it TV. Or music. Or Pilates hotties. No single distraction works for everyone, and studies suggest that multiple distractions may work best to improve exercise adherence. In one study, researchers assigned 56 exercisers to four groups: music only, television only, music and television, and no distractions. The music-and-television group had about half the dropout rate of the three other groups. (They also registered a significantly higher aerobic capacity after a 14-week period.)

THE WEDNESDAY WORKOUT

- Do 15 repetitions of each exercise in a circuit.
- Start with a warmup circuit, using one-half to two-thirds of the weight you'll use in your work circuit.
- Then do one work circuit.
- Finish by doing the cardiovascular workout detailed at the end of this article.

LEG PRESS

(1) Position yourself in a leg press machine with your feet slightly wider than shoulder-width apart and toward the top of the platform. (Use the position that's most comfortable for your knees.) Straighten your legs without locking your knees. (2) Release the supports, then lower the platform until your legs are just past a 90-degree angle. Keep your lower back against the pad throughout the movement. Push the platform back to the starting position.

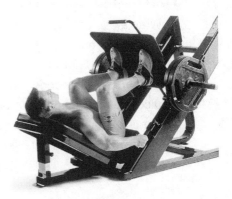

GOOD MORNING

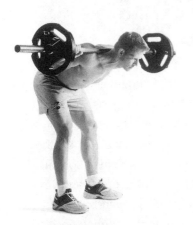

(1) Stand holding a barbell behind your neck so it rests evenly across your shoulders and upper-back muscles. Place your feet shoulder-width apart and bend your knees slightly. Keep your eyes focused forward and your lower back in its natural alignment. (2) Slowly bend forward at the hips until your torso is parallel to the floor. Keep your lower back straight throughout. Raise your torso back to the starting position.

WIDE-GRIP BARBELL BENCH PRESS

(1) Lie on your back on a flat bench. Grab a barbell with an overhand grip, your hands a bit farther apart than for the barbell bench press, and lift it off the uprights. Hold it over your chin at arm's length. (2) Lower the bar to your chest. Pause, then push the bar back up until your arms are straight and the bar is over your chin again.

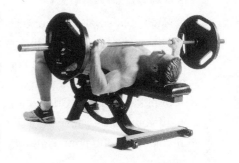

TOWEL PULLDOWN

(1) Wrap a pair of towels around the bar of a lat pulldown machine. Position yourself in the machine and grab a towel with each hand, keeping your hands just wider than shoulder-width apart. (2) Pull the bar down to your chest as you lean backward slightly, keeping your back straight. Return to the starting position.

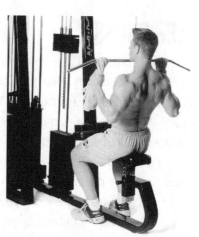

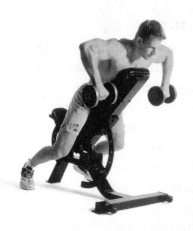

45-DEGREE LYING DUMBBELL ROW

(1) Set an incline bench to a 45-degree angle. Grab a pair of dumbbells and lie face-down on the bench, holding the weights straight down from your shoulders with your palms turned toward your feet. (2) Lift the weights up and out to your sides so your elbows are bent about 90 degrees and your upper arms are nearly perpendicular to your torso. Slowly return to the starting position.

TOWEL CRUNCH

(1) Roll up a small towel and lie faceup on the floor with the towel in the arch of your lower back. Place your feet flat on the floor, put your hands behind your ears, and point your elbows out. (2) Curl your rib cage toward your pelvis, lifting your head and shoulders off the floor. Return to the starting position.

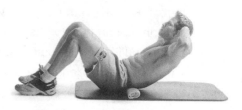

THE FRIDAY WORKOUT

- Do 10 repetitions of each exercise.
- Start with a warmup set, using one-half to two-thirds of the weight you'll use in your work sets.
- Do three consecutive sets of each exercise before moving on to the next exercise.

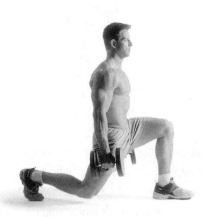

DUMBBELL SPLIT SQUAT

(1) Grab a pair of dumbbells and hold them down at your sides as you stand with one foot about a yard in front of the other, as if you've just taken a long forward stride. (2) Lower your body until the top of your forward thigh is parallel to the floor and your rear knee almost touches the floor. Return to the starting position. Finish the set, then repeat with your other leg forward.

WIDE-GRIP STIFF-LEGGED DEADLIFT

(1) Grab a barbell with an overhand grip that's about twice shoulder-width. Stand holding the bar down in front of you at arm's length and resting on your thighs. Set your feet shoulder-width apart and bend your knees slightly. (2) Slowly bend at the waist as you lower the bar to just below your knees. Lift your torso back to the starting position. Keep the bar as close to your body as possible when raising and lowering it.

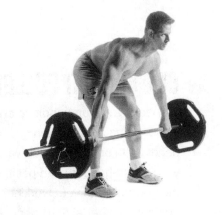

COMPARED TO A NORMAL-WEIGHT MAN, THE AMOUNT MORE MONEY THAT AN OVERWEIGHT MAN PAYS OVER HIS LIFETIME FOR MEDICAL CARE: $4,200

TWISTING DUMBBELL SHOULDER PRESS

(1) Stand holding a pair of dumbbells at the sides of your shoulders, palms turned toward each other, feet shoulder-width apart. (2) Lift the right dumbbell straight over your shoulder as you twist your torso to the left. Lower the weight as you twist back to the starting position, then repeat with your left arm, twisting to your right.

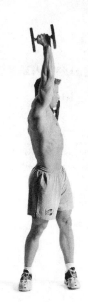

BRIDGE

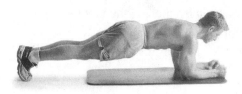

(1) Get into the pushup position on the floor, but rest your weight on your forearms and toes. Keep your back straight. (2) Pull in your abdomen as far as you can—imagine you're trying to touch your belly button to your spine. Breathe as you hold in your abs for 10 seconds. Release and rest for a few seconds. Try to do six repetitions. One set is plenty.

ONE-ARM LAT PULLDOWN

(1) Attach a stirrup handle to an overhead cable. Using an overhand grip, grab the handle with one hand (start with your left if you're right-handed) and position yourself in the machine with your working arm straight up and the other at your side. (2) Pull the handle straight down until it's in front of your chest. Return to the starting position and repeat for the designated number of repetitions. Then, without resting, do the same number with the other arm.

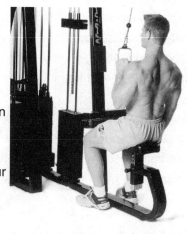

HOW FAT ARE YOU?

For years, obesity researchers used a standard called the body mass index to determine a person's chubbiness and health risk. It's a simple calculation of a person's weight-to-height ratio. To determine your BMI, divide your weight in pounds by your height in inches. Then divide the result again by your height in inches and multiply that number by 703. A number between 25 and 30 indicates you're overweight; a BMI over 30 signifies obesity.

But BMI has one big drawback: It doesn't account for weight distribution. A 5-foot-10-inch, 220-pound couch potato has the same BMI as most NFL running backs.

That's why researchers have begun using waist size—more specifically, the ratio of your waist size to your hip size—to determine health risk. Here's why it's more useful than BMI: Fat that pushes your waist out in front is the most dangerous kind of fat you can have in your body. Exercise attacks abdominal fat, so the more you have, the less likely it is that you get a healthy amount of exercise.

To figure your waist-hip ratio, measure your waist at the narrowest point and your hips at the widest (around your buttocks). Divide waist by hips. Your goal is to fall under 0.92.

CARDIOVASCULAR WORKOUT

- Do any type of aerobic exercise you like, one to three times a week after lifting.
- Warm up for 5 minutes by going at a very easy pace, gradually increasing your effort until you're at 50 percent of your maximum.
- Go as hard as you can for 15 seconds.
- Recover for 2 minutes, returning to the pace at which you finished your warmup.
- Start the next interval, and do a total of six to 10 of them.
- After your last 2-minute recovery, go at an even easier pace for 3 minutes to cool down.

Cut Out the Middle, Man

I weighed 360 pounds and was literally eating myself to death. I had one last chance to save my life: gastric bypass surgery

By Jonathan Wander

Make an "okay" sign with your thumb and index finger. You're looking at the approximate size of my stomach. That tiny circle, the result of gastric bypass surgery, has made an enormous difference in my life. It's taken me from 360 pounds to 180, from a 60-inch waist to a 36, and from a four-door sedan to a cherry red convertible.

My journey into fatness began around age 7, when I started stretching the seams of my Sears Husky Boys pants. My parents weren't heavy and I had no siblings, so I got the milk and cookies all to myself. I began reaching adult weight by the time I was in seventh grade, and I practically had to oil myself to squeeze into the school desk. Gym class was a nightmare—I couldn't run (the teacher used to make me race against a kid who had one leg), and just the anticipation of a game of basketball would make me break out in a cold sweat. At our school, the teams would be "shirts against skins," and if you're a 12-year-old boy with breasts, you'd rather die than suffer the embarrassment of running up the court topless.

By 10th grade, I was over 200 pounds. In addition to Hershey bars and Wendy's double burgers, I also lusted after girls. But as much as girls don't want to be fat, they absolutely don't want to date fat.

In high school and college (where I reached the magical 300-pound mark), I had a couple of girlfriends, but mostly I had girl friends who wanted advice on, of course, their boyfriends. Like many fat guys, I simply shut down the libidinous part of myself. One pathetic example: In college, I took a trip to Manhattan and had one night solo, the perfect opportunity to indulge in some primal pleasure. A night at Scores just wouldn't have done it. Instead, I was in my hotel room, alone with . . . a pastrami sandwich from the Carnegie Deli.

To be that fat was to be constantly self-conscious and uncomfortable. Never let 'em see you sweat? My thick casing of insulation meant I always felt trapped in my own personal sauna. At job interviews (wearing my too-tight

HOW GASTRIC BYPASS WORKS

First, a new, tiny stomach is cut away from the old feedbag. This will make a former gorger feel full after only a few bites. Second, the duodenum and jejunum—two segments of the small intestine—are bypassed, keeping extra calories from being absorbed and turned into belt-busting lard.

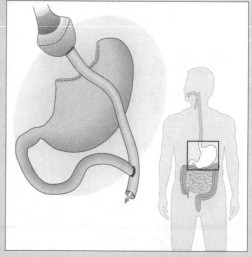

sport coat and tie), I'd feel sweat dot my forehead and occasionally run down my cheek, and I would instantly recognize the look from across the desk: "You are just not the image we want for our company." I got the same look when talking to women. Carrying around more than 100 extra pounds was a burden on my heart, physically and emotionally.

Of course, after depressing and humiliating experiences like these, a guy needs some comfort. So on the way home from an interview, or any other fat-related rejection, I would hit the drive-thru and get a Big Mac, a Quarter Pounder, two small orders of fries, and a chocolate shake. (Two small fries? I always hoped this would fool the drive-thru person into thinking the order was for two people.) When I got home, I would top off the tank with some ice cream and cookies. Anybody see a cycle here?

The only thing more frustrating than being fat was trying to get thin. I tried eating grapefruit before every meal, all carbs, no carbs, high protein, low protein, liquid diets (twice), and injection with the urine of pregnant women. (In the 1970s, injecting HCG, a hormone extracted from pregnant women's pee, was the latest groovy diet aid.) I ventured into more legitimate approaches, too—Weight Watchers, NutriSystem, and Overeaters Anonymous, where I tried, but failed, to admit I was Powerless over Pizza.

It was through one of these dieting attempts that I met my first wife. We were both at the lower end of our yo-yo weight patterns, and throughout our marriage our weight went up and down, sometimes in sync, sometimes not. As with any relationship in which both people are addicted to something (food, booze, cigarettes), attempts to get unhooked led to either support or sabotage. When both of us were determined to succeed, the teamwork was great. But when one of us was ready to fall off the wagon, we could drag the other off, too.

As the years ticked by, the scale clicked higher. But at least my health, for the most part, was good. A heart palpitation here, some pain in the knees there, but my blood pressure was surprisingly normal, and I wasn't having much shortness of breath, lower-back pain, or any of the other usual symptoms of being (I still hate this term) "morbidly obese."

My big wake up came during a routine visit to my doctor, Ed Miller, in 1998. I stepped on the standard doctor's scale, ready to watch the numbers climb once again . . . but this time the numbers couldn't climb any higher. The scale's 350-pound max wasn't enough to weigh me. When the nurse told Dr. Miller, the two of them went to another exam room and wheeled in a second scale (as others watched, of course). I was shocked, scared, and red-faced with complete humiliation. They put the two scales side by side and had me step up, one foot on each. The result wasn't exact, but it at least gave a rough idea of my weight. One thing, though, was perfectly clear: My run of moderately good health was sure not to last. I was approaching 40, heart disease and diabetes ran in my family, and I couldn't recall seeing many old men schlepping around 360 pounds.

"You've tried everything else, so you might as well go all the way," Dr. Miller said, and he recommended obesity surgery. He told me about the gastric bypass, a surgery that would forever alter my plumbing so that I absolutely had to lose weight and keep it off.

A DETOUR AROUND MY DUODENUM

How does a gastric bypass work? Two answers: restricted food intake and malabsorption. With Roux-en-Y (pronounced roo-en-wy), the most popular

HOW TO HANDLE A BIG LOSS

Gastric bypass surgery may be the most extreme answer to obesity, but it isn't the only option for the desperately fat. Here are five other weight-loss last resorts.

Prescription drugs. There are two: Meridia, which affects the brain chemicals serotonin and norepinephrine to help you feel full longer, and Xenical, which reduces fat absorption by blocking digestive enzymes. While Meridia seems to be more effective—researchers found it lowered people's body mass indexes (BMIs) 4 percent more than Xenical—the watchdog group Public Citizen recently asked the FDA to ban it because of dangerous blood pressure spikes. Xenical's own nasty side effect—oily anal discharge—can be minimized with Metamucil.

Very low calorie diets. These "crash diets" allow 800 or fewer calories per day—about a third of a man's normal intake—and are sometimes prescribed for people with BMIs of 30 or more who've failed at conventional diet and exercise programs. In a Dutch study, men following a very low calorie diet lost an average of 19 pounds in 6 months. Which is fine if you're just trying to fit into your tux on wedding day. But the honeymoon will be short. "Patients typically end up regaining all the weight they lose," says Matthew

Hulver, Ph.D., an obesity researcher at East Carolina University.

Liposuction. Fat men aren't the best candidates for liposuction. In fact, the American Society of Plastic Surgeons recommends it only for men with "localized areas of unwanted fat" and says, "It is generally not a suitable method for weight loss."

Vertical banded gastroplasty (VBG). With VBG, staples and a mesh band are used to cordon off a small area of the stomach. But unlike with Roux-en-Y gastric bypass, there's no intestinal rerouting involved. "Long-term data is showing too much regaining of weight, partly because there is no malabsorption factor," says Philip R. Schauer, M.D., director of bariatric surgery at the University of Pittsburgh Medical Center.

Laparoscopic adjustable gastric banding (LAGB). Like VBG and Roux-en-Y gastric bypass, LAGB restricts food intake by sectioning off part of the stomach. The big differences are that LAGB requires only 24 hours of hospital recovery time and that an adjustable band is used, instead of staples. If you're not losing enough weight, the surgeon can go back in and tighten the band to make your stomach even smaller. Still, LAGB isn't as effective as Roux-en-Y.

type of bypass, the stomach is divided into two sections: a tiny pouch for all future digestion and a larger area that will never hold food again. The idea is to make a patient feel full after only a few ounces of food. Next, a Y-shaped section of the small intestine is stapled and sutured to the new stomach to allow food to bypass the duodenum (the first segment of the small intestine) and jejunum (the second segment). Because most nutrients are absorbed by the small intestine, bypassing several feet of this digestive piping means fewer evil calories converted into fat. (There's also less opportunity for nutrients to be absorbed, making daily vitamin and mineral supplements a necessity.)

Due to the length of the operation, a pulmonary embolism—a blood clot in an artery to the lungs—is one rare but possible surgical complication. Intestinal leakage into the abdomen, resulting in an infection, is another. Overall, the risk of death with Roux-en-Y is 0.5 to 1 percent.

Obviously, this is a complex, major operation, a true last resort in the fight against fat. The way Dr. Miller described the surgery, I would have a long, painful incision down my middle, days and days in the hospital, and weeks laid up at home.

Despite my desperation, I balked at the scope (and pain) of the procedure. Not sure what else to do, I ate. Then I did some research online, where I discovered another option: A local surgeon was performing Roux-en-Y using a laparoscope rather than the more invasive "open method."

A laparoscope is a fiber-optic video camera that's inserted through a small incision to show a patient's innards on several television monitors. This makes it possible to perform a gastric bypass from "inside" the body; the surgeon simply makes five or six tiny incisions in the abdomen and inserts his surgical instruments through the holes, using the monitors to guide him. The result is minimal post-op pain, only a few days in the hospital, and a return to work in just 2 to 3 weeks. I made my decision. Dr. Miller checked out the surgeon, and I was on my way.

It turned out that the local surgeon I'd stumbled upon was one of the best. Forty-one-year-old Philip R. Schauer, M.D., is the director of bariatric surgery at the University of Pittsburgh Medical Center. With approximately 1,000 gastric bypass surgeries to his credit, he's a leader in his field. Tall, with dark hair and blue eyes, he's also the object of a crush for every female patient he's treated. And that's one big fan club: More than 80 percent of Dr. Schauer's bypass patients are women. "Women are usually first to try a method of treating obesity," he says. "Men tend to get in touch with us when they're older and the health problems of their obesity have caught up with them."

THE FEAST BEFORE THE FAMINE

The doctors tell you not to overeat during the days before the bypass. "Overeating prior to surgery can adversely alter glucose metabolism and lead to post-op complications," says Dr. Schauer. But how could I help it? Just the thought of that little stomach was enough to send me into food panic. Instead of looking forward to being thin, I obsessed about how in a few weeks the overeating that had given me comfort and pleasure for so many years was about to be gone for good. Unlike with a diet, a gastric bypass doesn't let you hop off the wagon for a Super Bowl binge or a cruise ship gorge-athon. It's a lifelong chastity belt around your gullet, and only your surgeon has the key. (The surgery can be reversed, but that's rarely requested.)

My 2 weeks before surgery became a fortnight of Last Suppers—Baskin-Robbins, steak and baked potato, pumpkin pie, Pittsburgh favorites like fries from the Original, pizza from Mineo's, and a Primanti's sandwich. And it even meant a pilgrimage, a trip from Pittsburgh to Corky & Lenny's, just outside Cleveland, for some real deli food. (Pittsburghers usually avoid the trip to Cleveland, unless it's Steelers fans going to "take care of" some Browns fans.) Yes, I spent hours on the turnpike just to gorge myself on a meal of stuffed kishke, corned beef, cheesecake, and matzoh balls. Now my stomach is about one-third the size of one of those matzoh balls.

The actual day of the bypass meant early rising, a shower, and off to UPMC and la-la land, for my life to be saved and changed. My operation took Dr. Schauer more than 5 hours to perform (including some extra time because I also had a diseased gallbladder to remove). That was 4 years ago. Today, hundreds of surgeries later, Dr. Schauer can complete a Roux-en-Y bypass in as little as an hour.

The few days after surgery were, amazingly, no big deal. As advertised, the laparoscopic method left me with little need for painkillers and just a few buttonhole incisions, instead of one as tall as this book's spine. Still, there was no denying that my gut had just undergone a major renovation. The replumbing, stapling, and stitching were so extensive that my new digestive system needed to be slowly eased back into eating. So Dr. Schauer prescribed a three-phase diet regimen: Phase 1 (first 2 weeks) was liquid; phase 2 (weeks 3 through 6) was pureed and soft stuff, like yogurt and canned fruit; and finally, phase 3 was real American solid food.

Phase 1 went pretty well, both physically and psychologically. I say psychologically because I tend to be a very visual person. It was easy for me to imagine chicken broth and iced tea sliding through my rerouted system. But when it came to the yogurt in phase 2, I was a little shaky. What's more, it had been so long since I'd eaten anything solid that simply holding a spoon was strange. It ended up taking me longer to eat a container of yogurt than it would have to eat an entire pizza just a few weeks earlier. Once I had finished phase 2, real food—chewing food—was on deck. Phase 3 taught me what I'd never known: You're supposed to chew your food before you swallow.

THINK YOU'RE BYPASS MATERIAL?

An estimated 65,000 men undergo gastric bypass surgery each year. To qualify for the procedure (and the insurance coverage), you need to have a body mass index (BMI) over 40, or a BMI of greater than 35 and a related medical condition, such as high blood pressure or diabetes. (See "How Fat Are You?" on page 19 for instructions on calculating your BMI.) You also must meet the following criteria.

• You're between the ages of 16 and 70. (There are some exceptions.)

• You've failed with diet plans and behavioral and medical therapy, including the use of prescription drugs.

• You have acceptable operative risks (that is, your body, including your heart, can withstand the rigors of surgery).

• You're committed to long-term medical follow-up and lifestyle changes.

If all of those apply to you, your next step is finding a surgeon who's done at least 75 bypasses. "Gastric bypass is a complex surgery, and there is definitely a learning curve," says Philip R. Schauer, M.D., director of bariatric surgery at the University of Pittsburgh Medical Center. "Reports are showing that after 75 to 100 surgeries, the complication rates go down." Also, find out if the surgeon is a member of the American Society for Bariatric Surgery at www.asbs.org/html/member/regmem.html; members have to be board-certified surgeons. Last, make sure the surgeon provides nutritionists, counselors, and patient-support groups to help you make the adjustment to life with less stomach and a lot less weight.

THE SEVENTH-INNING RETCH

One of the (many) ingenious aspects of gastric bypass surgery is that the surgeon makes the opening (the stoma) from the new stomach into the bypass much smaller—approximately the diameter of the tip of your pinkie finger. "A small stoma slows down the transit of food into the intestine," says Dr. Schauer. "This gives a sensation of being full for a longer period of time." It also forces you to chew your food completely or risk getting something lodged in the stoma. When your stoma is blocked, it causes a dull but significant pain square in the middle of your chest. (If you're morbidly obese, this can make you think your heart has finally had enough.) Actually, this blockage is usually no big deal. Often the piece will work its way through. But if it won't go down, of course, it must come up.

That's one of the things people hear about most when they start to investigate gastric bypass surgery. "You're having the surgery? I hear you puke your guts out!" The truth is, plenty of people don't vomit at all. Most do so very rarely. I didn't belong to either of those camps. I was a puker, and every wretched retch was my fault.

The best example of this was taking my 9-year-old son, Alex, to a Pirates game. I figured, ball game with the boy, gotta have a dog. But I was too busy concentrating on the action to think about chewing, and a piece of Hebrew National got stuck. This was a bad one. In fact, it was the worst case of stuck-in-the-stoma I ever had. I went to the busy men's room and tried to work it out. No go. I was too uncomfortable to stay at the game, so we headed home midway through. Alex was understanding about needing to leave. The part he didn't like was the drive home. I had one hand on the wheel and the other holding a Pirates souvenir cup, into which I was slowly coughing up my wiener.

One appeal of the surgery is that I can eat practically whatever I want, just not very much of it. The operative word is *practically*. Some foods, particu-

WHERE I LOST MY APPETITE

Before Bypass Surgery . . .	After Surgery . . .
Breakfast	
Sesame bagel with butter; large bowl of Golden Grahams cereal with whole milk	Balance Gold or Myoplex Lite protein bar or 8 oz Dannon Light yogurt
Midmorning snack	
Hershey bar with almonds; package of 6 mini doughnuts; large Diet Coke	Dutch hard pretzel
Lunch	
Big Mac; Quarter Pounder with cheese; 2 small orders of fries; large chocolate shake; large Diet Coke	Half a bagel sandwich with turkey, lettuce, tomato, and mustard, or I slice pizza; Diet Coke
Afternoon snacks	
Pint of toasted-almond-fudge ice cream; 2 or 3 large oatmeal raisin cookies; large bag of peanut M&Ms	Hershey bar with almonds or 4 Snackwell's cream sandwich cookies; fresh fruit
Dinner	
4 or 5 slices Pizza Hut Pan Pizza; salad covered with dressing; side dish of macaroni salad; large Diet Coke	Small piece of grilled chicken; vegetables; small serving of rice or pasta; Diet Coke
Nighttime snacks	
Large bowl of Golden Grahams cereal; bagel with peanut butter and jelly; pint of chocolate ice cream	Kid's scoop of Baskin-Robbins No-Sugar-Added ice cream or half a bag of light buttered popcorn
Supplements	
None	Centrum Performance multivitamin, 1,000 mg vitamin C, 500 micrograms vitamin B_{12}, 2 Viactiv calcium chews, 65 mg iron

larly sweets, can be hard to handle. "Sugars can move too quickly through the intestine to be properly digested, causing 'dumping syndrome,'" says Dr. Schauer. "The effects can include abdominal cramps, nausea, sweating, weakness, and diarrhea." Dumping isn't dangerous, but it is a horrible feeling, as if your entire body were melting and sinking into the ground. When I told Dr. Schauer that too many sweets made me sick, he smiled and said, "Great, I'm glad to hear that." The docs know you can't consume many calories, so they want you to avoid the empty ones.

Other foods, such as red meat and milk products, can cause problems for a few patients, and some vegetables (celery, asparagus, lettuce) can be hard to digest, too, partially because they're stringy and difficult to chew well. And with alcohol, a little bit goes a long way. "Alcohol is absorbed quicker, and relatively small amounts can have a big effect," says Dr. Schauer. He's right—and it can be embarrassing. Recently, I was dining at a fine Italian restaurant and ordered a vodka and tonic. I drank exactly half. When I woke up about 10 minutes later, my face was flat on the table, permitting a nice side view of my Penne Mediterranean.

LIFE WITHOUT THE LARD

Fortunately, puking stopped being a problem early on, and I haven't done it in the past few years. What I have done, though, is lose weight—every pound I had hoped to.

In anticipating the weight loss, Dr. Schauer had said to me, "The bigger you are, the faster you fall." As an example, he said a man who's 5 foot 9 and 350 pounds usually will lose 85 to 100 pounds in the first 6 months, and then 75 to 100 additional pounds over the next year. When I started, I hoped to eventually get under 200 pounds. I now weigh around 180, exactly half the man I used to be.

Of course, the effects of losing weight reach beyond the physical. People treat you differently when you're fat, and dealing with the world from a "normal" perspective takes some adjusting. To start with, women flirt (I never knew!), and that was fun and slightly intimidating at first. There's no more need for self-consciousness, especially when walking into people-filled areas I used to dread, like airplanes. What was never considered a possibility before, or even offered, is suddenly very reasonable. ("Yes, I *would* like to try on that shirt." "Parasailing? I'm in.") And some automatic thoughts need to be changed, like now hoping for a booth at a restaurant instead of a table with chairs.

The effect on the individual of losing so much weight can be profound, and the effect on couples, equally so. Dr. Schauer reports that he's seen couples go one of two ways after one or both lose a significant amount of weight. Some become much closer, and many divide. My wife and I, both of whom were successful patients of Dr. Schauer's, fell into the latter category. Fat can hide more than cheekbones and abs. It can hide years of fatal flaws in a marriage. It wasn't long after she and I lost the bulk of our respective weight that we split up.

I recently remarried. My new wife, Rachel, is an intelligent, beautiful, funny, sexy woman of my dreams. Would she have given me the time of day when I was fat? In her words, "Sorry, but no way. I would have said, 'You're fat. It's disgusting. Go for a walk!'" (You might think this would bother me, but it doesn't. It's the kind of funny, honest, to-the-point remark that's one of the reasons I love her.)

So, am I where I want to be? Not exactly. When you lose half your body weight, your skin can't exactly keep pace. I still have double chins plus (are there triple chins?). And while I'm pretty happy with the way I look in clothes, I'm certainly not thrilled with my appearance without them. The shar-pei look for the thighs—not cool. Basically, the bod is droopy, and no amount of gym time can tighten it to satisfaction. Like many who lose more than 100 pounds, I'll probably be turning to a good plastic surgeon to finish the job.

By itself, losing weight didn't change who I am. But the fat buffer between me and the public world is gone. To be thinner is to be more approachable, and some formerly fat people have difficulty adjusting to this. Some feel "the world" should have given them a chance even when they were fat. A few become intimidated, longing to have their fat back the way a newly released prisoner wishes to be sent back to the security of the cell.

But I was more affected by the expansion of possibilities in my life. Lying in bed at night, I think of spending more years with my wife; having less fear of heart attacks and strokes; and spending better, more active times with my 11-year-old son, my 6-year-old daughter, and the baby Rachel and I are expecting later this year. That child, unlike Alex and Aviva, will never know what it's like to have a fat dad. Buying normal-size khakis at the Gap is great. But these are the reasons why, when I meet now with Dr. Schauer, I feel a lump in my throat from gratitude.

The New Rules of Fitness

It's never been easier to get from where you are to where you want to be

By Lou Schuler

A lot of men know just enough about the rules of fitness to be scared away from starting a workout routine. No pain, no gain? No thanks. But that's why we prefer to do our rule breaking *in* the gym, where it does the most good.

The latest stuff coming down from the physiology labs and exercise eggheads shows that you can make big gains with a relatively small investment of pain and time. If the old rules have left you fat and tired, it's time for some new rules. For a new you.

CHANGE YOUR BODY BY CHANGING SPEEDS

Simply running faster for a minute, then going a little slower for a minute, helps you lose weight faster than moving at a steady pace, according to a 2001 study in *Medicine and Science in Sports and Exercise*. After 10 weeks, those in the study who changed speeds had lost more weight and more fat. Bonus: better thyroid function, too!

Follow the rule: Gradually increase your running speed to one you think you can maintain for 20 minutes or so. Go slightly faster than that pace for a minute, then run a minute at a slightly slower speed. Continue for about 20 minutes, then cool down for 5 minutes. In no time you'll be donating pants to the Home for Middle-Age Fat Runners.

20 MINUTES, TWICE A WEEK

That's all it takes for a major health upgrade, says Bert Jacobson, Ed.D., an exercise researcher and health professor at Oklahoma State University. Jacobson examined the absentee records of 79,000 workers and found that those who did a little exercise had fewer sick days than inactive guys. And here's the really cool part: The twice-weekly exercisers saw the same health gains as those who worked out a lot more. "You don't have to bust your butt to get benefits," Jacobson says.

Follow the rule: If you're not exercising at all, schedule two brisk 20-minute walks a week. Or four brisk 10-minute walks. You can achieve the same results with 10-minute chunks of exercise as you can with longer sessions. Just keep the total exercise time the same.

IF YOU HATE TO JOG, DON'T

Despite the benefits of aerobic exercise, you can reach the same goals through weight lifting and a healthy diet, with a few added dividends: bigger, stronger muscles and bones, a faster metabolism, less fat. In fact, a new study at the University of Wisconsin at La Crosse found that a single session of heavy lifting could increase a man's metabolism for the next 48 hours. (Metabolism goes back to normal half an hour after moderate aerobic exercise.)

PERCENTAGE OF MEN WHO CONSIDER THEMSELVES PHYSICALLY FIT: 69

PERCENTAGE WHO ACTUALLY ARE: 13

Follow the rule: Try strength training with limited rest between sets, which will improve endurance. If you want a fat-burning boost in metabolism, use the exercises that work the most muscle (squats, deadlifts, pullups, rows, and chest and shoulder presses) and rest about 2 minutes between sets.

WEAK ABS CAN KILL YOU

A Canadian study of more than 8,000 people discovered that over the 13 years of the study, those with the weakest abdominal muscles had more than two times the death rate of those with the strongest midsections. Our theory:

FOUR OLD RULES THAT STILL WORK

I. No single program works for everyone all the time. "There are a million experts out there, but no one has the fail-safe recipe that works I00 percent of the time," says Michael Mejia, C.S.C.S., *Men's Health* magazine exercise consultant. The best programs are a mix of styles and philosophies, and anyone who insists there's only one true path to exercise enlightenment—whether it's Tae Bo or Super Slow—is just plain wrong.

"On any new program, you'll make gains during your first month or two," says Mejia. "You just have to remember that nothing works forever. You have to expose your body to new methods, and that's how you keep making gains."

2. Improvements must be incremental. Many new or returning exercisers suffer from Superman syndrome. They run three times one week, then go out the next week and run 6 days. Or, for their second workout, they double the weights they used in their first. Soon they're felled by chronic injuries.

"The development of tendon and ligament strength lags behind the development of muscle strength," says Avery Faigenbaum, Ed.D., C.S.C.S., an exercise scientist at the University of Massachusetts. So your muscles may be strong enough to lift a weight or push you through a run, but your connective tissues may not be ready.

Faigenbaum stresses the I0 percent rule: Never increase volume, weight, distance, speed, or any other variable by more than I0 percent a week. Ignore the rule and you decrease activity to a big, fat zero.

3. Form comes first. No matter what type of exercise you're doing, perfect technique is the key to safety and efficiency. "Especially as you grow older, you have to pay more attention to your form. When you get hurt, your injuries take longer to heal," says John Raglin, Ph.D., an exercise researcher at the University of Indiana. He recommends an occasional tune-up session with a trainer or coach, no matter how long you've been working out.

In fact, a recent study at Ball State University found that men who worked out with personal trainers had bigger boosts in testosterone than those who worked out unsupervised. In other words, you just *think* asking someone for help makes you a weenie. It actually turns you into a sex machine.

4. The more you want, the harder you have to work. Sorry, but there is no safe, easy, fast, foolproof way to get in shape for a marathon, lose 4 inches around your waist, or build biceps like softballs. Those who do the work, and do it the right way, reap the most rewards.

A man who has his abs in balance has won the blubber war. There is no surer ticket to living long enough to enjoy that 401(k).

Follow the rule: A study at Springfield College in Massachusetts found that athletes who did abdominal and lower-back exercises on an exercise ball had much better midsection strength and overall balance than those who did crunches and back extensions on the floor. In other words, get on the ball.

THE HARDER YOU GO, THE HARDER YOU GET

You can attain great health benefits and lose weight without pushing yourself particularly hard. But if you crank it up a notch—turning those brisk walks into slow jogs—your body compensates by using more fat for energy in the hours afterward, according to a new study at East Tennessee State University. "As intensity increases, your body shifts to using more fat after exercise," says Craig Broeder, Ph.D., who conducted the study of men in their mid-twenties.

Follow the rule: The men in the study worked at 60 percent of their maximum aerobic capacity and burned 720 calories in the workout. You can tell you've reached 60 percent of your maximum when you're breathing steadily and deeply. You should be able to speak during these workouts, as long as you keep your comments brief. To burn 720 calories in a workout, a 180-pound man would need to jog for 53 minutes at a 10-minute-per-mile pace.

LIFT FREE OR DIE

The easiest strength exercises—the ones you perform on machines—involve movements that don't translate directly to real-life activities. A study at Georgia State University put older adults on a 2-year strength-training program using exercise machines. The seniors improved their strength an average of 34 percent in the 2 years, but their measures of physical function actually declined 3.5 percent. Over the long haul, machine exercise produces diminishing returns.

Follow the rule: If you're currently using machines, switch to free-weight exercises to improve flexibility and balance. Try these functional moves, suggested by Juan Carlos Santana, C.S.C.S., owner of the Institute of Human Performance in Boca Raton, Florida.

Instead Of . . .	Try . . .
Leg presses	Squats
Leg extensions	Lunges
Leg curls	Romanian deadlifts
Machine chest presses	Dumbbell chest presses while lying on a stability ball
Machine shoulder presses	Dumbbell clean and presses (lifting weights from just above knees to shoulders, then overhead)

Got a Minute? How About 15?

Here are six workouts that get the job done fast

By Lou Schuler

I've heard some good excuses for not exercising. "I'm too tired." "I don't want to get all sweaty." "I just gave birth." They're all understandable—especially the last one, which came from my wife. But there's one excuse you should never use: "I don't have time."

"People perceive that exercise is too low on the priority list. But then you realize that their priorities include watching television 3 hours a night," says John Jakicic, Ph.D., an exercise psychologist at Brown University Medical School.

But let's just say, for the sake of argument, that some of us truly don't have an hour and a half to go to the gym, change clothes, do a full-on workout with warmup and cooldown and three sets of everything in between, take a shower, and then go home or to the office. Let's say some men can't spare more than 15 minutes a day.

What can you do in 15 minutes? Keep reading and we'll show you.

THE 15-MINUTE FULL-BODY FLEXIBILITY WORKOUT

Flexibility doesn't have to mean stretching and yoga and inner peace. It can mean sweat and grunts and a heart-pounding workout. These moves will stretch your muscles in ways that will help you with real-world activities—like yanking lawn mower cords and extracting kids from car seats.

Perform these exercises as a circuit—one set of each stretch immediately after the other—as fast as possible, says trainer Juan Carlos Santana, C.S.C.S., owner of the Institute of Human Performance in Boca Raton, Florida. Do four or five circuits, 20 repetitions of each exercise. Use this as a stretch break on its own, or do two or three circuits to warm up for sports or weight lifting.

ROTATIONAL PRESS

(1) Start with a wide stance, your hands down at your sides. (2) Lift your right arm as high as you can straight above your shoulder and twist your body 90 degrees to the left, lifting your right heel as you turn. Repeat the movement to your left side.

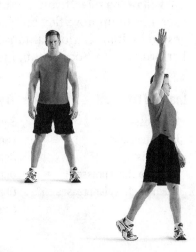

ALTERNATING UPRIGHT ROW

(1) Bend over slightly at the hips until your upper body is at a 30-degree angle from vertical. Look at the floor and let your arms hang straight down from your shoulders. (2) Then lift your left elbow as high as possible, as if starting a lawn mower. As you lower your left arm, repeat the movement with your right arm.

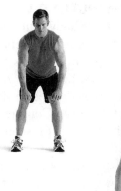
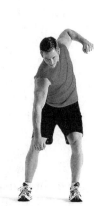

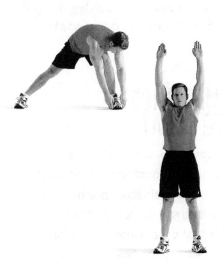

REACHING LATERAL LUNGE TO PRESS

(1) Step to the left with your left leg, keeping the toes of your left foot pointing forward. (2) Bend your left knee about 20 degrees and bend over to touch the toes of your left foot with the fingertips of both hands. Push back to the starting position, then reach as high as you can with both hands. Repeat the movement to your right side. That's one repetition.

PERCENTAGE MORE LIKELY THAT AN OVERWEIGHT MAN WILL DEVELOP HEART DISEASE: 50

PERCENTAGE MORE LIKELY THAT HE WILL DEVELOP DIABETES: 250

PERCENTAGE MORE LIKELY THAT HE WILL DEVELOP HIGH BLOOD PRESSURE: 70

THE 15-MINUTE NO-WEIGHT WORKOUT
Works: Lower body, upper torso

When Adam Archuleta first walked into Jay Schroeder's Evo Sports gym in Mesa, Arizona, he was a 17-year-old kid with average strength and speed and the quixotic dream of becoming a great football player. Last April, Archuleta was drafted in the first round by the St. Louis Rams after twice leading the Pac 10 Conference in tackles. The following no-weight exercises helped him wow NFL scouts by bench pressing 430 pounds and running the 40-yard dash in 4.55 seconds.

This program won't be a 15-minute workout the first time you try it. It'll take a few weeks to build up to that. Once you reach that point, you can add weight to make the moves even more difficult, try the exercises from different angles, or invent your own exercises, using the techniques described here. Schroeder suggests doing this workout 3 days in a row, resting a day, doing it 2 more days, then resting 2. Repeat for the rest of your life, if you want.

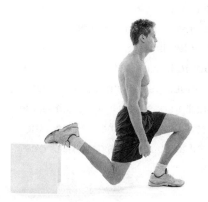

EXTREME-RANGE ONE-LEG SQUAT

Stand with your back to a box, place your right foot on it, and squat down. Hold for 2 seconds, release, then squat down further and hold as long as you can. Repeat until your leg can't take it anymore. Then repeat with your left foot on the box.

EXTREME-RANGE PUSHUP

Set two sturdy boxes 30 to 36 inches apart. Drop into a pushup position and lower your chest between the boxes for 2 seconds. Relax, then repeat, holding as long as you can. Rest a minute, then go down and hold again. Repeat until your upper body begs for mercy.

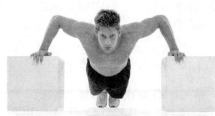

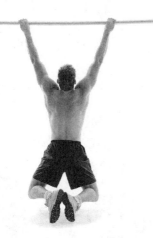

EXTREME-RANGE PULLUP

Using an overhand grip, hang from a pullup bar for 2 seconds. Drop from the bar and relax. Now grab the bar again and hang as long as you can. Drop and rest a minute, then go up and hold again. Repeat until your back refuses to do any more.

THE 15-MINUTE DUMBBELL WORKOUT
Works: Shoulders, triceps, upper back

Forget everything you learned from *Rocky IV*. Most Russian athletes and soldiers of the Cold War era trained with basic iron. But you shouldn't confuse low-tech with inferior results, says Pavel Tsatsouline, author of *The Russian Kettlebell Challenge* (kettlebells are balls of iron with handles; you see them being used in pictures of old-time weight lifters).

These three moves offer two big benefits. The side presses will build your arm strength rapidly, and the other two exercises will work your entire body so intensely you'll burn extra calories during and after your workout. "You'll lose your spare tire quickly," says Tsatsouline, who trained Russian special forces back in the day and now works with U.S. SWAT teams. He recently introduced kettlebells to the U.S. Marine Corps martial arts program.

Try the workout three times a week, using dumbbells (or kettlebells, to keep it authentic; order them at www.dragondoor.com). You can probably use the same weight for each exercise. To keep the workout to 15 minutes, rest as little as possible between sets.

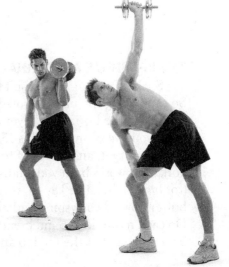

SIDE PRESS

(1) Hold a dumbbell in your left hand, beside your left shoulder. Step forward a few inches with your right foot. Lean over and forward slightly so your weight rests on your right leg. (2) Now push the weight straight up from your left shoulder, then lower it slowly. Keep all the muscles on your left side tensed as you raise and lower the weight. Do three to five sets of five reps.

ONE-ARM SNATCH

(1) Using an overhand grip, hold a dumb-bell between your legs, with your knees bent, back straight, head up, and abs pulled in tight. Your weight should start back on your heels. (2) Swing the weight up until it's straight overhead, assisting the movement by snapping your hips forward as if jumping up from a chair. Do two or three sets of 20 to 30 repetitions.

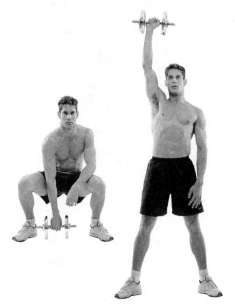

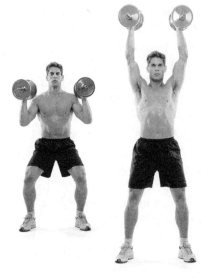

TWO-ARM JERK

(1) Hold two dumbbells at shoulder height, your palms facing your head. (2) Dip your knees slightly and then straighten them as you push the weights overhead. Lower the weights to your shoulders and repeat. Do two or three sets of 20 to 30 repetitions.

THE 15-MINUTE ABDOMINAL WORKOUT

Sucking in your gut doesn't fool anyone—not her, not you, not your tailor. So start using the natural corset you were born with: the transversus abdominis. It's the horizontal layer of muscle beneath your six-pack, and it can make your waist smaller. This 15-minute Pilates workout (no, Pilates is not just for girls—try it, and be ready to hurt) from Terrence Carey, a trainer in New York City, works both your transversus abdominis and your rectus abdominis (for bigger abs). The key to working that transverse layer is to pull your belly button toward your spine and hold it there for the duration of each exercise. Do each move slowly, and breathe slowly. Perform five repetitions of the roll-back and eight of the toe tap and pushup.

ROLLBACK

(1) Sit with your knees bent and your heels on the floor. Keep your torso upright, shoulders back, and arms extended forward, parallel to the floor. Inhale while keeping your belly pulled in. Roll backward, rounding your spine while you hold your chin to your chest. (2) Stop two-thirds of the way to the floor. Exhale and return to the starting position. As you gain strength, roll back closer to the floor.

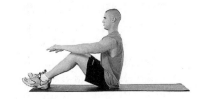

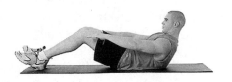

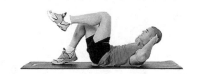

TOE TAP

Lie on your back and place your fingers behind your ears. Lift your legs until your knees are above your hips and your lower legs are parallel to the floor. Press your lower back against the floor and crunch forward until your shoulders are off the floor. (1) With your toes pointed down, lower your right foot as far as you can without lifting your back off the floor. (2) Return to the starting position and repeat with your left leg.

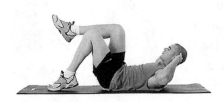

LEG LIFT PUSHUP

Get into the down position of a pushup, your hands in line with your shoulders, about 6 inches away from your body. Set your feet hip-width apart. (1) Push up by straightening your arms. Then raise your left leg as high as you can. (2) Keep your leg raised while you perform a normal pushup by lowering your chest to the floor. Keep your back flat and your body rigid. Switch legs on each repetition.

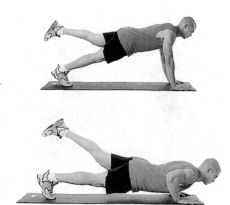

THE 15-MINUTE LOWER-BODY WORKOUT

We don't all need legs like those of America's top speed skater, Casey FitzRandolph. And we certainly don't need his alterations bill every time we buy pants. But we can all gain something from his lower-body training. His regimen is aimed at the muscles around the joints, making them stronger and stabler. "Big muscles don't do you any good if your joints can't support them," says FitzRandolph. So this phase of his workout concentrates on the smaller, stabilizing muscles around your knees. You'll be better equipped to make quick moves and cuts in basketball, soccer, and skiing—with lower risk of injury.

These exercises begin to build overall leg strength, flexibility, and endurance. If you're a beginner or haven't worked out in 6 months, use only your body weight for each exercise. If you've been working your legs weekly, keep the weight light—5- or 10-pound dumbbells, for instance.

Do the workout two or three times a week, with at least a day of rest between sessions. Perform three sets of 10 to 14 repetitions of each move; for the stepups, that means 10 to 14 with each leg.

FRONT STEPUP

Works: Quadriceps, hamstrings, gluteals

(1) The step should be high enough that your thigh is parallel to the floor when your foot is on the step. (2) Place your left foot on the step and push yourself up until your left leg is straight. Your right foot doesn't need to rest on the step. Step back down, right foot first, followed by your left.

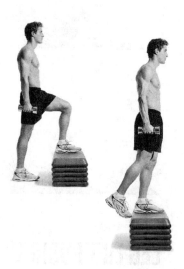

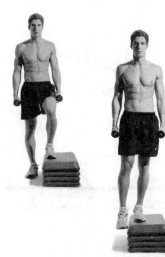

LATERAL STEPUP

Works: Groin, quadriceps, hamstrings, gluteals, calves

(1) Use a step that's about 12 inches high. (2) Follow the same procedure as for the front stepup, but stand sideways next to the step, instead of facing it.

BALL SQUAT

Works: Quadriceps, hamstrings, gluteals
(1) Hold a medicine ball or a basketball between your knees as you perform the exercise. (2) Keep your upper body as straight as possible and lower yourself until your thighs are parallel to the floor. Then return to a standing position. (Squeezing the ball incorporates the muscles of your outer thighs, which will improve your lateral movement.)

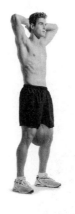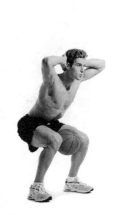

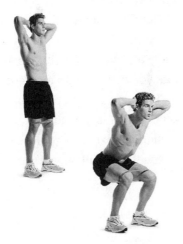

BELT SQUAT

Works: Quadriceps, hamstrings, gluteals
(1) Position a rubber belt, tube, or band just above your knees and push out as you squat. (2) Keep your body as upright as possible throughout the movement, and lower yourself until your thighs are parallel to the floor. Then return to a standing position. (Pushing out on the belt incorporates your hip adductors—the muscles of your inner thigh that help you move your legs toward your body—for better lateral movement.)

THE 15-MINUTE TOTAL-BODY WORKOUT

Do more work in less time at your job, and you get a raise. Follow the same principle in the gym, and you get more muscle. To get strong fast, try this 4-week full-body 15-minute workout from Charles Staley, a strength coach in Las Vegas.

Do five repetitions of the deadlift, immediately followed by five repetitions of the high-cable crunch. Do this a total of five times in less than 8 minutes. Do five repetitions of the bench press, immediately followed by five repetitions of the lat pulldown. Do this five times. Do the workout 3 days a week, using a variation of each exercise (except the high-cable crunch) each day. Each time you work out, add one repetition of each exercise.

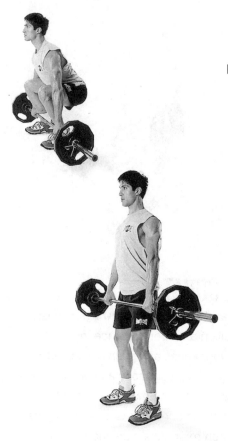

DEADLIFT

Works: Hamstrings, quadriceps, lower back, abs

Monday workout: Stand with the bar against your shins. (1) Then squat down, keeping your back flat, and grab the bar with an overhand grip, your hands slightly wider than shoulder-width apart. (2) Keep your shoulders pulled back and stand with the bar, thrusting your hips forward so the bar rests against your thighs. Return to the starting position.

Wednesday workout: Stand holding the bar as in the Monday workout (2), with your knees slightly bent. Bend forward at your waist by moving your hips backward while your back remains slightly arched. Lower your upper body as far as you can or until it's parallel to the floor. Return to the starting position.

Friday workout: Same as the Monday workout, but start the exercise from the (2) position and squat down into the (1) position.

HIGH-CABLE CRUNCH

Works: hamstrings, quadriceps, lower back, abs

Attach a rope to the high pulley of a cable station. Grab the rope and stand facing away from the machine. (1) Pull the rope down to your chest. (2) Curl your upper body toward the floor until your head is level with your knees. Return to the starting position.

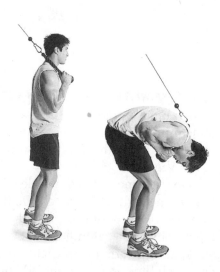

BENCH PRESS

Works: Chest, triceps, shoulders; middle and upper back

Monday workout: Lie on your back on a flat bench, with your feet on the floor. Grab the bar with an overhand grip, your hands about 8 inches beyond shoulder-width apart, and lift it off the uprights. (1) Hold it at arm's length above your chest so that your elbows are directly under the bar. (2) Slowly lower the bar to your chest. Return to the starting position.

Wednesday workout: Same as the Monday workout, but grab the bar about 4 inches beyond shoulder width.

Friday workout: Same as the Monday workout, but this time grab the bar at shoulder width.

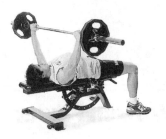

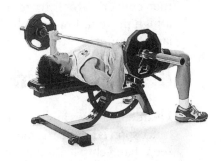

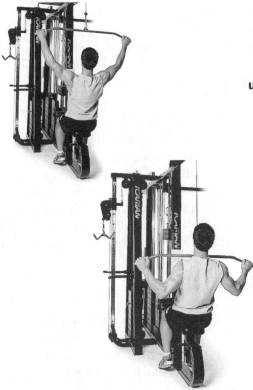

LAT PULLDOWN

Works: Chest, triceps, shoulders; middle and upper back

Monday workout: (1) Grab the pulldown bar with an overhand grip, your hands spread as far apart as possible. Keep your back slightly arched. (2) Pull the bar down to your collarbone as you squeeze your shoulder blades together.

Wednesday workout: Same as the Monday workout, but use a medium-width, underhand grip—about where the bar bends.

Friday workout: Same as the Monday workout, but use a close underhand grip.

KNOW THIS

Protein Power

A new study in the *American Journal of Clinical Nutrition* found that obese men convert carbohydrates to fat faster than lean guys do. This suggests that a high-protein, low-carbohydrate diet may be one of the best ways to shed large amounts of weight.

Get Rock Solid

Bearded Basques and skirted Scots have been lifting stones for ages. Now the fringe sport is found in some American gyms. "Maximum Bob" Whelan, C.S.C.S., keeps hand-chiseled stones and sandbags in his gym in Washington, D.C. "Odd-object lifting"—stones, sandbags, anvils, corpses—"takes a lot of coordination," says Whelan. "It works your back, abdominals, hips, thighs—the core muscles."

For more information, see www.naturalstrength.com. Want stones? At www.atomicathletic.com, you can buy a 100 pounder for $160, or a 365 pounder for just $430. (We saw a good one for free in a culvert off Route 128.)

The Skinny on Living Longer

According to a study from the University of California, the fewer calories you eat each day, the longer you can expect to live. Researchers found that mice on a low-calorie diet lived longer than those with a higher calorie intake. But more important, the researchers also discovered that switching a mouse from a higher-calorie diet to a lower-calorie one eliminated up to 70 percent of all genetic signs of aging that the animal had previously shown. "This suggests that much of the damage from a high-calorie diet isn't permanent and can be rectified by a simple change in the amount you eat," says Stephen Spindler, Ph.D., the study author.

Bodybuilders Beware

A study published in the journal *Annals of Emergency Medicine* found that the compound gamma-butyrocaltone (GBL), which is used as a bodybuilding supplement, causes men to go into severe withdrawal once they stop taking it. Withdrawal symptoms include paranoia, delusions, and hallucinations.

DOWN THE PIKE

No More Gut, No Sweat

Researchers in Scotland are developing a class of drugs capable of fooling your body into thinking it's exercising, even when you're watching TV. The drugs boost metabolism, helping your body burn off stored carbohydrates and fats. The medication could help promote weight loss and reduce diabetes risk.

Junk-Food Tax

In the future, you may have to pay $3 for a Snickers, thanks to a group of food reformers led by Kelly Brownell, Ph.D., director of the center on eating and weight disorders at Yale University. They believe the food industry is largely to blame for America's obesity epidemic.

"Healthy food costs more and is harder to get," Dr. Brownell says. "Unhealthy food is everywhere, and it's cheap. And that should be reversed."

To change the culture, Brownell and friends are fighting for sweeping changes: requiring restaurants to provide nutrition information, regulating food advertising, and imposing a "fat tax" on junk foods. Some rabid food reformers advocate that health insurers charge higher premiums for the obese, just as for smokers. They also support filing multimillion-dollar class action lawsuits against giant junk-food companies, much like those filed against the tobacco industry. One change that's already in the works: Lawmakers in four states are trying to ban soda and junk food from school campuses.

PERCENTAGE OF AMERICANS WHO FAVOR LEVYING A JUNK-FOOD TAX: **23**

PERCENTAGE WHO WANT FAST-FOOD ADVERTISEMENTS BANNED: **19**

PERCENTAGE WHO BELIEVE THAT PEOPLE WHO MAINTAIN A HEALTHY WEIGHT SHOULD RECEIVE DISCOUNTS ON THEIR HEALTH INSURANCE: **54**

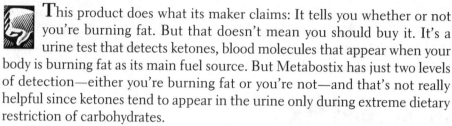

DOES IT WORK?

Metabostix

 This product does what its maker claims: It tells you whether or not you're burning fat. But that doesn't mean you should buy it. It's a urine test that detects ketones, blood molecules that appear when your body is burning fat as its main fuel source. But Metabostix has just two levels of detection—either you're burning fat or you're not—and that's not really helpful since ketones tend to appear in the urine only during extreme dietary restriction of carbohydrates.

You'd be better off judging your weight loss with a more tried-and-true method: stepping on a scale.

Jackie Chan's Cableflex

 The infomercial for this $120 rope-and-pulley device claims you can do abdominal and lower-body exercises with it as well as just about any exercise that can be done with free weights.

Our recommendation? Don't waste the ink to write out the check. Even at its most difficult setting, we didn't notice any more resistance than you'd get from using a 10-pound dumbbell. And the resistance felt lighter during the lowering portion of the lift, so you don't get the benefits of negative resistance. We say use that $120 to buy 200 pounds of dumbbells and a good jump rope. In our opinion, they'll do more to get you in shape than this gadget ever will.

Electric-Pulse Machines

 Like most lazy-man fixes, the idea behind electronic muscle stimulation (EMS) sounds logical. Strap electrodes to your gut, zap some electricity to cajole muscles to contract, and voilà! Awesome abs (for just 32 easy payments of $19.95). Problem is, EMS-induced contractions are so weak that there's no payoff. (Sort of like buying her dinner and getting a good-night handshake.)

In an 8-week study conducted by the American Council on Exercise, 29 college-age volunteers who used EMS devices experienced no significant changes in weight, body-fat percentage, strength, or overall appearance. We say get off your duff and sculpt your abs the old-fashioned way: Earn 'em.

WHAT'S THE DIFF?

Nutritionist vs. Dietitian

A nutritionist doesn't necessarily have formal training. When your wife tells you those pork rinds just took 17 minutes off your life, she's being a nutritionist. A dietitian has studied and earned the R.D. Still, some dietitians call themselves nutritionists to avoid sounding like someone who dispenses tapioca pudding to Aunt Ethel at the home.

Low-Fat vs. Reduced-Fat

By federal law, a product labeled low-fat must contain no more than 3 grams of fat per serving, and a reduced-fat product must contain at least 25 percent less fat than the full-fat version. But don't let a reduced-fat label fool you into thinking its contents are good for you. Take sour cream, for example. The reduced-fat brand we looked at has a mere 1.5 fewer grams of fat and 1 less gram of saturated fat than the full-fat stuff—plus it still packs a whopping 35 calories from fat.

Abductors vs. Adductors

If you thought abductors were guys who successfully make off with supermodels, you're wrong. They're the muscles along your outer thighs. And adductors are the muscles along your inner thighs. Without these two muscle groups, you wouldn't be able to open or close your legs. To exercise them, something or someone must provide resistance against your thighs as you attempt to either pull your knees apart (abduction) or push them together (adduction). While you could use your hand or an exercise machine to provide resistance, we suggest having a supermodel do it for you.

Ligaments vs. Tendons

Ligaments are tissues that run from bone to bone, holding your skeleton together (which is why a torn anterior cruciate ligament, or ACL, is so nasty). Tendons attach muscles to other body parts, usually bones (a torn biceps tendon sidelined former Angels first baseman Mo Vaughn for all of 2001).

TAKE ACTION

$\mathbf{A}$ great tip is an awesome thing. Whether it's an undiscovered restaurant, a sleeper stock, or a Sure Thing in the late double at Pimlico, savvy inside info imbues a man with confidence. Control. Strength.

Knowledge is power, baby.

It's also the secret to a lean, powerful body, as you're about to find out. In our never-ending mission to get you in the greatest shape of your life, we've grilled the world's top experts, combed our own archives, even eavesdropped on some cell phone conversations, to find 23 perfect fitness and weight-loss tips—small gems that will make a huge difference in any man's life.

Get ready: You're about to feel the power—and have the body to show for it.

I. Get up and at 'em. If you want to exercise before work but aren't a morning person, try this trick: For a set period—say, 4 weeks—force yourself to get up 15 minutes earlier than normal and do any type of physical activity (walking, for instance). "Make it so easy that you don't even have to change into your workout clothes," says John Raglin, Ph.D., an exercise researcher at the University of Indiana. As you near the end of the 4 weeks, you'll have a new habit and will then be able to progress to greater amounts of exercise.

2. Warm up the right way. Skip the treadmill warmup before lifting weights. Instead, do a warmup that targets the muscles you'll be using. For a full-body warmup, grab a bar (without weights) and do two sets of 10 repetitions each of the squat, deadlift, bench press, and bent-over row.

3. Manage your middle. Do your ab exercises at the beginning of your workout if you can't pass this test: Sit with your feet flat on the floor and your legs bent—as if you had just performed a situp. Then place your fingers behind your ears with your elbows pulled back. Lower yourself to the floor as slowly as possible. "If it doesn't take at least 5 seconds, you need to prioritize your abdominal training," says Australian strength coach Ian King.

4. Clock yourself. It takes your stomach 20 minutes to signal your brain that you're full. Stop eating when you've consumed 80 percent of what you normally eat, wait for 20 minutes to pass, and you'll feel satisfied with the amount you've eaten. You can chop hundreds of calories per day this way.

NUMBER OF AMERICAN MEN WHO DON'T PARTICIPATE IN SPORTS OR FITNESS ACTIVITIES: 20,800,000

5. Keep muscles limber. If you're under 40, hold your stretches for 30 seconds. If you're over 40, hold them for 60 seconds. As you reach your forties, your muscles become less pliable, so they need to be stretched longer.

6. Grow muscle, save time. Keep your weight workouts under an hour. After 60 minutes, your body starts producing more of the stress hormone cortisol, which can have a testosterone-blocking, muscle-wasting effect.

7. Exercise in order. Use dumbbells, barbells, and machines—in that order. "The smaller, stabilizer muscles you use with dumbbells fatigue before your larger muscle groups," says Charles Staley, a strength coach in Las Vegas. So as you grow tired, progress to machines, which require less help from your smaller muscles.

8. Strengthen your core. Don't be afraid of situps. We've changed our tune on these, and here's why: Situps increase your range of motion, making your abdominals work harder and longer. (Doing crunches on a Swiss ball or with a rolled-up towel under your lower back has a similar effect.) Just avoid situps with anchored feet, which can hurt your lower back.

9. Kill your excuse. If you think you're too busy to exercise, try this experiment: For one day, schedule a time to work out, and then stick to it—even if you can exercise for only 10 minutes. "At the end of the day, ask yourself if you were any less productive than usual," says John Jakicic, Ph.D., an exercise psychologist at Brown University Medical School. The answer will probably be no—and your favorite excuse will be gone.

10. Muscle up your back. When doing lat pulldowns, don't wrap your thumb around the bar. Instead, place it on top, alongside your index finger. This decreases the involvement of your arm muscles, so you'll work your back harder. Works for pullups, too.

11. Drink a pint, get ripped. If you're a beginner, train to failure—the point at which you absolutely can't do another repetition—then throw back a pint. In a new study, beginners who trained to failure with three sets of six exercises per day, then drank a supplement immediately afterward, gained more than 5 pounds of muscle in just 8 weeks. A pint of 1% chocolate milk will provide all the nutrients you need to achieve the same result.

12. Build better abs. Don't work your abdominal muscles every day. "Physiologically, your abs are like any other muscle in your body," says David Pearson, Ph.D., C.S.C.S., an exercise scientist at Ball State University. Train them only 2 or 3 days a week.

13. Turn heads with your legs. Do standing *and* seated calf raises. You'll get better results. "Your calves are made up of two different muscles, so you have to do the straight-leg and the bent-leg versions of the exercise to hit them both," says Michael Mejia, C.S.C.S., *Men's Health* magazine exercise consultant.

14. Test yourself often. Every 4 weeks, measure a variable—waist size, body fat, bench press—that equates to your end goal. "It'll show you the tangible results of your training," says Craig Ballantyne, C.S.C.S., Canadian strength and conditioning coach. And that translates into motivation.

15. Build big biceps. Bend your wrists to work your biceps harder. That is, extend them backward slightly—and hold them that way—while you do arm curls.

16. Ditch the weight belt. Over time, regular training in a weight belt actually weakens your abdominal and lower-back muscles. Wear it only when attempting maximal lifts in such exercises as squats, deadlifts, and overhead presses.

17. Stretch for strength. Between sets, take 20 to 30 seconds to stretch the muscle you just worked. Boston researchers found that men who did this increased their strength by 20 percent.

18. Drink up, slim down. Drink low-fat milk. Scientists in Canada found that people who consumed more than 600 milligrams of calcium a day—roughly the amount in 2 cups of milk, a cup of broccoli, and ½ cup of cottage cheese—had lower body fat than those who consumed less than 600 milligrams a day.

19. Multiply your muscles. Follow this simple formula to build more muscle: Multiply the amount of weight you lift for a particular exercise by the total number of times you lift it. Try to increase that number every workout by lifting heavier weights, increasing your repetitions, or doing more sets.

20. Sit back, squat more. Use a bench to squat with perfect form. That is, stand in front of the bench when you squat. Lower yourself as if you were sitting down. When your butt touches the bench, push yourself back up. Try it first with a light bar or a broomstick.

21. Get stronger legs. Do lunges in reverse. This forces your front leg to work throughout the entire exercise. Use the same movement pattern as in a traditional lunge, but step backward instead of forward.

22. Get a better grip. To strengthen your grip, wrap a towel around the bar when you do arm curls. It makes the bar thicker, which forces your forearm muscles to work harder.

23. Feed your muscles. Satisfy your sugar cravings immediately after your workout. Eat at least 20 grams, along with some protein. The sugar will help carry protein to the muscles you've just worked. So have a soda with your tuna sandwich, but limit your sugar intake the rest of the day.

NUMBER OF YEARS ADDED TO YOUR LIFE BY MAINTAINING A HEALTHY WEIGHT: 1.5

NUMBER OF YEARS ADDED TO YOUR LIFE IF YOU EXERCISE VIGOROUSLY THREE TIMES A WEEK: 2.1

ANY QUESTIONS?

Spread Yourself Thin

I'm working out to lose weight, but I'm getting nowhere. Most nights I arrive home late, eat dinner, have two light beers, and crash. Could this be sabotaging my effort?

—G. L., Blue Lake, California

Maybe. Try spreading those calories throughout the day, even if it means stashing an energy bar in your desk to curb hunger before you get home, suggests Chris Rosenbloom, Ph.D., chairman of the department of nutrition at Georgia State University. Try to eat your largest meal of the day at lunch, and lighten up on the nighttime meal. By eating a heavy meal with alcohol right before bed, you're more likely to store those extra calories as fat. And while a light beer contains only about 100 calories, try cutting back to one a night during the week. Cutting 100 calories out of your daily diet would be equivalent to 700 calories a week and could lead to nearly a 10-pound weight loss in one year.

Quick Fix

What's the absolute best way to lose a couple of pounds fast (like, within a few days)?

—K. B., Wichita, Kansas

Besides a guillotine, there's no way to do that, at least not safely. Starvation and fad diets can produce rapid and misleading results, but most people end up gorging later, says Janet Lepke Harris, R.D., a dietitian in North Carolina. Crash diets cause metabolism to slow, while the deprivation tempts you to binge.

If you need to look thin fast—for a wedding, reunion, or parole meeting—try changing clothes. "Wearing the right clothes is the easiest—and quickest—way to slim down," says Brian Boyé, fashion director for *Men's Health* magazine. Stick to grays and blacks for jackets and trousers (dark colors are slimming), and try for a close color match; head-to-toe continuity accentuates length over girth. Of course, the only way to look great *out* of your new clothes is to get in shape. Start with any of the 15-minute workouts from Got a Minute? How About 15? on page 32.

Taste Pattern

I'm trying to cut out snacking, but I crave chips or ice cream when I watch TV. How can I stop this? Any healthy snack ideas?

—E. C., St. Louis, Missouri

Your problem is not the mint–chocolate chip. Your problem is the mint–chocolate-chip–*West Wing* thing you've got going. For you, eating and TV watching are one activity. You need to uncouple the two. To get out of the Must-Eat TV pattern, designate one place where you're allowed to eat, preferably your dining room or kitchen table, says Jean Harvey-Berino, Ph.D., R.D., associate professor of nutrition at the University of Vermont. If you must have ice cream, turn the TV off, get up, dish out the ice cream, eat at the designated place, then go back and turn the TV on. Seem like a hassle? That's the point. You need to make long-term solutions, and munching on carrot sticks while still watching the tube will not break the habit.

Heart of the Matter

What's better for keeping my heart healthy: running or weight lifting?

—F. V., Grand Rapids, Michigan

That's like having to choose between ESPN and the Playboy Channel. You really want both. But if you had to choose one or the other, there's more research to support the heart-protecting benefits of aerobic exercise, says Barry Franklin, Ph.D., director of the cardiac rehabilitation program at William Beaumont Hospital in Royal Oak, Michigan.

Aerobic exercise has a greater impact on the overall efficiency of your heart and lungs, but Franklin is quick to add that you shouldn't underestimate the heart benefits of weight training as a complement to aerobic exercise. In fact, the American Heart Association now recommends pairing resistance training with aerobics to prevent and treat heart disease. Weight lifting is a key component of most post–heart attack therapy, for several reasons: (1) Resistance training makes the heart more efficient; (2) weight training may lower your resting heart rate and blood pressure; and (3) the stronger your muscles are, the less strain your heart experiences when you do something physical.

So try your best to do both types of training. Franklin recommends 30 minutes of moderate aerobic activity (the equivalent of a brisk walk) on most days of the week and 15 minutes of resistance training at least twice a week. Target the whole body by doing a single circuit of 10 to 15 repetitions of eight different weight-lifting exercises. "One set of each lift is all you need to do to reap musculoskeletal benefits," says Franklin. "Especially for beginners, 85 to 90 percent of strength improvement comes with the first set."

One Step at a Time

My only chance for exercise on weekdays is a quick walk at lunchtime. Will it really make any difference?

—J. J., Madison, Wisconsin

Stride on, J. J. Walking briskly for 30 minutes provides the same health benefits as running for 30 minutes, says Stanley Birge, M.D., of the Washington University in St. Louis School of Medicine. Walk this way: Warm up at an even stroll for 5 minutes, hold a brisk pace for 20 minutes, and then cool down for 5 minutes, says Sara Donovan, president of WalkSport America. Gauge your workout pace with the walk-and-talk test: You should be breathing hard, but still able to hold a conversation. By yourself? Talk anyway. You'll get plenty of extra sidewalk room during the lunch rush hour. Add light hand weights (no more than $1\frac{1}{2}$ pounds) to work your granny-flap arms, and buy a good pair of walking shoes.

If you've got a gut to lose, you'll have to go longer, or harder: A 165-pound man sheds about 150 calories during a 30-minute walk, compared with 225 if he jogs.

Speed Limit

The trainer at my gym keeps telling me that the best way to build muscle is by doing really slow repetitions. Is this true?

—B. E., Louisville, Kentucky

Several years ago, a study suggested that lifting weights slowly—at the snail's pace of 14 seconds per repetition—increases strength faster than lifting at regular speed. But there was a huge flaw in the study: It demonstrated only that the slow lifters gained more strength in slow lifts than the others gained in lifts done at normal speed. The study never compared the absolute strength of the two groups, says Alex Koch, Ph.D., C.S.C.S, an exercise scientist at Truman State University.

A more recent study at George Washington University medical center looked at slow versus regular lifting but compared apples with apples: how much the men could lift for one repetition before and after a 10-week training program. The results are a lot more believable: The men lifting weights at regular speed gained 24 percent more strength than the slow Joes. Hope that gets you back up to speed.

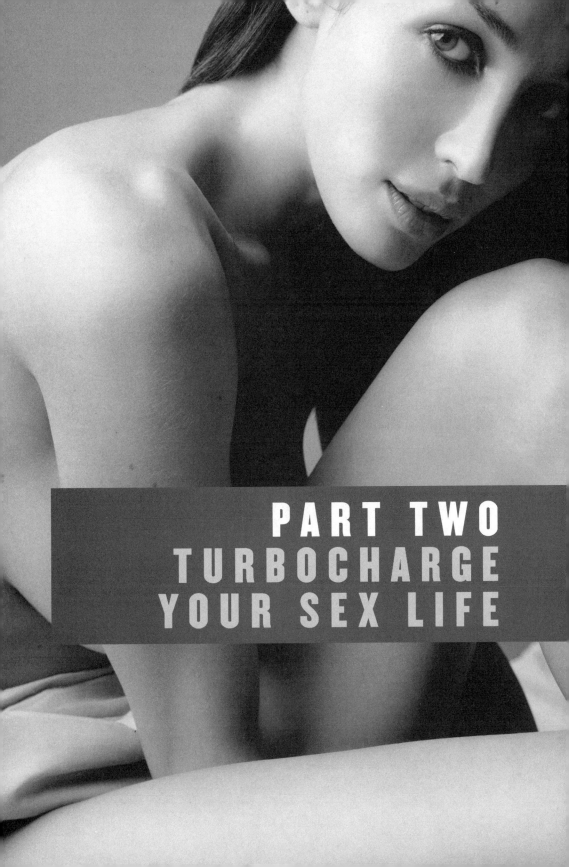

PART TWO
TURBOCHARGE
YOUR SEX LIFE

GAME SHOW

Who Will Be Impotent First?

Will one of these guys fall down on the job, or will you?

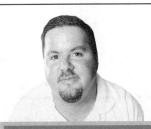

GEORGE ALLAN
Age: 31   Height: 5'10"
Weight: 230

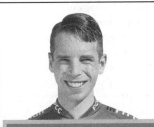

JOE PAPP
Age: 25   Height: 5'8"
Weight: 150

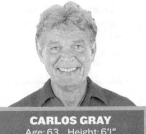

CARLOS GRAY
Age: 63   Height: 6'1"
Weight: 197

WHY HE'S AT RISK
• Fifty pounds overweight, doesn't exercise, eats high-fat food, and has a family history of high blood pressure and diabetes. A Harvard study found that men over 50 with 42-inch-plus waists are almost twice as likely to experience erectile dysfunction as men with 23- to 35-inch waists. Penile arteries are narrow, so plaque formation is likelier to compromise bloodflow there than elsewhere in the body.

WHAT HE'S DOING ABOUT IT
• Practically nothing. Two young children and working on commission leave him little time for exercise and nutrition. He contends that his cholesterol and blood pressure are normal, plus he says he has sex nearly every day. Regular erections keep the penis healthy by nourishing it with fresh blood and oxygen.

GEORGE'S PREDICTION
• "Not me! Junior's the only part of my body that gets a daily workout. I think biker boy will go limp first."

WHY HE'S AT RISK
• A bicycle road racer who rides 300 to 500 miles per week during the season. Has been cycling for 15 years (10 years competitively). Studies show that sitting on a hard, narrow bike saddle for long periods can compress penile arteries and nerves, eventually reducing bloodflow and sensation.

WHAT HE'S DOING ABOUT IT
• While he doesn't use one of the new anatomic seats designed to redistribute weight, he does make sure his bike fits properly and that he gets out of the saddle frequently. Despite a family history of high cholesterol, he's in excellent condition, with low body fat, low blood pressure, and favorable lipid levels. On average, he has sex four times per week.

JOE'S PREDICTION
• "If you're smart about how you ride, you don't have to worry about impotence. The benefits of cycling far outweigh the risks. I think the old guy is the one who's in trouble."

WHY HE'S AT RISK
• He's a grandpa, and an estimated 60 percent of men in their sixties have difficulty getting and maintaining an erection. The odds of trouble increase with every birthday as blood vessels naturally harden and lose their capacity to dilate. This inhibits bloodflow needed to produce an erection.

WHAT HE'S DOING ABOUT IT
• Following a health-obsessed lifestyle that includes daily exercise (swimming, strength training, 400 Kegel exercises) and a diet rich in fruits and vegetables. His life is filled with more play than work, so he has very little stress. Has sex three to five times per week, but he's hoping for more.

CARLOS'S PREDICTION
• "I'll outlast both of them! It's important to me never to let sex slip away, so I eat right and exercise. The out-of-shape guy will lose it first, then the cyclist."

And the Winner Is . . .
George Allan

We asked Laurence Levine, M.D., director of male sexual health and fertility at Rush-Presbyterian St. Luke's Medical Center in Chicago, to handicap the competition. He developed the scorecard on the opposite page to gauge impotency risk. The lower your score, the greater your chance of becoming impotent.

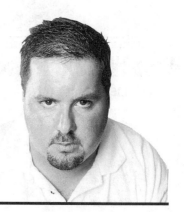

FINAL ANALYSIS

Although Allan doesn't have problems yet, his poor diet, sedentary lifestyle, and family history will eventually catch up with him. Fortunately, his fate isn't inevitable. Laurence Levine, M.D., director of male sexual health and fertility at Rush-Presbyterian St. Luke's Medical Center in Chicago, says if Allan exercises and eats right, he'll lose weight, control his blood pressure, and increase his sex-life expectancy. If not, he has about 10 years of erections left.

Despite Papp's bike riding, his risk of becoming impotent is only about 4 percent, says Dr. Levine. "Cycling can cause repetitive trauma to the blood vessels, but it's rare," he says. Papp has taken all the right precautions (adjusting his seat height so his knees bend just slightly at the bottom of each pedal stroke, angling the nose of the saddle slightly downward, and leaving the saddle every 10 minutes). The cardiovascular effects Papp gets from cycling far outweigh his slim risk of becoming impotent.

As for Grandpa Gray, he's doing everything possible to stay virile, and it's working. "His age does put him at risk," says Dr. Levine, "but he takes care of himself, and that counteracts his risk. If Allan would adopt Gray's lifestyle, the tables would turn."

Will You Go Limp?

IMPOTENCE FACTOR	POINT VALUE	GEORGE	JOE	CARLOS	YOU
AGE Arteries narrow and restrict bloodflow with age.	Over 60? −2			−2	
	Over 40? −I				
	Under 30? +I		+I		
HEALTH Diabetes, high blood pressure, and cholesterol are major "erection busters," says Dr. Levine. Being overweight increases your risk for these conditions.	Overweight? −2	−2			
	High cholesterol? −2				
	• family history? −I		−I		
	High blood pressure? −2				
	• family history? −I	−I			
	Diabetes? −2				
	• family history? −I	−I			
	Excellent health? +2		+2	+2	
STRESS Chronic high stress elevates blood pressure, which constricts bloodflow.	High? −I				
	Moderate? 0	0			
	Low? +I		+I	+I	
DIET Fatty foods contribute to arterial plaque. Fiber helps keep vessels clear.	High fat, low fiber? −I	−I			
	Low fat, high fiber? +I		+I	+I	
EXERCISE Regular exercise helps control weight, blood pressure, and cholesterol.	Fewer than 3 times/week? −I	−I			
	More than 3 times/week? +I		+I	+I	
ALCOHOL Binge drinking can cause an impotence episode that leads to performance anxiety.	2+ drinks a day? −I			−I	
	Fewer than 2 a day? 0	0	0		
SMOKING Dr. Levine calls smoking an erection buster. It constricts blood vessels throughout the body.	More than half a pack a day? −2				
	Occasionally? −I				
	Never? +2	+2	+2	+2	
TEMPER Chronic feelings of anger and hostility spike blood pressure.	Get mad? −I	−I			
	Stay calm? 0		0	0	
DEPRESSION Studies find depressed men are likelier to experience impotence.	Personal experience? −2				
	Family history? −I				
	None? 0	0	0	0	
SEXUAL ACTIVITY "You've got to use it if you don't want to lose it," Dr. Levine says.	Less than once a week? −I				
	More than once a week? +I	+I	+I	+I	
PERFORMANCE ANXIETY Worry over a past failure can cause future ones.	Past performance problems? −2				
	Smooth sailing? 0	0	0	0	
SADDLE SPORTS Cycling, motorcycling, wave running, and horseback riding can cause impact trauma.	Regular activity? −I		−I		
	Occasional activity? 0	0		0	
TOTALS		−4	+7	+5	

▶ **IF YOUR SCORE IS −3 OR LESS:** You're at high risk, and you need to change your lifestyle immediately.

▶ **IF YOUR SCORE IS −2 TO +2:** You've still got it, but maybe not for long.

▶ **IF YOUR SCORE IS +3 OR MORE:** Continue what you're doing and enjoy a long, hard life.

MUST READS

Be Superior in the Sack

We've snuck a peek at the average guy's sex life. Not because we enjoy being Peeping Toms. We did it for *you*. So you could know once and for all what's typical in the sack—and how to make your sexual performance far better than average

By Matt Marion

You'd think writing *The Great Gatsby* would have convinced F. Scott Fitzgerald that he measured up. But then, it is a very short novel. Maybe that's why he took it so hard when Zelda complained that he couldn't satisfy her. It was "a matter of measurements," she said. Scott confided all this to his friend Ernie. And, according to the account in *A Moveable Feast*, Hemingway bravely took a peek and then reassured him, saying in essence: "You're okay, but Zelda's nuts." What a pal.

And now we're here to do the same favor for you. We did some peeking of our own and discovered a lot about your neighbor's sexual measurements—how often he does it, who he's doing it with, what he's most likely to do when he's finished. This article is like a reality Web cam, telling you all there is to know about the average guy's sex life.

Best of all, we grilled America's top sex experts and learned how you can become anything but average. It's time to stop peeking—and start peaking.

THE AVERAGE GUY HAS SEX TWICE A WEEK

That's if he's married. If he's single and living solo, frequency drops to once a week. Single and shacking up? Three times a week. Hey, there's a reason they call it living in sin.

You Can Do Better

No need to cash in your 401(k) and hit every brothel in Reno. Touchy-feely relationship issues aside, the best way to guarantee return engagements is to do more of what she likes in bed and less of what she doesn't. For instance . . .

Bow to her breasts. You might think you focus too much on her breasts. You can't. According to Patti Britton, Ph.D., a clinical sexologist and the coach behind www.sexcoach.com, a woman's nipples are the best place to stimulate her, except for her genitals. But don't just grab and squeeze. Britton suggests first slowly circling your fingertips around the base of each nipple, then gently pushing down the tip and letting it spring back. "Like just about everything else, women need you to build toward the center of interest, and that certainly includes the nipples," she says.

Don't settle for the missionary position. "It's all about the angle of the dangle," says Alicia Saunders, Ph.D., a certified sex therapist in Short Hills, New Jersey. "In the missionary position, it's often difficult to stimulate the clitoris, and a man needs to have fairly strong arms and legs to be at all effective." If you must do it missionary style, put pillows under her backside to prop her up at a better angle; this will allow you to aim more effectively.

Use circular reasoning. Rather than roughly shoving your hand down there and frantically rubbing away, try slowly tracing the outer edges of her labia with your fingertips while gently parting the lips. "Stretched skin tends to have greater sensitivity, so this should send waves of pleasure through her," says Lou Paget, a sex educator and author of *The Big O.*

THE AVERAGE GUY'S EQUIPMENT IS 3.4 INCHES TURNED OFF AND 5.8 INCHES TURNED ON

A reassuring stat, but one that makes us look awfully one-dimensional. Truth is, when the average guy gets aroused, he also gets wider (girth goes from 3.8 to 4.9 inches) and hangs lower (testicle size increases by 50 percent).

You Can Do Better

There are all sorts of creepy surgical options, but we don't recommend you try any of them. Instead, play it safe and employ these simple no-scalpel strategies.

Get rid of your butt. Despite the length of his lasso, odds are the Marlboro Man was not hung like a horse. In one study at the University of California at Irvine, researchers measured the penises of smokers and nonsmokers and found that those men who liked to light up were of significantly smaller stature. One theory is that smoking somehow damages penile tissue, eventually making it less elastic and preventing it from stretching.

Thank Dr. Kegel. Everyone's heard of Kegel exercises, the repeated flexing of the pubococcygeus (PC) muscles, which control urinary flow. Well, of all the reasons to do them, including the ability to hold out longer during sex,

---

SEXUAL POSITION THE AVERAGE GUY MOST FREQUENTLY USES: MISSIONARY

HIS FAVORITE POSITION: DOGGY STYLE

this may be the most compelling: "Developing your PC muscles may increase the width of your penis a fraction of an inch," says Alex Robboy, a sex researcher at the University of Pennsylvania and the creator of the Web site HowToHaveGoodSex.com. It's not much, but we'll take it. To help your penis realize its full potential, Robboy recommends tensing and relaxing your PC muscles at least 20 times a day.

THE AVERAGE GUY LASTS 14 MINUTES DURING SEX

If that sounds like a marathon, you may be among the 30 percent of men who suffer from premature ejaculation.

You Can Do Better

It took nanoseconds when you were 17. Today you're up to a quarter of an hour. Tomorrow? The pinnacle of self-restraint, thanks to these slow-down strategies.

Use the Valsalva maneuver. Sounds exotic, but it isn't. The instant you feel like you're going to pop your cork, bear down as if you were trying to have a bowel movement (uh, don't actually have one). "Increasing your intra-abdominal pressure relaxes the muscles that contract during ejaculation," says Dudley S. Danoff, M.D., a urologic surgeon at Cedars-Sinai Medical Center in Los Angeles. "You can actually get a few more minutes."

Consider an antidepressant. If your trigger-happy tendencies are seriously affecting your sex life, Zoloft may help. This antidepressant can delay ejaculation. According to Michael O'Leary, M.D., director of the Men's Clinic at Brigham and Women's Hospital, the elevated blood levels of serotonin produced by Zoloft help neutralize the sexually stimulating effects of dopamine. "Whether you're unhappy or she is, it's safe to try it," says Dr. O'Leary.

Note: It usually takes a few weeks to start working. Ask your urologist if Zoloft is right for you and what other side effects you might experience.

AMERICAN MEN BOUGHT 5.39 BILLION ADULT VIDEOS LAST YEAR

And the most popular porn movie of 2001 was . . . *Fade to Black*, starring the amazing Taylor Hayes.

You Can Do Better

Think about it: What good is being a platinum member of X-plicit Video if your wife or girlfriend won't watch and get turned on with you? Not much, which is why we asked Linda De Villers, Ph.D., a sex therapist in Marina del Rey, California, and our panel of expert female judges to pick five seemingly innocent movies that'll have her undoing your belt before the credits roll.

Bull Durham: (1988) Baseball, sex, and Susan Sarandon.

What the judges said: "Seeing careless sex on the kitchen table, in the living room, on the bedroom floor, and in the bathtub—all within a 10-minute span of time—definitely put me in the mood to take my clothes off."

The Mask of Zorro: (1998) Sharp weapons and Catherine Zeta-Jones before Michael Douglas brainwashed her.

What the judges said: "The sword fight and the sexual tension didn't let me think about anything else but sex."

Henry and June: (1990) Artsy film set in 1930s Paris.

What the judges said: "This movie is just all-out hot. Since it's solely about sexual desire, it really gets you worked up by the end."

The Thomas Crown Affair: (1999) Remake of the classic Steve McQueen heist film.

What the judges said: "The sex scenes show Pierce Brosnan and Rene Russo laughing and playing together, which makes them more romantic and realistic than most movie love scenes. A big turn-on."

The Piano: (1993) Chick flick about, well, a piano.

What the judges said: "The sequences between Harvey Keitel and Holly Hunter are incredibly slow, naughty, and arousing. Watch for the stocking scene."

THE AVERAGE GUY HAS 12 SEX PARTNERS IN HIS LIFETIME

His wife or girlfriend? Just four.

You Can Do Better

To increase your LIA (lifetime intercourse average), try to identify your blind spots when it comes to romancing women. For instance . . .

Being sarcastic. While your buddies may not mind being called dumb ass, chances are she doesn't find your playful teasing half as clever as you do. "Sarcasm is for your guy friends. Women don't sit around and say 'you bitch' to each other," says Felicia Rose Adler, author of *Master Dating: How to Meet and Attract Quality Men.*

Saying, "I love you." Saying this anywhere in the vicinity of first-time sex is going to make it sound like a line. "Worse, if you start making love noises, she's likely to think of you as relationship material and want to wait to have sex," says Adler. Save your profession of love for when sex isn't an option, like when she's doubled over the toilet with a stomach virus.

Groping instead of kissing. You're close, really close, but you're forgetting what got you here in the first place. "Women get their greatest erotic pleasure from frequent, passionate kissing," says Britton. "If you get the sense that she's starting to lose interest, kissing is always the best way to bring her back

ETHNIC GROUP THAT GIVES AND RECEIVES THE LEAST ORAL SEX: CAUCASIANS

into it." Just remember that passionate kissing doesn't always mean frantically swabbing out her tonsils. Try to mix up your tongue play with the occasional closed-mouth kiss on her nose, eyes, and forehead.

THE AVERAGE GUY HAS SEX WITH THE LIGHTS OFF (BUT HE'D RATHER HAVE THE LIGHTS ON)

Note: Sex with strobe lights on is a separate category.

You Can Do Better

You'd rather not do it in the dark, but she's self-conscious about how her body looks in the buff. The compromise: lighting that complements her curves while hiding her flaws. Jeff Kent, a senior editor at *Professional Photographer* magazine, recommends that you first fit a desk lamp with a low-wattage "soft light" bulb, then tilt the shade away from your partner so the light reflects off a nearby wall. This technique, known as "bouncing," disperses light around the room, creating a subtler effect.

THE AVERAGE GUY STANDS A 1-IN-3 CHANCE OF GOING LIMP

Bifocals aren't the only side effect of middle age. The risk of erectile problems increases by 300 percent after age 50.

You Can Do Better

This is literally a case of use it or lose it. Most urologists recommend frequent sex—three or four times a week—to move enough blood into the penis's chambers to keep them pliable into your old age. And yes, masturbation counts toward your weekly quota. Other, less enjoyable forms of erection insurance include . . .

Eating an apple a day. Or a bowl of oatmeal. "Foods like oats and apples are loaded with soluble fiber, which pushes excess cholesterol through your digestive system before it can be deposited along artery walls," says Wahida Karmally, R.D., director of nutrition at the Irving Center for Clinical Research in New York. "Lower cholesterol means cleaner arteries and better bloodflow." Strawberries and kidney beans are also high in the cholesterol-scouring fiber.

Jogging a few miles daily. In a Boston University study of nearly 600 men, researchers found that burning 200 calories a day through aerobic exercise reduced the risk of erectile dysfunction by as much as 70 percent. The reason?

PERCENTAGE OF AMERICANS WHO HAD
MORE THAN ONE SEX PARTNER LAST YEAR: 11

PERCENTAGE OF MEN WHO CLAIM TO HAVE HAD TWO
OR MORE SEXUAL RELATIONSHIPS GOING AT ONE TIME: 31

"Exercise may help prevent the development and progression of atherosclerotic vascular disease, which eventually can lead to erectile dysfunction," says Irwin Goldstein, M.D., one of the study authors.

Using Viagra for insurance. Turns out the little blue pill may be able to prevent, as well as treat, erectile dysfunction. "Taking half a tab a week, especially for guys whose erections aren't always fully rigid, can stimulate bloodflow and cause nighttime erections," says Chris Steidle, M.D., an associate professor of urology at Indiana University School of Medicine. Typical candidates for using Viagra preventively include men with impotence risk factors such as a history of smoking, high stress levels, or diabetes. Your urologist can assess whether it's right for you.

THE AVERAGE GUY THRUSTS 90 TIMES PER SESSION

Sorry, but you still need to hit the gym; for all that friction, you're only burning 2 calories per minute.

You Can Do Better

Tap your finger 90 times. A bit much, isn't it? And for what? She may still not be satisfied. Here's how to be a model of efficiency.

Downshift. "Women get the most stimulation from slower thrusts," says De Villers. Don't worry—you'll have no problem figuring out when she wants you to start speeding things up.

Be a shallow guy. Going deeper than any man has gone before isn't the idea. The only thing you're going to do is hit her cervix, which could make her writhe—in pain. Instead, use shallow thrusts aimed at the outer one-third of her vagina; this area has the most nerve endings and is more engorged, so it creates more friction, says De Villers. "Many women haven't experienced shallow penetration, but odds are they'll like it a lot." To control the depth of each thrust, wrap your hand around your penis close to the base and use only the exposed portion.

THE AVERAGE GUY WHO LOOKS AT INTERNET PORN SPENDS A FEW MINUTES A DAY VIEWING IT AT WORK

Men may be the biggest Internet oglers, but the ladies fill up the porn chat rooms—twice as many women as men visit them.

You Can Do Better

You know that you shouldn't visit Internet porn sites at work, but who can resist "Nude Czech Gymnasts?" You, with these stay-employed strategies.

Kill the mood. You need the visual equivalent of a cold shower. First, click over to www.dol.gov/opa/media/press/eta/ui/current.htm. It features a weekly update of the country's jobless rate. Next, try moving the desk photo of your family right next to your monitor so you see their financially dependent faces as you surf.

Handcuff yourself. Fact is, if you're able to download porn at work, then your company's filtering software probably isn't up to snuff. Spring for Net Nanny 4.0 ($40) and install it on your company desktop (do it after work). Despite the name, this is one of the best porn blockers for adult surfers, too. "The neat thing about Net Nanny is that it dynamically tracks and blocks content based on URLs submitted by users. That's important because porn sites often change their meta tags and URLs to escape detection," says Rebecca Viksnins, associate editor of software and Internet services at CNET/ZDNet Reviews.

THE AVERAGE GUY'S PARTNER INITIATES SEX ABOUT 20 PERCENT OF THE TIME

That's counting your birthday.

You Can Do Better

With the right encouragement (and some deft manipulation), you really can get her into the habit of ripping your shirt open and pushing you onto the kitchen table.

Let her act the part. Next time you're having sex, suggest that each of you take on a role, with her playing a dominant figure like a teacher or a prostitute. "She'll be less nervous about taking charge because she'll think, 'It's not really me, it's the role I'm playing,'" says Max Fitz-Gerald, Ph.D., a sex therapist and codirector of the Fitz-Gerald Institute in Wilson, North Carolina. "Once she discovers her dominant side, it may help her to move forward in initiating sex in the future."

Use code words. Women are usually the better communicators, but not necessarily in the bedroom. "She might want to have sex but feel too shy to convey that to her partner," says Cynthia Lief Ruberg, a sex and relationship counselor in Columbus, Ohio. To find out if that's her, wait until she's in a playful mood, then ask her to help you come up with a secret code word or phrase for sex. "Creating your own language for sex helps intimacy and can get past her embarrassment," says Ruberg. Can't think of anything? Try *giddyap*.

Reward her bravery. When she does initiate the action, make an extra effort to please her sexually and to let her know how much you approve. "Tell her you really loved it that she initiated," says Fitz-Gerald. "Women aren't sure if you're going to perceive initiation as negative or if it might make you uncomfortable."

THE AVERAGE GUY WILL FIRE OFF 1 TRILLION SPERM IN HIS LIFETIME

For those of you scoring at home, that's 18 quarts of semen—worth $247,840 to your local sperm bank.

WHAT BELOW-AVERAGE GUYS SAY TO STAY THAT WAY

"I knew we'd get together when I saw you through my binoculars."

"I can't believe you're an accountant."

"It's amazing how different they looked under your sweater."

"No, I love your stuffed animals. They're really absorbent."

"Don't mind Rex. It's his bed, too! Isn't it, good buddy? Yeah, that's my boy! What's that? You want to kiss her, too? Well, we'll just have to ask, won't we, big boy? Hmm?"

"I find that if I leave Ted Koppel on, I last longer. Just knowing he's there."

"You're okay with the whole Web cam thing, right?"

"Behold! The light saber!"

"You know, from this angle you could be just about anyone."

"Why don't you put on these goggles?"

"I wasn't laughing. That was a snort of astonishment."

"Found it! I think . . ."

"Your skin is so soft and firm, it feels like cheese."

"I thought the church lifted the ban on that in Vatican II. . . ."

"Keep making that face. Just move back into camera range."

"She's gonna blow!"

"Time? Yeah, it was great. A personal best."

"There's no such thing as bad sex. Or so I've heard."

"I told you I could finish before the commercial ended."

"Are you my best lover ever? In the continental U.S., definitely."

"Whew, I feel like I should leave money on the dresser."

"Had to type a quick e-mail to your office to tell you how much I dug that twisted boinking we did last night. Specifically . . ."

"I'm not going to wash you off. Ever."

You Can Do Better

The important thing is having plenty of ammo for when you're ready to make babies. Increase the volume of semen you're pumping out, and you should be ready for the egg hunt.

Prime the pump. Masturbate a few hours before sex, but stop when you near the point of ejaculation, recommends Lyle Lundblad, M.D., director of Midwest Urology in Minnesota. "Your prostate and seminal vessels will produce a great deal of semen that's still going to be there a few hours later," he says. That means that when you actually have sex, you'll ejaculate your normal amount of semen, plus the extra you built up masturbating.

Ask her to wear that wig. Or any other prop that'll get you more aroused than usual. "The amount of fluid you ejaculate has a great deal to do with your degree of sexual excitement," says Dr. Lundblad.

Consider the patch. Testosterone supplements—like the patch, gel, or injections—can significantly increase your rate of semen production, particularly if you've demonstrated low testosterone levels in the past, says Dr. Lundblad. Ask your doctor to check your blood level of testosterone; it should be at least 280 nanograms per deciliter.

THE AVERAGE GUY IS READY FOR ACTION AGAIN IN 30 MINUTES

The 18-year-old you needed only 15 minutes; the 60-year-old version will need 20 hours.

You Can Do Better

You're a battery in need of charging, a gas tank in need of filling, a stapler in need of . . . You get the point.

Grab a bottle. Instead of falling asleep after your first orgasm, roll out of bed and pour two glasses of wine. In addition to its being a surprisingly romantic gesture, the alcohol will help increase the arousal signals between your brain and your penis, says James Barada, M.D., a urologist and director of the Center for Male Sexual Health in Albany, New York. Stop at one glass, though; more than that will actually depress your nervous system and make it harder to have an erection.

Don't reach for it. Daily masturbation may someday bring about world peace, but it won't shorten your refractory period. "The more you ejaculate, the longer your refractory periods," says Dr. Danoff. If you're planning a particularly big night of romping, try not to masturbate in the week prior.

THE AVERAGE GUY SPENDS 15 MINUTES ON FOREPLAY

No, not per year.

You Can Do Better

Improve the quality of foreplay and she'll never again bug you about the quantity. "If you act as if you're just going through the motions to get to the sex, she's going to notice, and it will take longer for her to get excited," says Michael Perry, Ph.D., a sex therapist in Encino, California. So do what you want to do. If you like how her calves feel, stroke them. If you like her butt, kiss it. "When a man is loving what he's doing, it's going to show through and turn her on, too," says Perry. Still taking too long? Try these time-savers.

Let her simmer. "You have to get her mind working on sex," says Gloria Brame, a clinical sexologist based in Atlanta and author of *Come Hither: A Commonsense Guide to Kinky Sex.* Maybe ask her to wear a thong in the morning, then whisper something dirty over the phone at lunch. She'll be so excited by the time dinner rolls around that she'll be willing to spend less time on foreplay.

Create touching moments. Don't wait until you're tearing open the condom wrapper with your teeth before making that initial physical contact. Whether it's resting your hand on her leg while you're driving, or carefully pulling that loose strand of hair away from her face, a touch here and there will pay off big later. "Do this enough and she'll be jumping on you and wanting to have sex," says Marilyn Fithian, Ph.D., a sex therapist in Long Beach, California.

Ignore her breasts for a moment. Ask her to roll over so you can work on her lower back instead. It's the one place you must rub/massage/fondle. Why? According to Brame, this is a major erogenous zone for most women. "It'll stimulate her pelvic muscles and make her feel more relaxed."

THE AVERAGE GUY HAS A 60 PERCENT CHANCE OF BEING INFECTED WITH A SEXUALLY TRANSMITTED DISEASE

And odds are it'll be human papillomavirus, a.k.a. genital warts; it's estimated that about 1 million men are infected.

You Can Do Better

Keep your eyes open for a no-excuse condom like the eZ-on from Mayer Labs. First, it's designed to unfold in both directions, meaning you don't have to slow down the sex by worrying about accidentally contaminating the business side with pre-ejaculatory fluid. Second, the eZ-on has a baggy fit for improved sensation. Finally, since it's made with polyurethane, latex allergies—hers or yours—aren't a concern. "This is a radical departure from traditional condom design," says Paul Blumenthal, M.D., director of contraceptive research and programs at Johns Hopkins Bayview Medical Center. The eZ-on received FDA approval October 2001 and is available in stores now.

THE AVERAGE GUY MASTURBATES ONCE A DAY

In case you were wondering what she does with all those D batteries . . . women masturbate once a week.

You Can Do Better

Masturbation isn't just DIY sex; it's also a "conditioning program" for guys who suffer from premature ejaculation. If that's you, try this.

Week 1: Masturbate with a dry hand until you can go 20 minutes before ejaculating.

Week 2: Add a lubricant such as baby oil or Astroglide, and masturbate until you can hold out for 20 minutes again.

Week 3: Keep practicing.

Week 4: Add your favorite porn mag to the mix and work on reaching 20 minutes once more. Stop when you can go the distance with the lube and the magazine.

THE AVERAGE GUY'S SEX LIFE STAYS THE SAME OR GETS BETTER AFTER MARRIAGE

We're not just talking about newlyweds. Eighty percent of married men remain sexually active after they turn 70.

You Can Do Better

Even if the sex is honeymoon quality, there's room for more wedded bliss.

Pop the question. Come right out and ask what she likes during sex. "Most women appreciate men who want to make sure they're satisfied," says Barbara Bartlik, M.D., a professor of psychiatry at Cornell University. "If she notices you're working hard to please her, she'll be more likely to return the favor." And tell us: Is there a better place to develop your work ethic?

Cut out the Internet porn. You'd think it would make things hotter, but according to a survey of Web porn viewers, 68 percent of couples have had their sex lives adversely affected by the glowing box in the next room. "The computer becomes a third person in the relationship," says Gerald Schoenewolf, Ph.D., a psychoanalyst and director of the Living Center in New York City. Try logging on less and ogling her more.

Tell her she hasn't lost it. As she gets older, she may begin to doubt her attractiveness, which could affect the quality of the sex, says Timothy Perper, Ph.D., author of *Sex Signals*. So tell her you still find her sexy, and make a point of frequently touching her face and hair, two places where women define their beauty. According to Perper, the more comfortable she feels with her body, the more likely she'll initiate sex and be more adventurous while having it.

The Master Craftsman's Guide to Sex

You already have the best tool for the job. Now you just need to hone your technique. Here, the proper method for whatever tonight's project might be

By Alix Strauss

Every woman wants a man who's handy around the house—a stud who can rewire a lamp, fix a leaky faucet, and restart her furnace on those damp, cold nights. As the saying goes, a man's work is never done: Come nightfall there's always one more job for her handyman, her Roto-Rooter guy, her Mr. Service-with-a-Smile.

Fortunately, men already come equipped with the right tool for the job. What you need is to learn its many uses, its wide variety of speeds, angles, and, yes, attachments. Simply identify the task you're looking to accomplish and

LET HER INTO YOUR TOOLBOX

A good handyman always has his tools, well, handy. So should you. Here are nine fine craftsman's tools to keep near your bed.

Misto sprayer. She may keep her olive oil in one, but you should store lube in this spray bottle. You can apply it—and reapply it—without making a mess. Find one in any cookware store.

Koosh balls. These rubber-tentacled toys are perfect for foreplay (think feather duster); or try stashing several of them under her back during sex for a rolling massage.

Doc Johnson I-Vibe. This is the perfect vibrator for first timers because it's small and friendly looking, says Susan Crain Bakos, author of *Sexational Secrets*. Order the vibrator for $30 from www.xandria.com.

Hot Sex. Our favorite sex manual. Tracey Cox, an Australian sex writer, packs her book with good, practical tips.

Herotica. You get turned on by pictures (keep those in a separate place); she gets turned on by words—the kind you'll find in this collection of sexual short stories. Order from www.xandria.com.

Car chamois. Not only does sheepskin feel great on naked skin, but the smell could also turn her on. "The skin of mammals has many musk glands that continue to emit odor after the animal's long gone," says David Givens, Ph.D., an anthropologist. "These scents often mimic human sexual steroids."

Trojan Pleasure Mesh Condom. Nothing against ribs, but most are too subtle to make much difference. This condom has hundreds of crisscrossed ridges you can actually feel. Get a free sample from www.trojancondoms.com.

Passion Dust. Sprinkle this chocolate-flavored powder on a few of her body parts, then help yourself. It's like sex with Nestlé Quik. Order from www.xandria.com.

Minivac. This electronics duster ($15 to $25)—the type used to clean keyboards and camera lenses—will feel as if it's giving her light kisses on the neck, breasts, and feet. Don't use your Hoover upright; it'll leave bruises.

use the technique we describe, and we guarantee you'll have just one project to tackle the next morning: fixing the headboard.

Your Task: GET HER TO ORGASM, PRONTO

Your Technique: The You-Sit-'n'-She-Spins

Grab the nearest handsaw and slice the arms off a dining room chair while she watches, admiring your biceps. Have a seat and ask her to take one, too—on your lap, facing you, her arms around your neck.

"This is a good position because you have clear access to her clitoris. While you penetrate her with your penis, you can stimulate her clitoris with your fingers, doubling her pleasure," says Gloria Brame, a clinical sexologist based in Atlanta and author of *Come Hither: A Commonsense Guide to Kinky Sex*. "Your scrotum is pressed up against her labia—the lips of her vagina—and you can penetrate deep within her, to hit her G-spot."

Master Craftsman's Tip: For advanced sex, says Brame, try the same trick with an armless rocking chair. "You get that extra lunging in on every rock."

Your Task: GET HER PREGNANT
Your Technique: The Advanced Missionary Position

Ignoring the advice of your college buddies ("You? Breed? Ew!"), you've decided to step up to the plate and take a whack at fatherhood. To fulfill this mission, you need to improve your standard missionary.

"If you want to get your partner pregnant, your goal is to have as much sperm move up through her cervix as possible," says Milton Haynes, M.D., a gynecologist at Lenox Hill Hospital in New York. "So a lot depends on the position of the cervix and the uterus."

Have her lie on her back. Insert tab A into slot B. Now gently lift her legs so they rest on your shoulders. "This allows the cervix to dip into the back of the vagina, where most of the sperm will accumulate." The closer her knees are to her chest, the deeper you can penetrate.

Master Craftsman's Tip: If 2 months' worth of dedicated tooling around doesn't produce the desired result, your partner may have the rare retroverted uterus: It points in a direction that makes it more difficult to conceive. Only her gynecologist can tell for sure; if the doctor deems it so, doggy style might be more reproductive for you.

Your Task: OPERATE HEAVY MACHINERY WHILE UNDER THE INFLUENCE OF ALCOHOL
Your Technique: The Modified Pushup

To begin, a brief lesson in hydraulics: Alcohol is a vasodilator, which means it sends blood out from your heart and into every other part of your body. But you need blood to concentrate in your penis, to make it erect and keep it hard until your work is done. So enlist the aid of gravity. "For a man who's having erection trouble, particularly in a case like this, the optimal position for him is facedown, or even standing," says Harris M. Nagler, M.D., chairman of the department of urology at Beth Israel Medical Center in New

DAY AND TIME THE AVERAGE GUY IS MOST LIKELY TO BE HAVING SEX: SATURDAY, LATE EVENING

WHEN HE'S LEAST LIKELY TO BE HAVING SEX: MONDAY, EARLY AFTERNOON

York City. Get on top, and once you enter her, push up with your arms so your upper body is supported above her, as though you were doing a pushup. This lets even more blood flow downhill while also keeping your stinking whiskey breath away from her delicate sensibilities.

Drunken Master Craftsman's Tip: Let her be the designated driver. To calm the spins, you lie across the bed with your feet planted on the floor and one hand against the wall. She hops into the driver's seat, engages the stick, and pilots the vehicle until you both arrive safely at your destinations.

Your Task: PROVE IT ALL NIGHT
Your Technique: The Sideswipe

"If you want to last through a sexual marathon," says Jacques Moritz, M.D., director of gynecology at Roosevelt Hospital in New York City, "the trick is to be in the position that's least tiring. The less body weight you have on you, the less energy you'll expend." Lie on the bed facing each other, legs intertwined. Keep the movements slow and small. "Right before the big moment, stop, slow down, let your penis relax, wait for it to get hard again, and continue," Dr. Moritz says. You can slow down emerging tremors by squeezing your butt cheeks together while tensing your PC muscles (not the ones you use to hurl a crashed computer through the bay window; we mean the pubococcygeal muscles—the same ones you'd use to stop the flow of urine).

Master Craftsman's Tip: Hold her and whisper, "In this position, we're like two waves coming together." She'll be reenergized and ready for more in no time.

Your Task: HIDE YOUR EXPANDING BEER BELLY
Your Technique: The Soft Supine

If you're on the heavy side, lie on your back. This flattens out your gut. Now have her straddle you and plant her hands on your chest. Presto—belly-be-gone! To add to this undercover operation, "invest in a supersoft comforter," says Brame. "Your out-of-shape body will sink right in."

Master Craftsman's Tip: The average 170-pound man burns 90 calories during 50 minutes of fooling around. The heavier you are, the more energy it takes to do your thing, and the more calories you'll burn.

Your Task: MASTER THE QUICKIE
Your Technique: The "Where's My Supper, Woman?"

"The typical American couple has sex at night, then they go to sleep," says Stephen Braveman, a certified sex therapist in Monterey, California. But sometimes life demands a more urgent response—like when you're really horny but late for a family reunion. "A kitchen table makes an ideal location because she's sitting on a high surface and you can enter her readily," Braveman says. The fridge is close, too.

Master Craftsman's Tip: To really add some spice to your sex life, Braveman suggests making a quick stop at a bank. "A safe-deposit-box room is quiet, the door is locked, and there's no camera." It's a great place to make a deposit and withdrawal.

Your Task: ROCK HER WORLD WITHOUT WAKING THE KIDS IN THE NEXT ROOM

Your Technique: Floor Exercises

"The floor is a nice place to be when you're trying to be quiet and have intimacy," says Braveman. "You can't hit your head on anything, and you have more space to spread out." And no squeaky mattress springs.

Lie on your back with a pillow or comforter underneath you, your knees bent, feet planted. This gives you leverage, balance, and control. "The more

FIX HER FAUCET

Perhaps the only thing more mysterious than a woman's mind is her body. You'll probably never really know what's going on up there, but you can get a pretty good idea of what's going on down there—in fact, maybe even better than she has.

1. Time her cycle. A woman has many ways of letting you know her period is coming, including pitching extended crying jags, throwing crockery, and, worse, sending you to the store to buy tampons. But a woman with irregular periods may not know when her time is coming—unless you use your superior handyman knowledge to forewarn her. If you notice an unusual thickness or tightness when you enter her, you can bet her period is only a few days away. That means you'll have to . . .

2. Treat her gently. When she has her period, her uterus tends to swell, which can make sex slightly uncomfortable for her, particularly if you're used to trolling in the deep water. Back off and use short, shallow thrusts.

3. Feel her pain. You just had vigorous sex, and now she's complaining of pelvic pain. Ask her

how many days it's been since her last period began. If it's been about 2 weeks, she's ovulating, and chances are Mr. Mojo ruptured a cyst—a small, fluid-filled sac that encloses the egg. The discomfort should abate in about an hour.

4. Explain that stain. Another result of rollicking sex can be a massive quantity of clear, watery liquid. She'll think she peed herself, but you'll know by the lack of odor that it's a by-product of the Skene's glands in her vagina. It's female ejaculate—uncommon, but produced during explosive orgasms. Take credit.

5. Take the blame. During intercourse, her vagina expands in width, and in length as the cervix lifts. When you pull out, air can get trapped in there, forming little pockets when she returns to normal size. These air pockets need to escape, so when she stands up, she may make a noise like a passel of cowboys after a chili-eating contest. Smile endearingly and explain that it's a normal by-product of sex. (Maybe she'll be more forgiving of you next time.)

physical control you both have, the less likely you are to moan and groan," says Braveman. Plus, in this position both partners can reach down and touch the woman's clitoris, which will increase her ability to reach orgasm.

Master Craftsman's Tip: If the kiddies wake up and see too much, don't rush to cover up anyone, or anything. "If kids don't see any action, they become disinterested," Braveman says. "If you get all hysterical, they won't leave."

Your Task: USE A TOOL THAT'S TOO SMALL FOR THE JOB
Your Technique: The High-Flying Flag

Not a problem for you, of course, but perhaps you have a friend who, in a moment of weakness, confessed this secret to you. Be supportive and share this method with him.

Lie on your back on a firm surface. Your body won't sink into the surface, and your penis will stay at its maximum elevation. Now have her climb on board, facing you. "This will allow you the most contact with her clitoris, which is more important in bringing her to orgasm than penetration, regardless of penis size or depth of thrusting," says Anna Marti, an intimacy coach in Portland, Oregon. Her professional assessment of the technique: "Yum."

Master Craftsman's Tip: With you still inside her, ask your gal to stretch her legs and squeeze her PC muscles. This contracts the vagina, makes her more orgasmic, and gives you a more taut feeling.

Your Task: DO THE WEEKI WACHEE UNDERWATER
Your Technique: The Weightless Wiggle

Male parrot fish have sex many times a day, with as many partners as they can find. Why should you be missing out? Dressed in scuba gear, and already immersed in water, have your little mermaid let out a bit of air from her buoyancy compensator (BC) device. "Now have her sit on top of your hips and wrap her legs around you while you support her with your hands," says David Taylor, an open-water instructor for Scuba Diving International. "Since she now weighs half a pound, this won't be hard." In fact, it's one time when she won't ask, "Do I look fat?"

Once you're inside her, add air to your BC so you'll both be weightless. "As always, keep the movements slow and easy," Taylor says. "If you need to, dig your feet into the sand for extra support."

Master Craftsman's Tip: Bring a little tube of lubricant. All that salt and rubber makes penetration a little tricky.

Your Task: TAKE OFF WITH AIRPLANE SEX
Your Technique: The Flight Attendant

Give your gal Friday a knowing nod and unbuckle her seat belt. Then wink. She heads to the rest room. After a moment, you follow to tend to her needs. "Once there, place her hands up against the wall as if you're going to frisk her. Pull her hips back and spread her legs," says R. Don Steele, author of *How to Date Young Women for Men over 35.* "Enter her gently from behind and enjoy the turbulence."

Master Craftsman's Tip: Find the lockbox. Rather than knock on the bathroom door, arousing the suspicions of *actual* attendants, add a moment of suspense by opening the door yourself. Look above the vacant/occupied dial for a small metal box about the size of an eraser. On some planes, this box contains a secret release that lets you in from the outside. Sneak in when no one's looking.

Swollen Gland

It's mysterious, it's agonizing, and it can screw up your sex life but good. Now new research may have the answers to the strange male illness called prostatitis

By Tom Zoellner

Clark Hickman's problems started one night when he was awakened by a ferocious need to pee and a burning at the core of his penis. The future professor, then just 25 years old, saw a doctor, who checked him for STDs, gave him some antibiotics, and told him he was fine. He wasn't. A nagging backache, a low-grade fever, and a perpetually swollen prostate soon joined his list of symptoms. He was unable to ride a bicycle, sit on a hard chair, or even lean to one side. "The pain was excruciating," he recalls. Six weeks later, a urologist found pus in Hickman's prostatic fluid and handed him the diagnosis: prostatitis.

It afflicts as many as 15 percent of men between ages 20 and 50, making it the most common ailment to affect a man's sexual plumbing. It's also one of the most painful. When prostatitis strikes, the walnut-shaped gland becomes inflamed and swells (not to be confused with benign prostatic hyperplasia, or BPH, in which the prostate literally grows larger as you age). As the prostate balloons in the already tight quarters it occupies, it begins to push against the bladder and the urethra. Crowd your bladder and you'll need to pee—bad. Squeeze your urethra and you'll feel as if someone had squirted lighter fluid into your penis and then struck a match.

The worst problem associated with the disease? Ignorance. About all that doctors know for sure is that a small percentage of cases are caused by a treatable bacterial infection. The rest—an estimated 90 percent—are labeled "chronic nonbacterial prostatitis," a condition that ranks right up there with fibromyalgia and chronic fatigue syndrome for sheer misery, mystery, and frustration.

"We're all over the place with this," says Jeannette Potts, M.D., a urologist with the Cleveland Clinic Foundation. "Most doctors take the strategy of giving the patient an antibiotic and hoping he'll go away. Most of these men wind up doctor hopping because nobody can tell them what's wrong."

According to a *Journal of the American Medical Association* report, some men even give up on conventional medicine: "Patients from across the globe have journeyed to the Philippines and to Ukraine to partake in undocumented cures, mail-ordered powerful magnets to sit on, and drunk gallons of carrot juice, all in hope of lessening pain and restoring a normal sex life."

But as bleak as things look, don't write off man's main gland just yet. There are a handful of researchers out there who have had the, well, balls to attack prostatitis with all the academic firepower at their disposal. The result? Two promising new theories that just may lead to a cure.

THE X GERMS

Somewhere in the not-so-exotic city of Fort Lauderdale, one guy's feeling remarkably optimistic about prostatitis. Daniel Shoskes, M.D., a urologist with the city's branch of the Cleveland Clinic, is one of a growing number of researchers who believe the key to solving the prostatitis riddle lies in questioning everyone's most basic assumption about the disease: that bacteria aren't to blame. "I believe some of these cases of so-called chronic nonbacterial prostatitis really are due to a bacterial infection," he says.

HOME GLAND SECURITY

There may not be a cure, but there is a guaranteed way to avoid coming down with prostatitis in the first place. It's called a radical prostatectomy. Or, if you'd rather reduce your risk without getting rid of your gland, you can try these strategies instead.

Drink two glasses of cranberry juice every day. A study review published in the journal *Urology* showed that tannins, phytochemicals found in cranberries, prevent bacteria from sticking to the lining of the urinary tract. "Theoretically, this should also inhibit the bacteria from setting up shop in the prostate," says Franklin Lowe, M.D., the study's lead author.

Don't hold back at the urinal. Next time you step up to pee, make a conscious attempt to relax your sphincter muscles. See, having a tense butt in the bathroom can keep you from draining all the urine out of your urethra and cause it to back up into your prostate, where it may leave behind bacteria and other waste.

Use a condom during oral sex? While he still lacks, er, hard evidence, John Polacheck, M.D., director of the Prostatitis Center in Tucson, believes some cases of chronic prostatitis are the result of unprotected oral sex. "It may be that bacteria in the mouth migrate up the urethra," he says. If you're the cautious type, you can at least make disease control fun for her by slipping a strawberry-flavored prophylactic on your Popsicle.

Like most urologists, Dr. Shoskes had always fallen back on a diagnosis of chronic nonbacterial prostatitis whenever a patient didn't respond to a course of antibiotics. But that line of reasoning went out the laboratory window last year with the publication of a study from the University of Washington.

In the prostate biopsies of several study subjects, researchers found the DNA of bacteria they had never seen before—in men who had been believed to be bacteria-free. Suddenly, urologists had to consider that the failure of antibiotics wasn't a sign of a nonbacterial condition but rather an indication that they weren't using the right drugs for this new strain of bacteria. The next step: identifying the mutant microorganisms and then developing the drugs to quash them. Studies are now under way at the University of Washington and the Cleveland Clinic Florida.

Such stealth bacteria may have been what invaded and inflamed Hickman's prostate. Even though previous courses of antibiotics had proved ineffective, the last urologist he visited (the ninth in a long string of shoulder shruggers) decided to put him on doxycycline. It seemed to work.

"The doctor stumbled onto something that I was sensitive to, and my symptoms cleared up," says Hickman, who's been mostly symptom-free for 8 years. But rather than being the magic bullet, doxycycline was probably just a lucky shot against an unclassified strain of bacteria. "It appears that the urologist just hit on the right antibiotic, but it could also be that the timing was coincidental and symptoms may have disappeared regardless," says Leroy Nyberg, M.D., Ph.D., head of urology research at the National Institute of Diabetes, Digestive and Kidney Diseases.

ARTHRITIS OF THE PROSTATE

But what about those men whose lab samples show no sign of infection whatsoever? Even in these cases, bacteria may be to blame, albeit in a roundabout way. In a recent study published in the journal *Urology*, researchers discovered elevated levels of cytokines—a classic marker of autoimmune response—in the prostatic fluid of some men. This finding—combined with the resemblance of prostatitis to other autoimmune disorders, such as rheuma-

HELP FIND A CURE

Call or write to your congressman and ask him to push funding for the International Prostatitis Collaborative Network at the National Institutes of Health. The network is a group of doctors and research centers working to find a cure for the disease.

Or, better yet, get in touch with the House and Senate Appropriations Subcommittee on Labor, Health and Human Services, and Education, the group that doles out the dough to the NIH. The address is 2358 Rayburn HOB, Washington, D.C. 20515-6024.

toid arthritis—has prompted researchers to theorize that the condition may also be the body's lingering response to an infection that was knocked out long ago.

"A lot of men are fixated on the idea that they have an infection and will stay on antibiotics for years," says Dr. Shoskes. "But their problems might be because their bodies are *acting* as though there is still something to fight."

If it turns out that some men's immune systems are swinging at bacterial ghosts, then medications used to treat rheumatoid arthritis should also work against prostatitis. This theory is being tested at the University of Maryland in a clinical study of Enbrel, a new anti-arthritis drug that works by "capturing" the excess cytokines believed to cause runaway inflammation.

"All of us are starting to realize that this disease is really several different diseases," says Richard Alexander, M.D., a urologist with the University of Maryland medical center.

In some cases these diseases may not be diseases at all but bad habits and bad coping strategies. One is known as dysfunctional voiding, an unconscious tensing of the sphincter muscles when you pee. This ill-timed pressure pushes urine back up through the urethra and into the prostate, where it causes irritation and inflammation, says Dr. Nyberg.

Another theory is that prostatitis is essentially a "headache of the pelvis," caused by stress and pent-up aggression. And there are a number of doctors who think that slight symptoms can escalate into big ones after the patient worries about them too much. In other words, it's all in their heads.

"I don't think patients create the pain," says Dr. Potts, "but treatment frustrations or the fear of underlying serious disease can magnify their perception of it."

IN THE MEANTIME, SOME RELIEF

Don't even think about telling Rich Ellenberger that the pain that pushed him into an emergency room was something he worried into existence. "It felt as if someone was stabbing my left testicle with a knife," says the 35-year-old NASA engineer from Houston. After a series of urologists brushed him off, Ellenberger flew to Arizona, where he'd heard a doctor was having success performing "prostatic massage," a procedure in which prostatic fluid is drained in an attempt to remove problem-causing substances—be they bacteria, cytokines, urine, or something else yet to be discovered.

When the massage was over, Ellenberger's symptoms abated, if only temporarily. But it was enough relief to convince him to stay in Arizona and telecommute to work for 3 months in order to continue to receive treatment. Today, back in Houston, he still goes for prostatic massages while he waits for a permanent solution.

"I've gotten it to a manageable stage," says Ellenberger.

And that's the trick, isn't it? Figure out a way to keep the pain at bay until you hear the researchers scream, "Eureka!" Prostatic massage is one way to go.

"A lot of men say they're miserable on the drive home, but then report the first pain-free days they've had in a long time," says Dr. Shoskes. (Go to www.chronicprostatitis.com/clinics.html to find a list of qualified urologists.)

Of course, there are less invasive methods you can try, like popping quercetin. A Scrabble-winning "Q" word, quercetin is an antioxidant that's been shown to have anti-inflammatory properties. In a study published in *Urology*, prostatitis sufferers who took 500 milligrams of quercetin twice a day for a month reported a 35 percent reduction in symptoms, compared with those who took a placebo. You can buy it in most drugstores.

Or you can ask your urologist about the prescription drug Proscar. Traditionally used to treat BPH, Proscar is showing promise against prostatitis. It's believed to lower levels of dihydrotestosterone, a hormone that can make your ever-expanding gland grow even bigger.

The simplest and cheapest remedy of all? Masturbation. This is essentially a DIY version of prostatic massage: You drain out some fluid, you get some relief. When Turkish researchers had men with chronic prostatitis masturbate twice a week for 6 months, they found that it improved the symptoms of roughly half the study subjects. Also works if your wife lends a hand.

Are You Ready to Get Fixed?

The decision to cut off your sperm supply, man's most prized possession, is complex. Here's how to simplify it

By Bill Stump

How about a little snip, snip?" my wife asked slyly, making a scissoring motion with the fingers of her right hand. I was naked, exposed, ready to step into the shower.

It was Saturday morning. The subject was contraception. The "snip, snip" was her way of telling me to get fixed. I can't imagine a more emasculating reference.

Surely she knew—she had to know—how sensitive a subject this was. Like most guys, I'd spent years, from teendom until age 30, establishing my virility. Weights, sports, cars, dates. Then came the ultimate proof: two of the cutest, smartest kids on God's green earth. And now, cutting off the ability to

NUMBER OF HOURS PER YEAR THE
AVERAGE GUY SPENDS THINKING ABOUT SEX: 730

NUMBER OF HOURS PER YEAR HE SPENDS HAVING IT: 22

SPLIT DECISION

By Joaquin Ramirez

I was the perfect candidate for a vasectomy. Mid-thirties, with three healthy boys, I was neck deep in that singular time of life when you're building a family and a career and don't have enough time for either. I was trying to make it work. It was a grind.

Sex with my wife was fine, and birth control was something I hadn't worried about in years. But she started forgetting to take her pill, and the last thing I wanted was another round of 2 A.M. feedings.

We talked about vasectomy, and I ran a quick personal inventory: I have three kids, I can't imagine having any more, I want sex with my wife, and I don't want any hassles. So I scheduled an appointment. It was quick and painless.

But my marriage wasn't. Over time, it became more and more complicated. She didn't like the frustrations life threw at her, and when I couldn't end them, I was let go so she could find someone who could. (She's still looking.) I was summarily dismissed as a husband, but my fathering duties and financial responsibilities remained intact.

I was relieved to have the burden of her expectations lifted, though, and I lived happily on my own, in a condo in a cool part of the city. The boys came twice a week and on weekends.

What I didn't expect was to get married again. Sex, sure. Relationship, sure. But I didn't want to get enmeshed again. Yet this woman was pretty, smart, and kind, and we got moving along that worn path quickly. Her husband had left her hurt and without children.

It took me 3 weeks—not long, you'd say, but long enough to know we'd be together—to tell her I'd had a vasectomy. She desperately wanted children but was supportive and hopeful with the what-ifs: We could reverse it, have in vitro, adopt.

I did have the vasectomy reversed, 2 years later. Cost me more than five grand. Didn't work. They took some sperm and froze it, though. We were disappointed, and it took a few years for us to regroup. So here I am, 45 years old, my wife 40. Our only option left for having our own children is to try in vitro fertilization with my cryogenic sperm. It will cost $10,000 a shot, and it's likely to take three or more shots, if it works at all.

I have three wonderful children, and my wife and I could buy a cabin upstate for the cost of an unsure thing. The key difference is, she has three wonderful stepchildren. Nice, but a cabin can't fill that void.

Adoption is still a possibility, but the clock is ticking for us both. I can't say I wish I hadn't had the vasectomy—who knew? Instead, I use it as a reminder that fate has an ironic sense of humor—don't tempt it.

reproduce at age 36 seemed such a waste. Not just for me, but for God's green earth, which can always use more cute, smart kids.

Factor in that I'd been trained since my earliest years never to put anything sharp near my testicles. My mind was made up.

No. The answer would be no. But then she upped the ante. She talked about sex, which she doesn't talk about, and hinted—kind of teased me—about the prospect of more, better sex. I think she used the word "spontaneity." I remembered I have a minivan. Why should birth control be solely her responsibility?

But on the heels of that thought came other, darker ones. What if something happened to one of our kids, or even my wife? What if someday I wanted more children? What, I thought, though not seriously, about my trophy wife when I'm 50?

"Umm, I'll have to think about it," I said, climbing safely into the stall and jerking on the cold water. "It's a big deal."

"Does it have to be?" she said. Then this: "Let me know. I'll be waiting."

Confused, I did what we *Men's Health* editors always do: I talked to our research department. They dug through tons of studies and consulted doctors who deal with this decision every day. Not just whether to have it done, but how, when, and why. The resources and information they offered follow here. My wife? She's waiting, and so am I. But neither one of us can wait forever.

THE SNIP DECISION

A vasectomy may be a minor procedure, but it's a major decision. True, microsurgical reversal has a 40 to 73 percent chance of leading to a naturally conceived pregnancy (versus test tube conception), but consider this: A vasectomy takes 8 to 30 minutes, can cost as much as $1,500, and may be covered (at least in part) by insurance. A reversal takes 4 to 5 hours, costs as much as $10,000, and is minimally covered by insurance if it's covered at all.

"Men need to go into vasectomy thinking it's permanent," says Marc Goldstein, M.D., professor of Reproductive Medicine and Urology and surgeon-in-chief of the Cornell Center for Male Reproductive Medicine and Surgery in New York City

Is it for you? Answer the following questions to find out.

- Are you married?
- Do you have two or more kids?
- Do you consider your marriage to be stable and happy?
- Are you 35 or older?
- Are you prepared for permanent contraception?

If you can answer yes to all of the above, you're a good candidate, says Dr. Goldstein. Even one no, however, and you should reconsider, especially if you're in a rocky or childless marriage. "The majority of men who divorce remarry, often to women 10 to 20 years younger with no children of their own," says Dr. Goldstein. "These are the men who come back for a reversal."

"I'VE BEEN NEUTERED" AND OTHER MYTHS

Vasectomy. Hear the word and thoughts naturally stray to that day Fido was fixed. Butts suddenly went unsniffed and couches unhumped; your wife started to call him "It." You never quite forgave yourself for neutering him, so how can you do it to yourself?

First off, it's a different procedure. Your best friend was castrated; you're just cutting off your sperm supply, and that has no effect on how horny you get, says Joel Feigin, M.D., an associate professor of family medicine at UMDNJ–Robert Wood Johnson Medical School in New Jersey.

Other urban legends . . .

You'll run dry. Actually, only 3 percent of a man's ejaculate comes from his testicles, but that's where 100 percent of his sperm originates. Not only will you still be erupting at full capacity, but there also will be no change in the semen's color, taste, texture, or smell, says Dr. Feigin.

You'll have scars. The two incisions made during a standard vasectomy are no longer than 1.5 centimeters and are sutured with one or two stitches. Within a few weeks of the procedure, all visible signs fade into the folds of the scrotum. The preferred, no-scalpel technique is even less invasive, requiring only a pinpoint puncture of the scrotal skin. The puncture virtually disappears from sight after surgery.

You'll get prostate cancer. A few years ago, researchers noticed that men with vasectomies had higher rates of prostate cancer. Is there a link? Absolutely not, says J. Stephen Jones, M.D., a urologist at the Cleveland Clinic Foundation in Ohio. "Men who get vasectomies go to urologists," he says. "Therefore they're also getting rectal exams and blood tests that detect prostate cancer." In fact, studies show that men who have vasectomies are more likely to have their prostate cancer diagnosed in its early stages, when it's still treatable.

DON'T GO UNDER THE KNIFE

Technically, you have two vasectomy options: scalpel and no-scalpel. Both are safe and medically proven, but if they were our eggs, we'd put them all in the no-scalpel basket. No-scalpel vasectomy (NSV) is up to 50 percent quicker, results in one-tenth the number of complications, and, because there are no incisions or sutures, involves less bleeding and postoperative pain. In 1995 (the last time the Centers for Disease Control and Prevention counted), NSVs made up roughly 30 percent of all vasectomies done in the United States.

The caveat? NSV requires considerable skill. Find a doctor who performs a minimum of 25 procedures a year, says Dr. Goldstein, who has himself performed 2,500 NSV surgeries since 1985.

PERCENTAGE OF PREGNANCIES THAT ARE UNINTENDED: 48

How a No-Scalpel Vasectomy Is Performed

During NSV, the scrotum is anesthetized with two injections. The surgeon isolates one of the vas deferens (the tubes that deliver sperm to the prostate gland) and with dissecting forceps makes a puncture 2 to 5 millimeters (mm) deep. The vas deferens is severed, cauterized, and returned to the scrotum. The opposite vas deferens is then extracted through the same hole, and the process is repeated. When it's all over, the puncture contracts to 2 to 3 mm in size, so no sutures are necessary. A dab of antibiotic ointment is applied, the puncture is dressed, and the patient is sent on his way. Total elapsed time: 20 minutes, tops.

The Pre-Op Checklist

- Schedule the procedure for a Friday. You'll be in, out, and back at work on Monday.
- Avoid aspirin. In the week before and after V day, avoid aspirin and anti-inflammatory analgesics like Advil (ibuprofen); they thin blood and can increase the risk of postoperative bleeding. Use a nonaspirin pain reliever, such as Tylenol.
- Eat light. The anesthetic (or the feeling of a needle piercing your privates) can induce nausea in rare cases.
- Shave yourself. That is, if you don't want to get mowed by a nurse. You'll need a silver-dollar-size bare spot in the middle of the scrotum, directly beneath the penis.
- Prepare to indulge yourself during recovery. Set up a recliner and a tray table in front of the TV with the essentials: list of shows, remote, magazines, and bell to summon pity food. Add a small cooler of beer and you'll wonder why you didn't get snipped sooner.

The Post-Op Checklist

- To minimize strain, replace your boxers with a jock strap.
- Keep your feet elevated for the first 24 hours after surgery.
- Ice the area with a bag of frozen peas (it'll conform to irregular shapes better than an ice pack).
- You can't participate in sex or sports for a week (watching is okay).
- To kill the itch when your hair resprouts—and believe us, it will itch—

AGE AT WHICH THE AVERAGE GUY LOSES HIS VIRGINITY: 17

AGE AT WHICH THE AVERAGE WOMAN LOSES HERS: 18

use a 50–50 mix of 1 percent hydrocortisone cream and Lamisil, both available over the counter.

KEEP THE CONDOMS

It's been a week, and your soldier's ready for deployment. Better strap on some protection. Why? There's still some ammo left in the barrel.

It takes approximately 15 postvasectomy ejaculations for a man to be azoospermic (fancy way of saying without sperm), says Richard E. Berger, M.D., a professor of urology at the University of Washington. Doctors perform a first semen analysis after 6 weeks, and a second 4 to 6 weeks later. After two consecutive samples come back sperm-free, you can trash your Trojans.

WHAT COULD GO WRONG?

The most common complication is hematoma, excessive post-op bleeding that causes the scrotum to swell, "sometimes to the size of a grapefruit," says Dr. Goldstein. Reoperation is sometimes needed to drain the blood. This is why you want a no-scalpel vasectomy. Hematoma is one-tenth as likely after NSV as after a standard scalpel vasectomy (one in 1,000 versus one in 100), says Dr. Goldstein.

WHY GENTLEMEN GET VASECTOMIES

If you really want to impress a woman, get a vasectomy. Bilateral tubal ligations (tube tying in women) still outnumber vasectomies by nearly two to one, despite the fact that tubal ligation can take three times longer than NSV and is 20 times more likely to lead to complications. The reasons? One, guys traditionally haven't been responsible for sterilization, and two, they're scared. Get over it. Statistics show that a woman's risk of dying from tubal ligation is small, but real. No one dies from a vasectomy.

WHERE DO ALL THE SPERM GO?

Every day, your body produces 72,000,000 sperm. On average, if you ejaculate every 3 days, that's about 6 teaspoons a week, a cup a month, a half gallon a year. You may have been fixed, but that doesn't cut your production. "All these millions of sperm make up only 3 percent of a man's ejaculate. They could fit on the head of a pin, but that's enough sperm to populate the United States," notes Dr. Goldstein. A vasectomy prevents these sperm from mixing with the ejaculate. With no outlet, the sperm sit in the epididymis. After a few days they die and are flushed from your system.

There's no risk that goes along with accumulating sperm—unless you decide to have a reversal of your vasectomy. After you get snipped, traces of sperm inevitably leak into the bloodstream. Your system treats them like viral invaders and starts concocting antisperm antibodies. The antibodies aren't dangerous, but if you have a reversal down the road, they may keep you infertile.

THE FRENCH CONNECTION

Thanks to an 18th-century Napoleonic law, vasectomy is outlawed in France. What's a Frenchman to do? Go to London. The birth control charity Marie Stopes International offers a vacation-vasectomy tourist package. Going rate for the procedure: $350—a good deal that should tempt any uninsured Americans traveling in Europe. You won't want to travel the day of surgery, and you will need to have your semen checked at least twice before the lab declares you "all clear." The French send their samples to Stopes, and you can, too. But if you don't want the FedEx guy to know what's in the bag, you may want to arrange testing locally. For more information, call Marie Stopes International at 44-171-574-7400 or go to www.mariestopes.org.uk.

KNOW THIS

The Long and Short of It

Taking a penis size survey is like asking Geraldo how important he is: You expect some exaggeration. Erection pollsters typically have trusted guys to measure themselves and tell the truth. *As if*. Recently, the condom maker LifeStyles set up a tent in Cancun during spring break, invited 401 college guys, provided girlie mags, and had two nurses measure (with a doctor supervising). The average length of an erect penis was 5.877 inches. That's ¼ inch to ½ inch shorter than in previous surveys. Average girth (crucial for condom making): 4.972 inches. Our favorite stat: 25 percent could not rise to the occasion.

Keep Things Up
When You're Feeling Down

Antidepressants help some men fight premature ejaculation, but for others they can spoil a night of sex. In a recent survey of 1,763 men taking antidepressants, 37 percent reported experiencing sexual dysfunction.

"Doctors have known for years about the relationship between these drugs and sexual dysfunction, but this is the first study to show how widespread the problem really is," says Anita Clayton, M.D., the study author. If you take an antidepressant and you've noticed a drop in sex drive or experienced erectile dysfunction, delay of orgasm, or inability to achieve orgasm, talk to your doctor about Wellbutrin or Serzone. They function differently in the brain than other antidepressants and trigger fewer sexual side effects. Or ask about Buspar, Symmetrel, or Viagra, which are up to 60 percent effective at reversing the sexual side effects of antidepressants.

**NUMBER OF MEN WHOSE
ERECT PENIS IS 9 INCHES OR LONGER:** 1 IN 100

Kick That Cold Sore Fast

The problem with cold sores isn't just that they look ugly and hurt like hell—they also mean a break from all your favorite oral activities (since the herpes virus that causes the sores could be transmitted to your partner's lips or genitals via contact). A new study shows that aspirin may help cold sores heal in half the time. When researchers gave 42 patients with cold sores either 125 milligrams of aspirin daily or no treatment, the aspirin subjects recovered in 5 days, compared with 9 days for the others. Aspirin may block proteins that fuel the herpes virus. "More research is needed, but if you can tolerate aspirin, it's worth trying," says Stephen Tyring, M.D., Ph.D., at the University of Texas.

Count Your Swimmers

The first FDA-approved home fertility test for men is now available in the United States. The product—called Fertilmarq—allows men to check their sperm levels at home and provides results within minutes. The test consists of a color-coded strip. Once a sample of semen is applied to it, the strip changes color. The darker the color, the greater your potency. Fertilmarq has been available in Europe for several years.

Fertility Finds

The journal *Human Reproduction* suggests that a common virus may be the cause of many men's infertility. In a study of 95 men, eight times as many infertile men had sperm with traces of latent viruses that can cause upper respiratory and eye infections. Researchers hope finding a medication that kills the virus will protect some men against infertility.

Another apparent sperm sapper: repeated exposure to organic solvents. Canadian researchers found that men who were frequently exposed to paint, ink, and building materials were three times as likely to have low sperm counts as men who weren't.

In related news, researchers at the National Institute for Child Health and Development (NICHD) analyzed sperm samples from nearly 1,500 men and found that many who were diagnosed as "borderline infertile" actually had few problems conceiving children. The study suggests that the medical guidelines used to classify men as infertile are often inaccurate. Meaning: Many men who are undergoing fertility treatment may be doing so unnecessarily, while men who've stopped trying to have children may actually be able to do so.

DOWN THE PIKE

No Cut, No More Kids

Researchers are in the early stages of developing a new no-cut vasectomy. With this new method, doctors clamp the vas deferens (the tube through which sperm travel out of the testicles) from *outside* the scrotum, then seal it shut with pulses of ultrasound. The vas deferens clogs up with dead cells and scar tissue, blocking the sperm.

Condom-Free Contraceptives

A new form of male birth control is currently in development in the United Kingdom. The implantable rods, which are inserted under the skin of the arm, contain a hormone that blocks sperm production—without altering the intensity of orgasms. The rods remain effective for up to 3 years.

In related news, scientists hope a new gel will do double duty as a contraceptive and as protection against sexually transmitted diseases. "BufferGel" reinforces the vagina's natural acidity to kill bacteria and sperm. Clinical trials are already under way.

AIDS: A Way to Stop the Spread

There's a new line of defense in the treatment of AIDS. Researchers at MIT have designed a protein that prevents HIV from entering cells, even after the virus has sneaked into the body. "The protein, called 5-helix, is carried in the bloodstream and prevents HIV from breaking through the outer walls of cells," says Michael Kay, M.D., Ph.D., one of the lead researchers. A drug based on 5-helix—which would be especially valuable for the treatment of people who have recently been exposed to the virus—could be available within 5 years.

PERCENTAGE OF MEN WHO WERE COUNSELED ON SEXUALLY TRANSMITTED DISEASES THIS PAST YEAR DURING A DOCTOR'S VISIT: 14

Help for Herpes

An experimental drug called resiquimod appears to significantly reduce symptoms of genital herpes. In a 6-month trial, patients taking the new drug experienced an average of one herpes recurrence, compared with patients on a placebo, who averaged 5.5 recurrences. Resiquimod also increased the time between outbreaks—from an average of 57 days to 169. Further clinical trials are currently under way.

Libido Booster in a Bottle

A nasal spray developed by Palatin Technologies that was initially intended to treat women with low-libido problems is currently undergoing clinical trials in men as well. The chemical targets "desire receptors" in the brain and, in tests on animals, was shown to arouse both sexes. Some men taking part in the preclinical safety trial experienced spontaneous erections. Brut's days may be numbered.

The Next Viagra?

University of Pennsylvania researchers have discovered a key enzyme responsible for causing sexual dysfunction. "In trials, we found that an enzyme called arginase decreases levels of nitric oxide in penile tissue," says David W. Christianson, Ph.D., the study author. "Without nitric oxide, the penis is unable to fill with blood, which can make getting an erection difficult, or even impossible," he says. A drug that blocks the production of arginase is in development but may not be widely available for up to 10 years.

Be a Straight Shooter

An estimated 1.3 million American men suffer from Peyronie's disease—a painful curvature of the penis caused by the formation of scar tissue within the organ. Treatment options used to be limited, but a medication currently in development may change that. In clinical trials, 50 percent of men with Peyronie's disease who were given Collagenase ABC experienced a significant reduction in penile curvature. The drug works by dissolving scar tissue, thereby freeing the penis and allowing it to straighten naturally.

DOES IT WORK?

Sex Selector

Researchers in Virginia have developed a machine that's capable of separating sperm cells based on whether they have an X or a Y chromosome. Once separated, the sperm samples give couples undergoing fertility treatment up to a 90 percent chance of being able to opt for a daughter and a 72 percent chance of choosing a son. The machine has been used in almost 300 pregnancies.

Does Viagra Go the Distance?

The little blue pill may not be a long-term solution for all men. A University of Alabama survey of 150 men found that after 2 years of using Viagra, 20 percent of the men had had to increase their dosage to achieve an adequate erection, while an additional 17 percent said even larger doses of the drug were no longer effective.

Sex on a Half Shell

Oysters and aphrodisiacs have been linked so long in the annals of aphrodisia that it's hard to say one without thinking the other. Sorry to disappoint, but there's no evidence that oysters will add any kind of magical boost to tonight's rocket ride. That's not to discount their erotic appeal. They're often part of a romantic evening filled with candles, wine, and lingering glances. But any boost in your sex drive is merely thanks to your *expectations* for the delicacy, not from any mysterious aphrodisiacal ingredient.

WHAT'S THE DIFF?

Prostate vs. Prostrate

Prostate is the gland that helps produce ejaculatory fluid. Prostrate is the prone position you end up in after you've released your ejaculatory fluid.

Orgasm vs. Ejaculation

An orgasm is the whole-body rush that swells over you at the culmination of a sex act. In short, it's the reason we keep, er, coming back for more. Ejaculation is the projection of the fluid (called semen) that almost always occurs simultaneously with an orgasm. It *is* possible to have an orgasm without ejaculating (although it's not very common).

PERCENTAGE OF MEN WHO THINK IT'S SEXIER FOR A WOMAN TO WEAR AN ARTICLE OF CLOTHING DURING SEX THAN TO BE COMPLETELY NAKED: 43

TAKE ACTION

The first thing they taught you in school, besides that bit about glue not being food, was the alphabet. Why? Because once you had that down pat, the rest of the English language was at your fingertips.

Sex is the same way: Once you know the basics, you can string small tricks together to guarantee your partner a triple-letter-scoring orgasm. Here are 26 good reasons (strangely, in alphabetical order) to learn the ABCs of S-E-X.

I. Areola. The Pointer Sisters had it half right. Women want a man with a slow hand. But an easy touch? Not necessarily. Turns out her nipples and areolas, the dark circles around them, aren't as sensitive as you think. In fact, they're two to three times less sensitive than her index finger, say researchers at the Boston University School of Medicine. While we're not suggesting you start "tuning the radio," you might want to use a firmer touch than usual. What feels strong to your fingertips might not even be registering on the ol' nipple meter.

2. Blade. Switching to an electric razor could transform not just your face but your coital prowess as well. In a recent survey, lather-'n'-scrape guys said they last an average of 5 minutes in the sack, while those who use an electric razor last 10 minutes more. Hard to tell how conclusive this is, or even what the heck it means, but we're guessing that there will be a few extra Norelco and Braun logos under the Christmas tree next season.

3. Camels. If the stinking clothes, yellow fingers, and chunks of lung hacked into your palm haven't convinced you to stop smoking, what about coming up soft in bed? A study from the New England Research Institutes in Watertown, Massachusetts, shows that around 30 percent of smokers experience impotence. The good news? Quitting now may lower your flop risk to where it was in your presmoking days.

4. Dr. Vibe. Arch supports, stinky-feet powder . . . vibrators? The guy who's been taking the musk out of men's shoes might be returning it to women's bedrooms with a new rechargeable vibrator, made by the fine folks at Dr. Scholl's. Although marketed as a back massager and sold at drugstores, it shockingly resembles the Hitachi Magic Wand—the most popular vibrator at Good Vibrations, a San Francisco–based sex shop. Wonder if those shoe inserts are actually panty liners.

5. Excuses. Next time she claims a headache, you can just chuckle and say (in your worst Barry White voice), "I've got just the thing, baby." According to

Beverly Whipple, Ph.D., a professor at the college of nursing at Rutgers University, stimulation of the G-spot has been shown to be an erotic Advil. "The pressure and stimulation make women feel pain much less intensely," says Whipple. Technically, orgasm isn't even necessary for a woman to benefit. (The sound of male cheers fills the auditorium.) The best way to hit the G-spot is manually or in the woman-on-top, rear-entry, or kneeling missionary position. Don't worry if you can't find the exact spot; stimulation anywhere along the front wall of the vagina is generally appreciated.

6. Fear. What's the number-one reason you're going home from the bar alone? Could be your delicate rectal odor. Or it could have something to do with white-haired women—that is, paranoid grandmothers warning their grown-up granddaughters to be careful of men slipping "roofies" (Rohypnol) into their drinks. As funny as it is to imagine 87-year-old women saying "roofies," this is no laughing matter. Women hear enough horror stories about the nice-guy-as-sexual-predator to be wary of even the tamest men. Next time you're at a party and see a woman you'd like to meet, don't approach her alone. Find a mutual acquaintance to introduce you, preferably a female one. How about your grandmother?

7. Guacamole. The firm, forever touchable skin of an avocado isn't half as erotic as what's inside. The fleshy green fruit is high in vitamin E, magnesium, potassium, and zinc, a combination that not only boosts libido but increases sexual stamina as well, says Barnet Meltzer, M.D., author of *Food Swings*. And the unsaturated fat won't kill you either. Peel and mash two avocados and stir in a chopped onion, a tomato, the juice of one lime, a clove of garlic (minced), and the love of a good woman. Season with salt and pepper. Apply liberally.

8. Happy hour. What strange force drives men to bars every Friday at 5:30 to cruise for women? Cheap beer, of course. Or could it be that deep down you know that when you push back those batwing doors—and the whole saloon stops to gape at you—you're packing 27 percent more sperm in your holsters than earlier in the day? According to a study at the University of Modena in Italy, quittin' time is the starting gun for your boy bullets. "Your best chance of conceiving is in the late afternoon or early evening," says the study's author, Angelo Cagnacci, M.D., of the university's department of obstetrics and gynecology. Just watch where you point that thing, Tex.

9. In your hands. Remember, there is no "I" in sex. But there is in masturbation, thank goodness.

10. Janitor. Not only is cleanliness next to godliness, but for some it's also a close second to sex. A majority of people claim they derive more satisfaction from a clean house than from their sex lives, says a national survey by Home and Garden Television. Which really throws a toilet brush in the works if you're a slob *and* a sloppy lover. So you should (a) invest in a housecleaning service and (b) put her feather duster to better use elsewhere.

11. Kindness. Or what you could be experiencing more of if she switches to the new birth control pill Yasmin. It not only prevents pregnancy if she remembers to take it every night but also defuses the symptoms of PMS, which serves as a helpful reminder. A miracle drug, you say? Could be. According to research presented to the American College of Obstetrics and Gynecology, Yasmin alleviates water retention, moodiness, and the increased appetite often associated with PMS. Which would make you more attractive, less irritating, and an even greater all-around great guy. And you don't even have to take the Pill!

12. L-arginine. Ditch the candles and champagne. To really put her in the mood, feed her a peanut butter sandwich. L-arginine, an amino acid found in peanuts, increases bloodflow in the body and acts as a signal for sexual arousal. "This is the only nutrient that has been proved to increase sexual satisfaction in women," says Mary Lake Polan, M.D., Ph.D., chairwoman of gynecology and obstetrics at the Stanford University School of Medicine. Which means your penis's official new nickname is Skippy.

13. Mrs. Robinson. Tired of striking out with your sister's friends? Try picking up your next date at Mom's bridge club. Before you laugh, think about this: Not only are older women closer to their sexual peaks, but chances are they'll think you're hotter, too, even as you age. Blame it on failing vision, but a survey of middle-aged Americans found that the percentage of people who view their partners as physically attractive actually increases with age. Can't imagine dating an older woman? Just think of all the beautiful actresses in the over-40 set, like Michelle Pfeiffer, Kim Basinger, Sophia Loren, . . . and Frances Sternhagen.

14. Needy. If there's one thing more pathetic than a man who thinks he can bed every woman he meets, it's a man who thinks he can't get any woman— and resorts to begging for sex. Despite what the rest room poetry says, whining does not lead to dining and sixty-nining. Women rank confidence as one of the sexiest qualities in a man. "Stand tall and make direct eye contact," says William Fitzgerald, Ph.D., a therapist specializing in relationships and sexual therapy. "And above all else, smile. A smile goes a long way."

15. Olfactory. Next time you want to get her in the mood to play blanket bingo, dust off your cologne bottle and spritz a few drops on her pillow. (That's drops, not glops.) A new study conducted by Indiana University researchers shows that women who smelled men's cologne while fantasizing about sex became more aroused than those exposed to a neutral odor.

NUMBER OF HUSBANDS WHO ARE AT LEAST 2 YEARS YOUNGER THAN THEIR WIVES: 1 IN 8

16. Percentages. It's like money—only 15 percent of the adults in America are having 50 percent of the sex. But we live in a free-market society here, fellas. Make it a goal to talk to one new woman every day. (In fact, make it a rule.) We know a guy who did this for 100 days straight and was blown off only a third of the time—a .667 batting average. That's better than Wade Boggs's. Heck, that's better than Wilt Chamberlain's.

17. Quickie. Sometimes women like quickies as much as we do. So how do you know when she's up for fast and furious? There's no perfect model for sex, even with a familiar lover, so take her lead. "She might not say, 'Push me down and take me now,'" says Fitzgerald, "but if you're firmer and more impulsive and she responds, go with it." Preferably before the light turns green.

18. Ringer. Next time you hit the local public house in search of true love, bring a ringer. Attracting women is easy. Just place a female friend at your elbow and tell a few jokes. Researchers at the University of Louisville found that a man was 50 to 100 percent more desirable to women when other ladies said they liked him. Just be sure to pay your friend up front in small, unmarked bills.

19. Surprise. There's nothing a woman hates more than a wham-bam-always-the-same-way man. Scientists at Emory University and Baylor College think the pleasure sensors in the brain react more strongly to pleasure when it's unexpected. Next time you're in the sack, have her close her eyes. Or, better yet, blindfold her with a scarf and then randomly touch and taste different areas of her body. Emphasize "no peeking!" That way you can simultaneously watch *RPM2Night* on mute with the closed-caption subtitles.

20. Toilet paper. A recent survey of 1,500 Americans found that those who have no toilet paper brand preference had sex at least twice as often as brand loyalists. We don't know what that means, but we've already replaced all the Charmin in the *Men's Health* job johnnies with randomly placed rolls of Scott, White Cloud, and 100-grit sandpaper.

21. U-spot. You finally located her G-spot and thought you'd found the Grail. (Ha! And you thought it was named for Graffenberg.) Not so fast. There's another female erogenous zone that needs your attention, and you don't need a mining lamp to find it. The U-spot resides at the opening of the urethra, just in front of the vaginal opening. "There are rich nerve endings surrounding the urethra," says Fitzgerald. "Many women enjoy gentle stimulation in this area with fingers and tongues." Call us if you get lost. Or, what the hell, go ahead and ask her for directions.

22. VHS. Don't think your partner wants to join your screening of *Up Your Auntie?* Think again. It's long been said that men are more aroused by visual stimuli than women are. But there's one type of visual stimulation that garners a greater response in women than in men: porn. Australian researchers found that when men and women watched the same scenes from adult films, women got a bigger adrenaline rush. Just beware of the raunch level. To pick a flick she'll like, visit Good Vibrations, which offers some videos geared toward women. (That means they probably have a plot.) See their selection at www.goodvibes.com.

23. Weekly. That's how often 48 percent of women are tinkering with their own toys, according to *The New Hite Report: The Revolutionary Report on Female Sexuality Updated.* So where do you come in? Hopefully before it's over. Most women prefer direct clitoral stimulation during masturbation, so taking a tip from her technique will ensure she has orgasms more frequently and will be ready for action more often. Fitzgerald suggests sliding a pillow under her back during missionary position sex. This will allow your pubic bone to stimulate her clitoris.

24. XOXOXO. You're ready to take the big plunge . . . drop the L-bomb . . . tell her that you (deep breath, cough, snort) love her. The last thing you want her to do, besides laugh in your face, is forget about it, but if you're whispering your sweet nothings into her right ear, she might do just that. Researchers at Sam Houston State University in Texas found that people are more likely to remember emotional words like "love," "adore," and "Porsche" if they hear them through their left ear. Port, ho!

25. Your ticker. Sex is the best thing for your heart since quadruple bypass surgery, and doesn't stain the sheets as much. Researchers at the University of Bristol in England found that men can cut their risk of dying of cardiovascular disease in half by having sex three or four times a week. Sex is just as good an exercise as walking for reducing the risk of stroke, according to a university spokesman. This doesn't excuse you from going to the gym, though. You burn only about 27 calories during a 15-minute session in the sack, which will leave you fat and happy.

26. Zzz. If you snore, you might not score. According to Mansoor Madani, D.M.D., a sleep apnea expert, roughly half of men who snore also have problems with erections. When you snore, tissues in your throat vibrate and can block your windpipe, temporarily stopping your breathing. This can impair bloodflow to other vital areas, says Dr. Madani. Thankfully, snoring can usually be cured by outpatient laser surgeries that take 15 minutes and reduce snoring by more than 70 percent. Now, if they could only do something about night drool. . . .

AMOUNT OF BLOOD
PUMPED BY THE HEART PER SECOND: **3.2 OUNCES**

AMOUNT PUMPED
PER SECOND DURING SEX: **13 OUNCES**

ANY QUESTIONS?

Size Things Up

I've heard that circumference is more important than length when it comes to penis size. Is this true?

—L. A., Estes Park, Colorado

A woman's vagina can be one very elastic organ: It can accommodate most any plane that pulls into the hangar—and even the widebody that pulls out 9 months later. You don't need to have the diameter of a tuna can, but where her pleasure is concerned, there may be some truth to the belief that girth is more important than length. The lower third of the vagina has the highest concentration of nerve endings. So when a woman is excited, this is where she'll experience the most stimulation. The wider you are, the more you'll fill the area. Recent research puts average girth at 4.97 inches, or about that of the average ballpark frank (after plumping).

If you want to enhance your girth, try using a penis ring. (Please, get one that's adjustable; you don't want to risk strangulation.) "It's like tying a string around your finger," says Ernie Green, Ph.D., a human-sexuality educator in Pennsylvania. "The blood gets trapped, and the appendage expands." For added effect, assume this position: Initiate the action missionary style. Now arch your back and support your weight with your arms. Have her raise her legs and rest them on your shoulders. This tightens and shortens her vaginal canal, making for a snugger fit.

Handle with Care

Sometimes when I grab a condom in the dark, I accidentally try to put it on inside out. Of course, I don't get far. I usually just flip it over and proceed. Is this safe?

—J. M., San Rafael, California

You must be more careful, young man. If you've touched the condom to your penis, you should consider it ruined. (The condom, that is.) Your erect penis has probably already released a small amount of semen, which you've now placed at the tip of your sheathed erection, and this can be enough to get your lady friend pregnant. We'll assume you don't want this. Yes, we know, they put spermicide on condoms nowadays. But that's no guarantee. Next time, unravel it a bit on your finger before putting it on.

Fast Asleep

After sex, I'm spent. I fall asleep in seconds, yet she's still wide awake. Why? Am I not satisfying her sexually?

—A. K., Santa Barbara, California

That depends. Do you do other things in seconds, too? Actually, there's a biological reason you want to hit the sack after getting her into it—and it has nothing to do with her level of satisfaction, says Marc Goldstein, M.D., professor of Reproductive Medicine and Urology and surgeon-in-chief of the Cornell Center for Male Reproductive Medicine and Surgery in New York City. When you reach orgasm, your adrenal glands release a burst of epinephrine— a chemical that accelerates pulse, elevates blood pressure, increases bloodflow to muscles, and in some men prompts phrases like "Who's your daddy?" This rush depletes your muscles of glycogen (an energy-supplying carbohydrate that converts to lactic acid during strenuous effort), causing that "spent" feeling. Women experience the same phenomenon, but because they generally have less muscle mass than men, the effect is less pronounced.

Fluid Check

When I ejaculate, why doesn't the same amount of sperm come out each time? How do you know how much comes out?

—J. R., Seattle

First of all, it's semen, not sperm. Only 1 percent is sperm; the rest is fluids that nourish the sperm on their exciting journey. The differences you notice probably are caused by two factors: the amount of time since your last orgasm and the level of your arousal. Your body is constantly producing semen. After

TOP THREE THINGS THE AVERAGE GUY WILL DO AFTER SEX:
1. GO TO SLEEP
2. WATCH TV
3. GRAB SOMETHING TO EAT

ejaculation, it takes about 3 days for your body to reach full capacity again. With more frequent ejaculations, the amount of semen coming out will be less. Now then: When you become aroused, your body begins pumping fluid into the back of the urethra. This, as Jon Pryor, M.D., chairman of urology at the University of Minnesota, likes to say, is like loading a gun. At a certain point, your muscles begin to contract and force the fluid out, firing the gun. The longer the buildup during arousal, the more ammo is ready to fire.

Hidden Pleasure

I can't find my girlfriend's clitoris. I know where it's supposed to be; it's just not there.

—J. D., Jackson, Mississippi

It could be hiding, but don't take it personally. About one in four women has a clitoris that doesn't fully poke out from under the foreskin—a condition called phimosis—and she may have trouble becoming aroused. All is not lost. If you can't push her button directly, give it plenty of indirect stimulation, says Laura Berman, Ph.D., codirector of the Female Sexual Medical Center at UCLA. During sex, shift your body forward so the base of your penis brushes against the skin that obscures her clitoris. Instead of thrusting, which affects only the vagina, concentrate on rocking, which causes the kind of rubbing that can stimulate a hidden clitoris.

Beauty and the Yeast

Can she give me her yeast infection?

—R. K., Chicago

Absolutely. Use a condom if she has an infection, and don't even think of going south—you can also get it in your mouth (a condition called thrush). If she has a yeast infection, believe us—she'll know it. She'll be itching down below and will experience redness and inflammation in her vagina. You'll know it because of the other symptoms: She may have a discharge that looks

PERCENTAGE OF MEN WHO THINK
SIMULTANEOUS ORGASM IS
NECESSARY FOR GRATIFYING SEX: 24

PERCENTAGE OF WOMEN WHO THINK SO: 14

like cottage cheese, or her vagina may smell a bit like bread that's just come out of the oven.

If the infection has made a move on you, your symptoms will be similar to hers: You'll likely get redness, inflammation, and a burning sensation. Also, look for a red rash on the shaft of your penis, or a white fungus growing on the tip or in the skin folds of your foreskin. It can also spread to your scrotum and inner thighs, a condition better known as jock itch. Yeast likes warm, dark, moist places, so your groin is the perfect sprouting ground, says Marjorie Crandall, Ph.D., a microbiologist and founder of Yeast Consulting Services in Torrance, California. But fear not: *Candida albicans* (the fungus behind the condition) causes a relatively harmless infection that you can treat yourself with over-the-counter antifungal creams, such as Monistat, Gyne-Lotrimin, or Mycostatin. If it doesn't go away within 2 weeks, see your doctor for a prescription antifungal medication.

Pregnant Pause

My wife gave birth weeks ago and still has zero interest in sex. How long do I have to wait?

—P. O., Yonkers, New York

Unfortunately, Cinemax may be your only sexual companion for the next few weeks. A woman's libido plummets after childbirth because her system flushes her sex hormones within 24 hours of delivery, says Bryan Jick, M.D., an obstetrician at Huntington Memorial Hospital in Pasadena, California. This triggers the onset of lactation, and as long as she's nursing your baby, expect her primary concern to be the little guy, not you and yours. "Her estrogen levels drop, and the vaginal walls are thinner and drier, meaning intercourse is likely to be uncomfortable," Dr. Jick says. Women who bottle-feed halt lactation and get their hormones—and libido—back as early as 3 weeks after delivery. Regardless of how Junior is fed, however, most couples find their way back to the sack after 6 or 7 weeks.

When she's ready, ease in with a position that's comfortable for her. Lie on your sides and gently spoon her from behind, or let her take the top position, which allows her to control the depth and vigor of the action, says Greg Phillips, M.D., of the American College of Obstetrics and Gynecology in Washington, D.C.

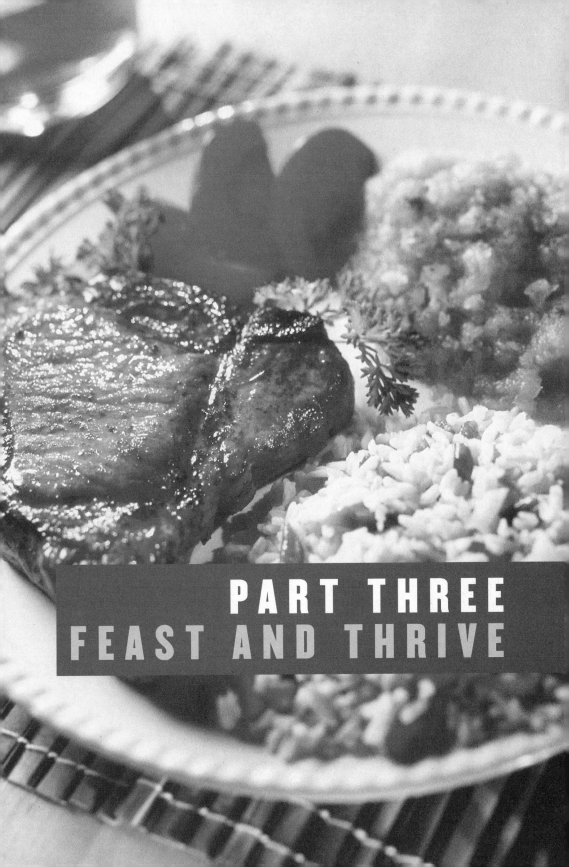

PART THREE
FEAST AND THRIVE

Who Will Keep You Healthy?

One of these health-conscious ladies, or the woman in your life?

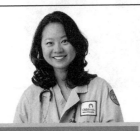

JULIE WEI, M.D.
Age: 32   Surgeon
Chicago

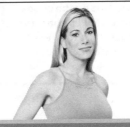

THERESA HESSLER
Age: 32   Personal trainer
Venice Beach, California

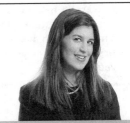

RANDI KONIKOFF
Age: 28   Nutritionist
Boston

HER LIFESTYLE

• Dr. Wei is a physician doing a fellowship in pediatric ear, nose, and throat surgery at a children's hospital. She typically works 10 to 12 hours daily.

• Dr. Wei meditates to relieve stress and gets 7 hours of sleep every night.

ADVANTAGES

• She loves tennis, and if you're her beau, you've got to play. That kind of motivation is a plus for you.

• As a physician, Dr. Wei is keenly aware of the importance of a healthy lifestyle. It's possible she'd be able to catch a health problem early, before it became serious.

DISADVANTAGES

• Her long hours as a surgeon (and her being a slave to a beeper) could tax the health of the relationship. Would the strain of her job get to you? If not, maybe her income would. A long-term study found that the higher a woman's income, the worse her husband's health.

JULIE'S PREDICTION

• "If my boyfriend had something he was ignoring, I would do whatever it took to make sure the problem was addressed and resolved."

HER LIFESTYLE

• A former champion fitness competitor, Hessler trains clients in the mornings, inline skates 13 miles every day, and lifts weights two or three times a week.

• She stays active with snowboarding, surfing, and scuba diving.

ADVANTAGES

• Hessler's love of fitness is likely to rub off on her partner. A study found that 39 percent of people say their significant other would be the strongest influence in persuading them to exercise.

• Studies show that fit women have greater sex drives than women who are out of shape. A healthy sex life has a profound effect on a man's happiness and, consequently, his health.

DISADVANTAGES

• Hessler spends a lot of time in tight outfits in front of men. Would your jealousy counter the physical benefits of having a very personal trainer?

THERESA'S PREDICTION

• "I don't like to just sit around. I would definitely be good for a man's health and influence his fitness."

HER LIFESTYLE

• Konikoff works in public relations at a nutrition school and research center and is a registered dietitian.

• She runs nearly every day and competes regularly in marathons.

ADVANTAGES

• Konikoff is aware of the latest nutrition news and practical tips for healthy eating. And she practices what she preaches. She claims that all of her boyfriends over the years lost weight and became fitter while dating her.

• She cooks nearly every night and makes even the healthiest meals taste great, which would bode well for the man in her life. People who eat more meals at home tend to have healthier diets than do people who eat out often.

DISADVANTAGES

• You can't live without cheeseburgers? Konikoff's cooking and eating habits are pretty darn healthy. Will your stress hormones rise proportionate to the number of tofu cubes on your plate?

RANDI'S PREDICTION

• "You are what you eat! I think of myself as an enabler of healthy choices. It's a total life discipline."

And the Winner Is . . .
Randi Konikoff

Fred Tudiver, M.D., a professor and research director for primary care at East Tennessee State University, helped us devise the quiz on the opposite page to gauge which woman would be best for a man's health over the long haul. Take it yourself to see how much your partner in life may affect your health.

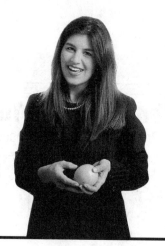

FINAL ANALYSIS

Make one of these women your wife and you'll be doing yourself a big favor. Simply having a long-term partner delivers strong health benefits. "Men do a lot better health-wise if they're hitched," says Fred Tudiver, M.D., a professor and research director for primary care at East Tennessee State University. "Research shows that men get most of their emotional strength and their support for health concerns from their partners, and very little of either from peers."

On average, married men are 30 percent more likely to live to 65 than life-long bachelors or men who have been divorced. And single men tend to have the worst overall health habits when compared with married men and women in general.

Okay, so you know that a long-term relationship is good for survival. And we're also going to assume that there's sexual chemistry, love, and respect in this partnership. Happiness, after all, plays a huge role in physical well-being. A 2000 study from the University of Toronto showed that the blood pressures of unhappily married men increased over a 3-year period, while happily married men watched their blood pressures drop. So, on a level playing field, why does Konikoff have the advantage over the others?

"She has the best shot at keeping a man healthy because good nutrition plays such an important role in the prevention of disease," says Dr. Tudiver. "Plus, she has an active lifestyle, so she's probably just as likely to help a man stay physically fit as Hessler."

Dr. Wei places third due to her career, in Dr. Tudiver's view. "She might not be as available (to support her partner's health), compared with the other women," he says. "Being married to a physician—I don't assume that's a major health benefit." While Dr. Wei may be quite fit, doctors in general don't tend to practice much healthier habits than other people do, Dr. Tudiver says.

Life Lines

FACTOR	POINT VALUE	JULIE	THERESA	RANDI	YOUR MATE
LOVE, COMPATIBILITY Love, sexual chemistry, respect, and compatibility are the cornerstones of any healthy relationship.	Brings all four to the relationship? +3	+3	+3	+3	
	Lacks one or more? Don't bother.				
DIET You're likely to eat what she eats, especially if she's doing the shopping.	Always eats a balanced, low-fat diet high in vitamins? +2			+2	
	Usually eats a healthy, balanced diet? +1		+1		
	Unstructured eating habits? 0	0			
	Eats an unbalanced and/or high-fat diet? −1				
COOKING You're less likely to snack and consume fatty and processed foods if you eat meals cooked at home.	Prepares one to three healthful meals daily for the two of you to eat together? +2			+2	
	Often prepares balanced meals for both of you? +1	+1	+1		
	Rarely cooks? 0				
	Often cooks unhealthful meals? −2				
EXERCISE If exercise is important to her, she may motivate you to work out as well. Plus, you're less likely to skip workouts if you exercise with a partner.	Exercises daily at high intensity? +2		+2	+2	
	Follows a moderate exercise program? +1	+1			
	Rarely exercises? 0				
	Encourages you to exercise on your own or with her? +1	+1	+1	+1	
	Doesn't care whether you exercise or not? −2				
PREVENTIVE MEDICINE A woman who takes care of herself and goes to the doctor for yearly checkups is more likely to encourage her partner to do the same.	Goes for yearly medical checkups? +1	+1	+1	+1	
	Calls attention to your health problems? +1	+1			
	Encourages you to get regular medical checkups? +1	+1	+1	+1	
	Doesn't go for medical checkups? −1				
	Lets you take care of yourself even if you're ignoring a potential health problem? −2				
BAD HABITS You're well aware of the dangers of secondhand smoke, but did you know that men who live with smokers typically eat less healthful diets than do men who live with nonsmokers?	Doesn't smoke? 0	0	0	0	
	Smokes? −2				
	Drinks more than two alcoholic beverages per night on average? −2				
TOTALS		+9	+10	+12	

IF YOUR PARTNER'S SCORE IS +6 OR MORE:
You'll grow old together.

IF YOUR PARTNER'S SCORE IS +2 TO +5:
She's better than a multivitamin.

IF YOUR PARTNER'S SCORE IS +1 OR LESS:
You love her, she's perfect—now change her.

MUST READS

Breakfast to Go

Is your commute a dash and dine? Here are eight morning meals that top the Pop Tart

By Brian Good and Kimberly Flynn

Two thousand pounds of cereal. Six hundred sixty gallons of milk. When these two forces of nature collided on April 17, 1998, in the piece of desert better known as the United Arab Emirates, the record for the world's largest breakfast was instantly set.

Nice story, except for one thing: Men without oil wells in their front yards don't have enough time in the morning to sit down and eat one bowl of cereal, let alone 14,000. What's more, the average working guy has to squeeze in breakfast under more trying conditions than dining in the Sahara. He's up against miles of stop-and-swallow traffic, a car with jackhammer shocks, and a clean suit that desperately needs to stay that way.

That's why an attempt at a more practical record seemed in order: the one for the world's fastest, healthiest, and most commuter-friendly breakfast. And we did it—eight times. We took the convenience and speed of prepackaged supermarket meals, combined it with all of our nutrition know-how, and then tossed out anything that either tasted lousy or had a fair chance of dripping, dribbling, or otherwise depositing itself on your self. The final record setters are listed below. Try 'em; we'll bet you start showing up at work well-fed, stain-free, and always on time.

PILLSBURY TOASTER BAGEL SHOPPE BAGELS
Prep time: 3 minutes

The Frankensteins of the breakfast food aisle, these holeless wonders combine the best features of Pop Tarts—a prefilled middle and a perfect fit for the toaster—with the authentic doughy flavor of a traditional New Yawk bagel. Look for strawberry, blueberry, cinnamon, and cream cheese flavors. A winner despite the spelling "Shoppe."

Make them better by . . . turning two bagels into a lox sandwich. Three ounces of lox—thinly sliced smoked salmon—is packed with 16 grams of protein and 70 percent of your daily requirement of omega-3 fatty acids. A morning hit of omega-3's will help protect you from heart disease and depression.

Per two bagels plus lox: 360 calories, 24 grams (g) protein, 48 g carbohydrates, 7 g fat

QUAKER INSTANT OATMEAL EXPRESS
Prep time: 2 minutes

If oats can help power Thoroughbreds around the track, imagine what the stuff'll do for you at the office. This version comes in its own bowl, which means you just stir in boiling water, then grab a plastic spoon and your keys. (Down a spoonful at every red light or when traffic hits a standstill.) The taste? It has the same grainy, slightly buttery flavor as regular instant oatmeal, with a choice of apple, peach, or brown sugar doctoring.

Make it better by . . . swapping in 1 percent milk for the water. The oatmeal will turn out creamier and have double the protein. After coffee, protein's the nutrient a man needs most to achieve maximum morning alertness.

Per serving with 1% milk: 310 calories, 14 g protein, 55 g carbohydrates, 5 g fat

HONEY NUT CHEERIOS MILK 'N CEREAL BARS
Prep time: None

When the folks at General Mills zapped a bowl of Cheerios and milk with their top-secret Dehydro-Beam, they successfully removed the ingredient for wetness (and front-seat spillage). Fortunately, they left behind the cereal's cholesterol-lowering power; in one study, eating a daily bowl of Cheerios lowered LDL cholesterol by 4 percent. And in case you're wondering what getting healthy on the way to work tastes like, think Rice Krispies treats.

Make them better by . . . eating more than one. A single bar is as nutritionally balanced as a bowl of milk and cereal, but who eats just 1 cup of cereal? If you want to feel full, shove a couple more bars into your briefcase.

Per three bars: 480 calories, 18 g protein, 78 g carbohydrates, 12 g fat

EGGO BLUEBERRY TOASTER DELIGHTS
Prep time: 3 minutes

Exactly like a blueberry muffin—that's been violently smashed into the shape of a slice of bread. The fresh berry flavor and moist, cakelike texture are similar to bakery muffins, with one road-worthy difference: They're virtually crumb-free.

Make them better by . . . turning three toasted slices and 2 tablespoons of fat-free cream cheese into a triple-decker sandwich. You get an extra 2 grams of protein per tablespoon of cream cheese.

Per three slices with cream cheese: 420 calories, 12 g protein, 65 g carbohydrates, 12 g fat

AUNT JEMIMA MINI PANCAKES

Prep time: 3 minutes

Like the silver dollar kind you never have time to go and order at IHOP, these frozen pancakes have a rich, biscuitlike flavor. Even better, they're low in calories; one pancake has just 18 calories and less than a gram of fat.

Make them better by . . . sandwiching a slice of Canadian bacon between two frozen pancakes, spearing the whole thing with a toothpick, and microwaving it on high for close to a minute. Since these sandwiches are small, you can eat up to five.

Per sandwich: 81 calories, 7 g protein, 8 g carbohydrates, 3 g fat

PEPPERIDGE FARM CINNAMON FRENCH TOAST

Prep time: 2 minutes

The best thing Pepperidge Farm has grown since goldfish. Thick slabs of bread are topped with an egg coating that doesn't peel off after it's been warmed.

TWO FOR THE ROAD

Need to whip up a quick breakfast? Try one of these recipes and hunger no more.

Minute Breakfast Burrito

    2 eggs

    2 tablespoons salsa

    I slice reduced-fat American cheese

    I soft flour tortilla

Do this: Spray a cereal bowl with nonstick cooking spray. Crack the eggs into the bowl, add the salsa, and stir. Microwave on high for I minute, stir, and cook for another minute or until the mixture firms up. Place the cheese in the center of the tortilla and top it with the egg mixture. Wrap it all up like a burrito and head for the car. (Don't worry; the salsa won't drip. It's cooked into the eggs.) Makes I serving

Per serving: 438 calories, 24 grams (g) protein, 45 g carbohydrates, 17 g fat

International Breakfast Sandwich

    I reduced-fat English muffin

    I slice Canadian bacon

    I small Italian plum tomato, sliced

    I slice reduced-fat American cheese

       Salt and pepper

Do this: Toast the English muffin. Top the bottom half of the muffin with the Canadian bacon, some slices of tomato, and the cheese. Cover with the top half of the muffin and microwave the whole thing for 20 seconds, or until the cheese starts to melt. Makes I serving

Per serving: 221 calories, 16 g protein, 29 g carbohydrates, 4 g fat

Make it better by . . . spreading on some peanut butter. One teaspoon of re-duced-fat peanut butter slathered between two toasted slices ups the protein by 2 grams.

Per sandwich: 427 calories, 13 g protein, 56 g carbohydrates, 16 g fat

KELLOGG'S EGGO WAF-FULLS

Prep time: 2 minutes

Drop two in the toaster, and 2 minutes later a complete waffle breakfast will pop up. How? Kellogg's grabbed a regular Eggo, jabbed it with a hypo-dermic needle, and injected the waffle with maple syrup, strawberry jelly, or apple-cinnamon filling. (At least that's how we like to imagine it happened.) The result is a surprisingly light and crisp waffle with just the right amount of filling for maximum flavor with minimum drip.

Make them better by . . . washing down your waffles with a pint of milk. It'll give you 16 more grams of protein and, if you do it right, a really stupid-looking milk mustache you can pretend you don't know is there.

Per two waffles plus 1% milk: 520 calories, 22 g protein, 76 g carbohydrates, 15 g fat

QUAKER TOASTED OATMEAL SQUARES

Prep time: I minute

Sweetened oatmeal cereal—brown sugar– or cinnamon-flavored—packed in a single-serving tube similar to a snack-size Pringles can. The only down-side: no room for a Pokemon toy inside.

Make them better by . . . stirring in a cup of low-fat vanilla yogurt. You'll probably need to eat a handful of cereal before you can squeeze the yogurt in, but once you do, you'll get more protein than you would from adding milk, without the risk of a slam-on-the-brakes drenching.

Per tube with yogurt: 455 calories, 17 g protein, 88 g carbohydrates, 5 g fat

Multiple Choice

Hankering for a multivitamin? Make sure you buy the right brand for the job

By Elizabeth M. Ward, R.D.

Do something good for yourself that takes just 3 seconds: Swallow a multivi-tamin before you go to work. "It's good insurance on days when your diet's less than perfect," says Roxanne Moore, R.D., of the American Dietetic As-sociation. In other words, taking a multivitamin is great for those days when you eat no fruit and too much grease.

But choosing the right vitamin can be a pain in the neck. Have you gone to the store and tried it? You practically need a degree in nutrition to know the right combination of beta-carotene and thiamin and vitamin C. (I should know. I have the degree, and it's still tough.)

"Today's multis are custom-formulated for specific conditions," says Moore. "To get the most health benefits, you have to pick the one that has the right mix for your needs. And that can be hard to find."

So we'll make it easy for you, as usual. No matter what your lifestyle, here's the right multivitamin to take if you want to . . .

BEAT A FAMILY HISTORY OF HEART DISEASE

Key nutrients needed: Vitamins B_6 and B_{12}

Why: Cleveland Clinic researchers found that men with diets that were low in B vitamins were more than twice as likely to develop heart disease as men with higher levels of the vitamins in their systems. These Bs lower blood levels of homocysteine, a rogue amino acid that irritates the linings of your blood vessels, making them more prone to clotting.

Brand to buy: Protegra Cardio Vitamin & Mineral Supplement, which contains more than four times your dietary reference intake (DRI) of B_6 and B_{12}, plus nine times your DRI of vitamin E, another proven heart disease fighter.

PROTECT YOURSELF FROM SUN EXPOSURE

Key nutrients needed: Vitamins A and C, and lutein

Why: Ultraviolet rays in sunlight break down vitamin A in your skin. Without that protective shield, you risk looking like Jack Palance by 40. But a steady diet of vitamin A can help you build up a reserve of the skin cancer–fighting nutrient. You'll also need a solid hit of vitamin C; your body uses C to produce collagen, a connective tissue that keeps your skin and facial muscles taut. The lutein? It's for your eyes—helping to repair damage from the sun so you won't have to squint while checking out the talent on the beach when you're 70.

Brand to buy: Centrum Silver. It's got your entire daily dose of vitamin A— and 20 percent of that vitamin A is in the form of beta-carotene, which your body converts into vitamin A as it needs it. Think of it as an automatic application of sunscreen.

FIGHT THE EFFECTS OF FLAB

Key nutrients needed: Vitamins C, D, and E

Why: Carrying around a few extra pounds isn't like doing the military press; it makes your bones weaker, not stronger. That's because excess fat blocks your body from absorbing vitamin D from sunlight, a crucial source of the bone-strengthening vitamin. Getting your D from a multi can help.

SHOULD YOU SUPPLEMENT YOUR SEX LIFE?

Men spend more than $2 billion a year on over-the-counter sex-enhancement supplements. But because the Food and Drug Administration doesn't regulate supplements, "you can't ever be sure of what you're getting in those pills," says Wayne Hellstrom, M.D., a urologist at Tulane University.

To come to some useful conclusions about what works and what doesn't, the Sexual Medicine Society appointed six of the nation's top researchers to look for hard science behind the claims of some common over-the-counter erectile dysfunction remedies.

Here's what they found.

Ginkgo Biloba

The claim: Improves bloodflow in the body, including, supposedly, the penis.

The facts: While good research proves that ginkgo biloba does increase bloodflow to the brain, no studies have shown that it will do the same for the penis. But ginkgo may still help if your problem is psychological, says Ira Sharlip, M.D., president of the Sexual Medicine Society. "The placebo effect for men with erectile dysfunction is as high as 40 percent." If you're on a blood thinner, be extra careful about ginkgo.

L-arginine

The claim: It's used by cells in your artery walls to manufacture nitric oxide—a molecule responsible for relaxing the smooth muscle of your penis, resulting in increased bloodflow.

The facts: A 1999 study in the *British Journal of Urology* found that 31 percent of men with erection problems who took 5 grams of L-arginine daily for 6 weeks improved their sexual function, compared with only 12 percent on a placebo.

Androstenedione and DHEA

The claim: The combination boosts libido by increasing testosterone.

The facts: It also elevates estrogen, the female sex hormone, and too much estrogen can give you gynecomastia—man boobs. Even worse, the combo can slash your HDL (good) cholesterol by as much as 12 percent.

Yohimbe

The claim: Acts on the area of the brain that controls arousal.

The facts: Supplementing three times daily with 5.4 milligrams was more effective than a placebo in treating erectile dysfunction, according to studies in the *Journal of Urology*. The problem is that very few over-the-counter supplements contain enough real yohimbe. "Getting a prescription for yohimbe from a doctor is the only way to ensure that it'll have enough of the active ingredient," says Dr. Hellstrom.

Finnish researchers found that men who took vitamin D reduced their bone fracture risk by 25 percent.

Being overweight also increases your risk of diabetes. That's where vitamins C and E come in. Both protect blood vessels when your blood sugar levels are out of whack.

Brand to buy: CVS Daily Multiple Plus Extra C, E, and B Vitamins for Men. It's got your DRI of C, D, and E—plus zinc, which has been shown to reduce the risk of a type of blindness associated with obesity.

COUNTERACT A NIGHT OF PARTYING

Key nutrients needed: Vitamins C and B_1

Why: Cigarette smoke—whether it's your own or someone else's—quickly burns up vitamin C reserves in your body, increasing your risk of lung cancer. Booze purges folate (folic acid), vitamin B_6, and zinc from your body. And we all know what a diet of vodka and wasabi peas can do to your liver. So down some vitamins C and B_1 before a night of drinking; they'll help neutralize alcohol by-products in your system, significantly reducing the potential for liver damage when you imbibe heavily.

Brand to buy: CVS Achieve Mature Adult. In addition to delivering 4.5 milligrams (mg) of B_1 and 120 mg of vitamin C, Achieve Mature Adult also packs your entire DRI of folate, vitamin B_6, and zinc.

SAVE YOURSELF FROM STRESS

Key nutrients needed: Choline, magnesium, and vitamin K

Why: Researchers at the University of North Carolina found that choline improves memory and helps cells in the brain communicate better. A good multi can also make up for the magnesium and vitamin K deficiencies you can get from living on take-out food.

Brand to buy: Rainbow Light Just Once. It packs the motherlode of stress fighters, including choline, magnesium, and vitamin K—plus nearly three times your DRI of vitamin C, which fights the effects of stress on the body. You'd normally get enough of these nutrients from vegetables and whole grain breads—if you had time to eat them.

BUILD MORE MUSCLE

Key nutrients needed: Chromium and vitamins B_6 and B_{12}

Why: Chromium improves your body's ability to convert amino acids into muscle. A University of Maryland study found that men who exercised regularly and took 200 micrograms of chromium a day added more muscle weight and lost significantly more body fat than lifters not taking the supplement. Hard workouts deplete your B vitamins.

Brand to buy: Solaray Men's Golden Multi-Vita-Min. It has all the chromium you need and megadoses of vitamins B_6 and B_{12}, plus your entire daily allotment of endurance-boosting zinc.

INCREASE YOUR ODDS OF BECOMING A DAD

Key nutrients needed: Folic acid (folate) and zinc

Why: USDA researchers studied 50 men and found that not only did those with low levels of folate produce fewer sperm, but their sperm cells were also more likely to have damaged DNA. Zinc is important for keeping sperm cells strong. And studies show that infertile men are often low on zinc.

Brand to buy: Stresstabs High-Potency B Complex plus Zinc, which contains all the folic acid you need, 159 percent of the DRI of zinc, and 500 mg of vitamin C—six times your necessary daily dose.

Fill Your Food Prescription

20 easy-to-swallow medical treatments you won't find in a pharmacy

By Kimberly Flynn

Dr. Harvey Kellogg invented cornflakes, but during the late 1800s he was more famous as a physician. The good doctor claimed he could cure virtually any disease, from ulcers and schizophrenia to acne. All it took, he said, was a dose of yogurt. Well, more specifically a yogurt enema. Dr. Kellogg, of course, was a flake. But he did make good cereal. And he did have the right idea. Research has shown that some foods can be just as effective as prescription drugs in treating medical conditions. Best of all, unlike his cure-all, our remedies slide into the portal of least resistance: your mouth.

Problem: YOU'RE WORRIED YOU'LL START WANDERING AIMLESSLY THROUGH THE CITY

Prescription: A bag of almond M&Ms

Chocolate-covered nuts may prevent or delay the development of Alzheimer's disease. It's not the chocolate that protects you, though; it's the E in the almonds. A National Institutes of Health study found that the antioxidant properties of vitamin E reduce deterioration in the brain as you age. Just 2 ounces of almonds contains your entire recommended daily intake of E.

Problem: YOU CAN'T BREATHE

Prescription: A few fish fillets each week

"Magnesium helps to improve lung function and reduce the frequency of asthma attacks," says Michael Dacey, M.D., a critical care physician in Rhode Island. "Emergency rooms use magnesium to treat patients having acute attacks," he says. Plus, recent research found that asthmatics with magnesium deficiencies spent more time in the hospital than those whose diets were rich in the stuff. For men with severe asthma, Dr. Dacey recommends eating at least one serving of fish, seafood, or spinach each day.

**NUMBER OF YEARS ADDED TO
YOUR LIFE BY EATING NUTS FIVE TIMES A WEEK:** 2.9

**NUMBER OF YEARS ADDED TO
YOUR LIFE BY EATING A VEGETARIAN DIET:** 2.4

Problem: YOU HAVE SORE JOINTS

Prescription: Half a cup of cooked mixed vegetables

The more cooked vegetables you eat, the lower your risk of developing arthritis, according to a recent Greek study. Researchers studied the diets and health of 330 people and found that those who ate the most cooked vegetables were 75 percent less likely to develop arthritis than those who consumed the least. One possible reason: Heat destroys the vegetables' cell walls, allowing your body to absorb more of the nutrients that would otherwise pass through your system.

Problem: YOUR GUMS BLEED WHEN YOU BRUSH YOUR TEETH

Prescription: An A.M. grapefruit

Inflamed gums hurt, and they can also mean you aren't getting enough vitamin C, says Cyndi Thomson, Ph.D., R.D., an assistant professor at the University of Arizona. When you don't get enough C, collagen in your body starts to break down. And that process starts in your gums. "One grapefruit provides your entire daily requirement of vitamin C," she says.

Problem: YOUR BREATH STINKS

Prescription: Eight glasses of water throughout the day

Instead of sucking on breath mints, keep a bottle of water by your side. "Bad breath is caused by sulfur compounds in your mouth, and sipping water frequently helps wash away those compounds and trigger the production of breath-neutralizing saliva," says Anthony Dailley, D.D.S., founder of the Center for Breath Treatment in San Francisco.

Problem: YOU HAVE DIARRHEA

Prescription: A glass or two of wine

It's not Pepto's pink color that makes you feel better; it's a compound called bismuth subsalicylate, which is also found in high levels in both red and white wine. According to one study, drinking a glass or two of wine is just as effective at controlling diarrhea as taking a single dose of most over-the-counter remedies. The bismuth compound appears to prevent diarrhea by slowing or stopping the growth of bacteria like Salmonella and *E. coli*, before they can make you any sicker.

PERCENTAGE LESS LIKELY YOU WILL GET HEART DISEASE IF YOU EAT BEANS, PEAS, OR LEGUMES AT LEAST FOUR TIMES A WEEK: 22

Problem: YOU DRANK TOO MANY BLOODY MARYS

Prescription: Lots of virgin Marys

Only time and aspirin can heal the effects of crazed celebration, but for a major hangover, reach for the red stuff—tomato juice. "If you're throwing up, it's likely you're low on potassium, calcium, and sodium," says Linda Van Horn, Ph.D., R.D., a professor of preventive medicine at Northwestern University. "That combination is what leaves you feeling sick and exhausted." Tomato juice is a good source of all those nutrients, along with additional water to make up for the fluids you've lost.

Problem: YOU'RE WORRIED ABOUT HEART DISEASE

Prescription: Drink a beer (but just one)

Beer may lower your risk of heart attack, according to a University College of London study. Researchers followed men in the Czech Republic and found that those who drank an average of one beer a day had the lowest risk of heart disease. But men who drank an average of two or more beers a day lost that extra protection. Doctors theorize that ethanol in the beer thins the blood and helps protect the heart.

Problem: YOU'VE GOT HIC-, HIC-, HIC- SPASMODIC CLOSING OF THE GLOTTIS

Prescription: A spoonful of sugar

If the thought of Dick Cheney's heart health doesn't scare away your hiccups, try this: "Pouring a spoonful of sugar under your tongue can cure a bad case of the hiccups," says Marla Tobin, M.D., a family physician in Higginsville, Missouri. Like the cause of hiccups themselves, the science behind the cure isn't clear, but Dr. Tobin theorizes that the sugar granules excite nerves in the back of your throat. Once stimulated, the nerves block other nerve signals within the body, including the one that might be causing your hiccups.

Problem: YOU HAVE HIGH BLOOD PRESSURE

Prescription: An 8-ounce glass of orange juice

A recent study in the *New England Journal of Medicine* reports that increasing the amount of potassium and calcium in your diet will significantly lower your blood pressure, whether it's elevated or not. "The minerals protect your kidneys from high levels of sodium, a known hypertension risk," says Van Horn. Calcium-fortified, not-from-concentrate orange juice is a good source of both calcium and potassium, along with vitamin C. Another plus: According to English researchers, people with the most vitamin C in their bloodstreams are 40 percent less likely to die of heart disease than people with lower levels of the nutrient.

Problem: YOUR LEGS SEIZE UP AFTER YOU LEAVE THE GYM

Prescription: A banana

You try to take care of your body by working out. It thanks you by cramping up. In most cases, though, those cramps don't mean you overdid it at the gym. "Muscle cramps after a workout tend to be a sign of a deficiency," says Thomson. "Exercise depletes the nutrients your muscles need to function properly." The alternative to pain and cursing: Replenish your magnesium and potassium immediately by eating a banana and drinking a glass of water to fight off dehydration. "That should be enough to eliminate cramps before they occur," says Thomson.

Problem: YOUR LDL HAS GONE TO HELL

Prescription: An 8-ounce glass of apple juice

Natural antioxidants in apple juice help reduce your risk of heart disease, according to a University of California study. Researchers at the school had 25 men and women drink a glass of apple juice every day for 6 weeks. At the end of the trial, it took 20 percent longer for bad LDL cholesterol in the volunteers' bloodstreams to oxidize and cause trouble. "The longer it takes for cholesterol to oxidize, the lower your overall risk of heart disease," says Dianne Hyson, R.D., the study author.

Problem: YOU'RE STARTING TO GO BALD

Prescription: Dinner at a steak house

Researchers may have discovered why Patrick Stewart lost his hair: one too many cheesesteaks. Order top round steak instead. It's the leanest cut of meat available on most menus. Going lean instead of eating fatty cuts of meat won't keep you from going bald, but it may slow down the process. According to a study in Australia, men who ate lean cuts of meat were less likely to go bald than those who ate fatty cuts of meat. Another plus: "Beef is an excellent source of zinc," says Thomson. "And not getting enough zinc can lead to sudden hair loss."

Problem: YOUR TEETH HURT

Prescription: A cup of tea

Although you wouldn't know it from looking inside the average Englishman's mouth, a cup of tea with a meal may help to prevent cavities. "Tea is a natural source of tooth-protecting fluoride," says Shelby Kashket, Ph.D., a senior investigator with the Forsyth Institute for Dental Health Research in

PERCENTAGE OF AMERICANS WHO REPORT THEY JUST "CAN'T HELP SNACKING ON SALTY SNACKS": 17

FOUR PROBLEMS YOU CAN CURE WITH FOOD (BUT NOT BY EATING IT)

This list doesn't include anything with whipped cream and a naked woman. (If *that's* your problem, you're in the wrong section of this book.) But it does give you permission to play with your supper.

Disinfect a wound. Pour a dab of honey on a cut before covering it with a bandage. "Studies show that honey has powerful antibacterial properties," says James A. Duke, Ph.D., author of *The Green Pharmacy*. One New Zealand study found that honey was capable of destroying almost all strains of the most common wound-infecting bacteria.

Repair dry skin. Baste yourself. "Try rubbing a small amount of corn oil over dry skin on your hands or feet, to add moisture and seal it into the area," says Cyndi Thomson, Ph.D., R.D., an assistant professor at the University of Arizona.

Treat poison ivy. Got itching? Get milk. Soaking a rag in cold milk and then holding it on your skin will dry out the rash of poison ivy and help ease the itch, says John Romano, M.D., a professor of dermatology at Cornell Medical Center in New York City.

Soothe a sunburn. To stop the itch and burn, mix together a bit of dry oatmeal and cool water. Make it slightly slushier than if you were going to eat it, and spread the mixture carefully on your sunburned skin. "This will relieve the pain and help reduce swelling," says Patricia Farris, M.D., a professor of dermatology at Tulane University.

Boston. Tea also contains polyphenols, the same stuff that keeps gum from sticking to your teeth. Drinking a cup before a meal will give your teeth a Teflon-like coating that'll keep cavity-causing sugars from sticking to your chops.

Problem: YOU'RE BLACK-AND-BLUE ALL OVER

Prescription: A couple of sides of broccoli

That excuse about walking into a door lasts only so long before people start asking questions. "If you're constantly getting bruises or turning black-and-blue, it may be a sign that you aren't taking in enough vitamin K," says Thomson. Although asparagus and some kinds of lettuce are good sources of vitamin K, broccoli is better. One serving of cooked broccoli has 250 micrograms, more than twice what you need each day. Eating at least a couple of cups of broccoli throughout the week will help strengthen your blood vessel walls, making it harder for them to break—and for you to bruise.

Problem: THE WORLD IS A CONSTANT BLUR

Prescription: Half a cup of cooked greens

Just opening your eyes can make you susceptible to disease. "Basic elements like light and oxygen increase a person's chances of developing vision problems such as cataracts," says Joanne Curran-Celantano, Ph.D., R.D., a professor of nutrition at the University of New Hampshire. "But eating half a cup of cooked greens every few days gives you enough antioxidants to delay the formation of vision problems by years."

Problem: THE FBI WANTS ANSWERS, NOW

Prescription: A cup of coffee

Caffeine does more for you than wake you up in the morning. According to Dutch research, taking as little as 32 milligrams of caffeine (the amount in just 2 ounces of coffee) before a test helped volunteers improve their memory, as well as their overall reading speed and level of mental alertness. To maximize the benefit, down the coffee at least half an hour before you really need to be thinking clearly. Need to be sharp for more than a couple of hours? Keep drinking coffee or caffeinated soda, but pass on the artificial sweetener. A recent study suggests it may impair short-term memory levels.

Problem: YOU'RE A FEW SWIMMERS SHORT IN THE FALLOPIAN TUBE RELAY

Prescription: A bowl of cereal

There may be a link between low sperm counts and folic acid intake. In a study conducted at the USDA Western Human Nutrition Research Center, researchers found that men with the lowest sperm counts also had the least folic acid in their diets. "It appears that men who are trying to conceive need folic acid for proper DNA synthesis and sperm production," says Lynn Wallock, Ph.D., a research chemist and the lead study author. Cereals are one of the best sources of folic acid. One bowl of Wheaties or raisin bran, for example, has 25 percent of your daily requirement.

Problem: EVERYONE BUT YOU HAS A COLD

Prescription: As much garlic as you can stomach

The second you notice that familiar tickle in your throat, drop everything and head to your nearest Italian restaurant for a plate of garlic bread and shrimp scampi. "Garlic has powerful antiviral properties that fight infections," says Thomson. "Just a couple of cloves of garlic, mixed into food, will jumpstart your immune system and improve your chances of fighting off an illness." If you have to continue the garlic-heavy diet for more than a few days, stick to tomatoey Italian foods, or drink a glass of tomato juice with each meal. Acids in the tomatoes will neutralize the odor-causing oils in the garlic, just as they do other scents—like skunk spray.

Problem: YOU HAVE A FAMILY HISTORY OF PROSTATE CANCER

Prescription: Low-fat vanilla ice cream

Can't stomach another tomato, no matter how much cancer-fighting lycopene it has? Cancel the pizza delivery and head for the freezer instead. In a study recently presented at the Society for Experimental Biology's annual conference, researchers revealed that the more boron there is in your diet, the lower your overall chances of developing prostate cancer. Vanilla ice cream is one of the very best sources of boron, with 25 micrograms per cup.

Gadgets Galore

We tested an amazing 11 infomercial kitchen products to see whether they're worth their weight in shipping

By Brian Good and Mike Zimmerman

Saturday morning on the couch. You search valiantly for SpongeBob but instead find Ron Popiel, the king of infomercials. You try to change the channel. But you can't help it. A countertop rotisserie . . . fascinating. You must watch. The chickens are seasoned, skewered, slid in, slammed shut. Another excruciating microsecond before Popiel grins, flips a knob, and cries—you know it's coming—wait for it—

"Set it . . ."

"*And forget it!*" you scream with the audience.

Ah, but should you buy it? Millions of men like you have guiltlessly bought into the "As Seen on TV" dream: the Turbo-Cooker, the Air Core, the Veg-O-Matic (and many more!). Cynics among us bellow dismissive mantras like "It's a piece of crap," and, "What a waste of my fine cash."

And yet Popiel and his company, Ronco, have sold 3 million Showtime Rotisseries so far. That's the entire population of Chicago setting and forgetting. That's compelling stuff. Compelling enough for us to reverse the mantras, asking, "Are they really pieces of crap?" and "Are they really a waste of our fine cash?" And what about more important questions, like "Do they really reduce fat? Save time? Improve your health?"

We tracked down America's most wanted—and most maligned—kitchen gadgets. We worked them over. And we discovered some amazing things. . . .

GEORGE FOREMAN GRILL
$59.99 from www.biggeorge.com

The pitch: "The lean, mean, fat-reducing grilling machine!"

How it's supposed to work: Slap almost any cut of meat between the grill's two electric surfaces and knock out a low-fat meal in no time.

How it worked for us: Like George (pre-Ali and post-Reagan), the machine is a champ. It offers everything a guy could want: speed, convenience, and an outdoor-grilled taste without the hassle. Plus, it cooks on a slant, so fat drains off. The only drawback comes after your meal. Even with a nonstick coating, George's grill is a lean, mean pain to clean.

Bottom line: Great if you cook burgers a lot. Not so great if you leave it sitting long enough for the grease to harden.

Health benefits: A

Performance: A

Ease of use: B +

Cleanup: D

Get it or forget it? GET IT!

AIR CORE
$299.99 from www.salton-maxim.com

The pitch: "Restaurant-quality cookware that does the cooking for you!"

How it's supposed to work: The thermal lining holds heat for hours, cooking food even after you take the pot off the stove (a great concept: brew food while you drive out to the stadium!).

How it worked for us: Not great. The lasagna noodles came out mushy. The chili beans, crunchy. The meat disintegrated into a soupy mush.

Bottom line: We'll bet the Air Core creators never foresaw the following scenario: You cook chili on the way to the Penn State–Michigan game with six buddies depending on you for lunch. You get there with your crunchy meat soup and you're the laughingstock of the parking lot. Humiliated. In front of girls of the Big Ten, no less.

Health benefits: B

Performance: D

Ease of use: B +

Cleanup: B +

Get it or forget it? FORGET IT!

VEG-O-MATIC
$19.95 from www.smdistributor.com

The pitch: "The original multipurpose food cutter!"

How it's supposed to work: Place the item you want to slice on the blades with the "food plunger" directly above it. Then, according to the instructions, you put your hands on the food plunger and "*ram* down fast and hard," forcing the food through the blades.

How it worked for us: This device is a classic, but we can't explain why. We *rammed,* baby. The carrot slices scattered to the four corners of the kitchen, the potato had to be custom-cut to fit into the mechanism, and the lemon had to be massaged into the blades before *ramming*. And when it was *rammed*? It blasted lemon entrails all over our tester.

Bottom line: A waste of cash and counter space.
Health benefits: C
Performance: F
Ease of use: C
Cleanup: C
Get it or forget it? FORGET IT!

TURBO COOKER
$79.90 from www.turbocooker.com

The pitch: "Cook a four-person, three-course meal at the same time!"
How it's supposed to work: Pour water into the skillet, and cover. The lid seals the steam inside, finishing your meal in just a fraction of the usual time.
How it worked for us: Fine, as long as you don't deviate from the Turbo Cooker recipe cards. As an added pain, you must constantly watch the clock to know when to lock steam in and when to release it. And forget cooking an entire meal at once. Every food, from broccoli to pork chops to chocolate cake, takes a different amount of time, a different amount of water, and a different setting.

Bottom line: It works, but the novelty will wear off faster than the time it takes to actually cook something in it.
Health benefits: C
Performance: D+
Ease of use: D
Cleanup: C
Get it or forget it? FORGET IT!

MAKIN BACON
$10 from www.makinbacon.com

The pitch: "Cook bacon better . . . above the fat, not in it!"
How it's supposed to work: Like a tie rack for your bacon. You drape the raw strips over a plastic T, then stick it in the microwave. As the bacon cooks, fat drips, making breakfast healthier for you.

PERCENTAGE MORE LIKELY THAT MEN WHO FREQUENTLY EAT BACON, HOT DOGS, SAUSAGE, BOLOGNA, AND OTHER PROCESSED MEATS WILL DEVELOP DIABETES: 46

NUMBER OF HOT DOGS AMERICANS CONSUMED IN 2000: 20 BILLION

How it worked for us: Just as it says. Our bacon came out crisp and delicious. And that drip tray accumulates a nauseating amount of goo. We collected 50 percent more fat, compared with microwaving bacon on a plate. The catch: You still have to cover the pig strips with a paper towel to save your microwave from spatters.

Bottom line: Truly a better way to cook bacon. Our only complaint is that we didn't think of Makin Bacon on our own. An 8-year-old girl did. And now she's richer than all of us.

Health benefits: B
Performance: B
Ease of use: A
Cleanup: C
Get it or forget it? GET IT!

SHOWTIME ROTISSERIE
$159.80 from www.ronco.com

The pitch: "Eat healthy! Cut the fat naturally!"

How it's supposed to work: The rotisserie spins your food while a drip pan catches the falling fat.

How it worked for us: That's some damn fine chicken. If you've never used a rotisserie before, this is the one to try. The spit impales meat with ease, and the fat runoff was impressive. Plus, watching the bird as it turns is an oddly fascinating way to pass the time before dinner.

Bottom line: A terrific guy-friendly appliance. Unfortunately, even with the drip pan, you'll still have to clean up a thin layer of grease throughout the machine. But hey, better in the machine than in your gullet.

Health benefits: B
Performance: B +
Ease of use: B
Cleanup: F
Get it or forget it? GET IT!

CITRUS EXPRESS
$17.95 from www.asseenontv.com

The pitch: "Perfect fruit slices, every time!"

How it's supposed to work: Core the fruit and press it onto the wedge cutter. As you rotate the fruit, the blade sloughs the peel away smoother than Hannibal Lecter ever could.

How it worked for us: After finally figuring out how to turn the flimsy plastic cutter, we did cut half an orange from its peel—while simultaneously crushing the rest and spraying juice all over the counter. The harder we pushed, the better the slices came out—but too much force would likely demolish the Citrus Express.

Bottom line: We're for anything that makes eating fruit easier, but you're better off using a knife. You'll save time that can be better spent scaring children with the Don Corleone peel-in-the-teeth trick (death throes included).

Health benefits: C
Performance: F
Ease of use: D
Cleanup: D
Get it or forget it? FORGET IT!

EGG WAVE
$14.95 from www.youcansave.com/eggwave.html

The pitch: "Perfect eggs in seconds!"

How it's supposed to work: Crack an egg into the cooker and nuke it. In less than a minute, you'll have poached, soft-yolk, sunny-side up, or scrambled eggs. Add cheese, ham, or other ingredients for an instant omelette.

How it worked for us: Perfectly cooked eggs? Good luck. Every egg we cooked came out differently. Some were runny, some rubbery—few were just right. And all that time you're allegedly saving? You'll need it. The Egg Wave is incredibly hard to clean—even in the dishwasher.

Bottom line: If you want to nuke some eggs, put them in a cereal bowl lubed with nonstick spray. Your eggs come out just the same, but the bowl will be much easier to clean.

Health benefits: D
Performance: F
Ease of use: B
Cleanup: F
Get it or forget it? FORGET IT!

V/SLICER
$27.95 from www.kingmarketing.com/slicer.htm

The pitch: "One of the most versatile kitchen tools ever invented!"

How it's supposed to work: Use the safety holder to slide fruits and vegetables against different blades, depending on your needs.

How it worked for us: Effortlessly, efficiently, euphorically—once we figured out how to use it, which took a while. The julienne blade consistently yielded slices the length and thickness of a matchstick. "Until I saw the pile of sliced potato, I didn't even know the thing was working," said one of our testers. "It's that easy."

Bottom line: This is the ideal tool for lots of chopping, with blades so ominous they look as if they could slice human flesh off the bone. That's a warning, by the way. Or maybe a selling point.

Health benefits: B
Performance: A

Ease of use: D
Cleanup: B
Get it or forget it? GET IT!

TOASTMASTER ULTRAVECTION OVEN
$99.99 from www.amazon.com

The pitch: Cooks everything from pizza and steak to fries and pastries "up to 60 percent faster than conventional ovens!"

How it's supposed to work: A combination of heating elements holds in juices while cooking your food super quickly. You get deep-fried taste without the nasty frying.

How it worked for us: Indeed, frozen and raw foods cooked in half the time they'd need in an oven. But the machine has to preheat, which negates the benefit. And the grilling basket is too small. Pizzas have to be less than 6 inches across. The handful of fries you can fit in the oven will taste great, but unless you put them in the basket carefully, they fall through to their death.

Bottom line: Good food, small servings, and zero time savings.

Health benefits: C
Performance: B
Ease of use: B
Cleanup: C
Get it or forget it? FORGET IT!

EXPRESS GOURMET
$18.99 from www.productsfromtv.com/expressgourmet.htm

The pitch: "The kitchen miracle that cuts, chops, and mixes in seconds with no mess!"

How it's supposed to work: Like a regular food processor or blender powered by brute arm strength.

How it worked for us: The Hindenburg of all the products we tried. According to the packaging, the tool is strong enough to chop ice. We had problems chopping a banana. Our attempt at a milkshake was worse: Even after we followed the manufacturer's recipe, each crank of the handle sent a wave of milk and melted ice cream squirting out from under the lid.

Bottom line: Considering the amount of emotional torment this product put us through, just buy a friggin' blender.

Health benefits: D
Performance: F
Ease of use: F
Cleanup: F
Get it or forget it? FORGET IT!

KNOW THIS

Have Your Steak and Eat It, Too

Surprise! The saturated fat in a strip of steak is better for you than the trans fatty acid in a serving of fries. Researchers in the Netherlands put 29 healthy adults on a 2-month-long diet in which 10 percent of calories came from either trans fats or saturated fats. Compared with the saturated fat regimen, the trans fat diet led to a 29 percent greater loss of blood vessel function and a 20 percent greater decrease in levels of HDL cholesterol (the good stuff), says Nicole M. de Roos, Ph.D., the study author.

They've Cracked the Case

Eggs are a mystery. They're packed with cholesterol, but eating them in moderation has little impact on cholesterol levels in your blood. Now researchers at Kansas State University may have discovered why: "In animal studies, we found that a compound called lecithin, found in eggs, reduces cholesterol's absorption into the bloodstream," says Sung Koo, Ph.D., a coauthor of the study. Since eggs are also high in protein and vitamins, Koo says you can safely eat one or two a day without worrying about damaging your heart.

Choc a Lot

Here's your license to stock up on Hershey bars. An 8-week study found that eating a few ounces of chocolate every day could raise HDL (good) cholesterol levels by 4 percent.

Mighty Mug

A study in the journal *Annals of Neurology* suggests that drinking coffee may reduce your risk of Parkinson's disease, a nervous system disorder that affects

THE AVERAGE NUMBER OF CUPS OF COFFEE CONSUMED PER DAY: 3.3

more than 1 million Americans. Caffeine appears to prevent the disease's destruction of brain cells.

Postpone the Picnic

According to a new USDA study, hamburger has less bacteria in the winter than in the summer. Between June and September, one out of every 600,000 servings of ground beef contains traces of *E. coli* or other bacteria, but researchers found that the odds dropped to one in 1.6 million between October and May. The change was attributed to cooler winter temperatures, which make it harder for bacteria to spread from one cow to another. To further reduce your chance of getting sick, toss freshly chopped onion or garlic into your patties before cooking them. Both contain bacteria-killing compounds.

Pop Some Produce

Berries, oranges, and peppers are loaded with fiber, antioxidants, and something else: salicylic acid—one of the active ingredients in aspirin. Researchers in Scotland compared blood samples from vegetarian Buddhist monks, who rarely use medication, and a group of healthy men who took aspirin regularly. To the researchers' surprise, they found that the monks had just as much salicylic acid in their systems as the frequent aspirin takers. "This may explain why eating lots of fruits and vegetables provides the same heart-healthy benefits as taking a daily aspirin," says John Paterson, Ph.D., the study author.

Hit the Sauce

Vegetable haters, rejoice. According to University of Scranton research, the food with the highest number of disease-fighting substances isn't broccoli—it's the cranberry. "Gram for gram, cranberries appear to be the absolute best food for fighting cancer, heart disease, and stroke," says Joe Vinson, Ph.D., the study author. Fresh and dried cranberries have the greatest protective powers, followed by cranberry sauce. Cranberry juice is a distant fourth.

DOWN THE PIKE

Cart Wash

Raw meat and babies' diapers can contaminate shopping carts, infecting your groceries when you go shopping. But a store in Louisville may have found a way to solve the problem—by installing the first shopping cart sanitizer. The machine works like a drive-thru car wash and will be available to more stores in the future.

Super Spuds

Researchers in Washington are developing red and purple potatoes that taste just like regular potatoes but pack up to four times the levels of disease-fighting antioxidants. The potatoes contain such high levels of nutrients that eating them is comparable to eating brussels sprouts, kale, or spinach, says Charles Brown, Ph.D., a USDA researcher.

A Great White

Israeli researchers have found a way to boost antioxidant levels in white wine—giving it the same health benefits as red wine—without altering its taste. The first versions of the new wine should soon be available in the United States.

A Boost for Your Bones

Plant biologists at Baylor College have identified the gene that controls the amount of calcium that plants absorb from the ground. By adjusting levels of the gene, they hope to naturally fortify foods like corn, potatoes, and oranges with extra doses of the bone-saving mineral.

PERCENTAGE OF PEOPLE WHO HAVE HEARD THAT GENETICALLY MODIFIED FOODS ARE SOLD IN GROCERY STORES: 55

DOES IT WORK?

Snack Bag Sealer

Historians concur that the invention of jumbo clips for keeping chip bags closed was a breakthrough of transcendent magnitude, up there with twist-off bottle caps. Now behold the EuroSealer, a battery-powered tool that reseals plastic bags with heat. We opened two bags of pretzels, sealed one, and clipped the other. Two weeks later, the winner was clear: the EuroSealer. It gets our seal of approval. Buy it for $10 from www.asseenontv.com.

Lettuce Life Extender

The makers of Green's Extra Life cartridge claim the plastic disk keeps fruits and vegetables fresher longer. The cartridge contains potassium permanganate—which eliminates the ethylene gas released by many fruits and vegetables, the stuff that makes apples rot and lettuce get slimy. Fruit storage companies have used similar packets of potassium permanganate powder for years, says Mark McLellan, Ph.D., a food science expert at Texas A&M University.

We say buy it, especially if you're constantly tossing out rotten produce. "The disk should help you stretch the life spans of most fruits and vegetables," says Mary Ellen Camire, Ph.D., a professor of food science and human nutrition at the University of Maine. Purchase it for $4 from www.dennisgreenltd.com.

Grape Seed Supplements

When it comes to grapes, the sum is apparently greater than the parts, according to John D. Folts, Ph.D., a University of Wisconsin heart specialist. "We compared grape seed extract and grape skin extract, and neither supplement appeared to provide any protection against the causes of heart disease," he says. The bottom line: Drinking two glasses of red wine or purple grape juice a day is better for your heart than taking a grape supplement.

WHAT'S THE DIFF?

Grilling vs. Barbecuing

You're grilling when you cook a steak on your (you guessed it) grill. You're barbecuing when you get up at 5 A.M. to start a smoldering fire in a pit and turn slabs of ribs or a brisket into falling-apart wonderfulness by dinnertime. And you live in Texas. And have two first names.

Salt vs. Sodium

Salt is a seasoning made of sodium chloride. Sodium is an element that can still exist in foods marked "no salt." Check the label.

Yam vs. Sweet Potato

A yam is a big honking tuber grown in Africa, Asia, and the Caribbean, and you've probably never eaten one. Grandma says she serves candied yams every Thanksgiving? She's a big honking liar. You're eating sweet potatoes, a smaller, sweeter, orange-colored native American root—high in beta-carotene and vitamin C.

Extra-Virgin vs. Virgin Olive Oil

The oil from the first pressing of olives is called extra-virgin. Its full flavor is best for dressings or dipping. Virgin olive oil is made from the second pressing, yet still gets to call itself a virgin. If you cook—you know, with that stove thing—pure olive oil works fine, and it's cheaper.

TAKE ACTION

Ah, men and our cars. We buff them, polish them, insure them, and, of course, drive them. We wouldn't dare fill our modern-day chariots with cheap gas. And risk their spitting, choking, and bucking? No way.

Yet we give little thought to the fuel we feed our bodies. To keep *your* frame running for the long haul, you need to start treating it with the respect of a Ferrari. After all, it's the only one you'll ever park in the garage. So step up to the service station you call a kitchen. Then follow these tips to start improving things under your hood.

1. Nibble away at fat. Eating several small meals throughout the day may lower your lipid levels. In a study of 15,000 men and women, researchers at the University of Cambridge in England found that people who eat six or more meals a day have cholesterol levels up to 5 percent lower than those of people who eat just one or two meals a day. Even better, the frequent eaters have lower cholesterol levels, though they consume more total calories and fat. "Eating frequently appears to influence your metabolism by preventing spikes in insulin production and reducing cholesterol production in the body," says Kay-Tee Khaw, M.D., the study author.

2. Spice things up. Tossing some oregano in your supper might help fight a bacterial infection. Researchers at Georgetown University recently found that the natural oils in oregano can kill dangerous, and sometimes even drug-resistant, forms of bacteria—including staph. "In animal trials, we found that a small amount of oregano oil diluted with olive oil was just as effective at preventing bacterial growth as some standard but more potent antibiotics, such as penicillin," says Harry Preuss, M.D., the study author.

3. Eat an apple, breathe easier. An English study of more than 2,600 people found that people who ate an apple a day had better lung capacity than people who rarely ate apples. The study also found that eating apples might reduce the risk of lung cancer while boosting resistance to respiratory illnesses. "Apples contain a huge number of protective compounds called flavonoids, which are absorbed by the body and help make lung tissue healthier and more resistant to disease," explains John Britton, M.D., the study author.

4. Beat cancer with berries. Nearly 10,000 men die every year from esophageal cancer. The disease primarily strikes smokers and drinkers, but unlike with other cancers, your odds of beating this version aren't good. Fewer than 12 percent of patients live more than 5 years after diagnosis. However, a new study suggests there may be a way to reduce your risk of the disease. Researchers at Ohio State University found that eating a cup and a half of berries a day may cut your risk of esophageal cancer in half. "Berries—especially strawberries and raspberries—are loaded with phytochemicals that may prevent development of the disease," says Gary Stoner, Ph.D., a study coauthor.

5. Load up on lycopene. This powerful phytochemical—found in tomatoes, watermelon, pink grapefruit, ketchup, and tomato juice—is not only great for your prostate; it can also do a lot for the rest of your body.

Lungs. A group of men who drank 12 ounces of V8 daily for just 2 weeks showed 20 percent less damage to lung cell DNA from ozone air pollution, an EPA study showed.

Heart. Middle-aged men with low lycopene levels are three times more likely to have heart attacks or strokes, researchers in Finland found. Lycopene keeps LDL (bad cholesterol) from oxidizing into a form that injures arteries.

Skin. A German study found that eating 1.4 ounces of tomato paste daily could reduce skin damage from ultraviolet rays by 40 percent.

Eyes. Lycopene lodges in eye pigment and deters macular degeneration, research at the University of Maryland shows.

6. Sidestep a hangover. According to research from the National Headache Foundation, a couple of spoonfuls of honey immediately before or after drinking may help prevent a hangover. "Honey contains fructose, a type of sugar that helps your body process alcohol more quickly," says Merle Diamond, M.D., a headache expert in Chicago. Surprisingly, she says, tomato juice is another good source of fructose—partially explaining why a Bloody Mary in the morning is sometimes considered a hangover remedy.

7. Use up leftover booze. We know what to do with most leftovers—turkey sandwiches, cold pizza for breakfast. But what do you do when the party's over and there's a fifth of a fifth left in the bottle? Add it to your food for more flavor. Some examples:

Add leftover white wine to an omelette. Wine gives eggs a little acidity and makes them whip up lighter and fluffier, says Alain Sailhac, senior dean of the French Culinary Institute in New York City.

Add leftover bourbon to baked beans. Add a splash of bourbon and two splashes of leftover black coffee to a can of baked beans. Toss in a teaspoon of chili powder and dry mustard, then cook for an hour. The whiskey will leave a toasted, caramel flavor.

PERCENTAGE OF AMERICANS WHO DRINK ALCOHOL EVERY DAY: 7

PERCENTAGE OF AMERICANS WHO SAY THEY SOMETIMES DRINK MORE THAN THEY THINK THEY SHOULD: 20

Add leftover sweet vermouth to shrimp. Sauté shrimp, diced tomatoes, and garlic, and add a dash of hot-pepper sauce and ½ cup of sweet red vermouth, suggests Linda Gassenheimer, author of *Low-Carb Meals in Minutes.*

8. Go to plan B. Some things—like slathering on sunscreen before ever stepping out of the house—are simply too much of a hassle. That's when you try a somewhat healthy alternative. Here's your plan B:

If you don't eat fish twice a week . . . You're not missing out on much, just a little puddle of oil that can reduce your risk of heart disease, ease post-workout muscle soreness, help you fight depression, and possibly even protect you from Alzheimer's. It's omega-3 fatty acids that make fish oil magic, and fortunately they've bottled the stuff. "If you don't like fish or don't get to eat it, fish oil supplements are just as good," says Mary Ellen Camire, Ph.D., a professor of food science and human nutrition at the University of Maine. But don't just grab any guppy grease. Look for omega-3 supplements that haven't passed their expiration date and that list vitamin E as the second ingredient. (The antioxidant effect of E will keep the oil from turning rancid.) The supplement's also available as a new orange-flavored food additive called Coromega. Sprinkle the ketchup packet–size servings into pudding, yogurt, softened vanilla ice cream, or a smoothie.

If you won't spread on SPF-15 sunscreen before you step outside . . . Wash down your morning multivitamin regimen with a bottle of iced green tea. In a recent Rutgers University study, mice given green tea had 51 percent fewer incidences of skin cancer than control mice, even after prolonged exposure to damaging ultraviolet rays. "The research looks very promising that green tea may protect humans against skin cancer, too," says James Spencer, M.D., an associate professor of dermatology at Mount Sinai School of Medicine in New York City. Researchers suspect that antioxidants in green tea fight skin cancer by neutralizing the free radicals that damage skin cells.

If you can never remember to clean out your refrigerator every 3 months . . . Hit the hardware store and pick up a refrigerator thermometer (about $10). Here's the logic: A crumb here or a drip there (okay, numerous crumbs and drips) won't hurt you as long as the temp is low enough to prevent bacteria and mold from turning your fridge into a greenhouse. "If you do nothing else, make sure the temperature always stays below 40°F," says Don Schaffner, Ph.D., a food safety expert at Rutgers University in New Jersey. But why the retrofit? Because many refrigerators don't come with their own thermometers, and even with those that do, there's a good chance they're off by a few critical degrees. Note: You can stick your thermometer anywhere but on the inside of the fridge door; odds are this spot is a few degrees warmer than the rest of your icebox.

ANY QUESTIONS?

Top It Off

What's the smartest topping to order on my pizza?
—G. M., Hermosa Beach, California

Bar none, your best bet is green peppers, says Franca Alphin, R.D., a clinical associate with the department of family medicine at Duke University. Nutritionally, they beat out the other traditional toppings—mushrooms, onion, sausage, pepperoni, and olives—by a long shot. Half a cup of sliced green bell peppers delivers 50 milligrams of vitamin C (that's more than half of what you need daily), 1 gram of fiber, and a decent dose of potassium, a nutrient that can lower blood pressure.

For an even smarter pie, ask the pizza baker to use just half the cheese and to add extra peppers to fill the crust. To load up on flavor, restaurants tend to dump on more cheese when they make pizzas with vegetable toppings than when they make meat-topped ones. So, if your goal is to boost nutrition and make a dent in calories and fat, you've got to cut the cheese.

Mineral Deposit

My wife takes calcium supplements to help prevent osteoporosis. Is this something I should be doing?
—R. P., Las Vegas

Osteoporosis, which thins bones and makes them vulnerable to breaks, isn't just an old-lady disease—about 2 million American men have it.

To keep bones strong, men under the age of 50 need 1,000 milligrams (mg) of calcium a day, and older men need 1,200 mg. You should be able to get that much from your diet alone, says Robert Heaney, M.D., a professor of medicine at Creighton University in Omaha, Nebraska. One glass of skim milk contains 300 mg of calcium, and a cup of nonfat yogurt has 215 mg. Women generally eat less overall, so it's harder for them to get sufficient amounts of calcium without a supplement.

Best Burger
What's the healthiest fast-food burger?
—B.Y., Katonah, New York

Pound for pound, the winners are (in a split decision) Wendy's and Burger King. Their 4-ounce burgers weigh in at about 350 calories and 16 grams (g) of fat. And while the 2-ounce McDonald's hamburger is the leanest (280 calories, 10 g fat), it's so small you might be tempted to eat two or three. To help curb your urge to eat fat-soaked fries, load a quarter-pound burger with lettuce and tomato.

Veg Out
I keep hearing that vegetables lose their nutrients when they're cooked. Is that true?
—C.K, Kaneohe, Hawaii

Not necessarily. Vegetables do lose a small percentage of their water-soluble nutrients (like vitamins B and C) when cooked, but cooking also makes cancer-fighting ones, like beta-carotene and lycopene, more absorbable, says Joan Carter, R.D., a spokeswoman for the American Dietetic Association. The key to maximizing nutrients is minimizing cooking time. In a microwave, heat vegetables until you can smell them, usually 7 to 10 minutes on high per pound of leafy vegetables, and 5 to 10 minutes on high per pound of denser vegetables, like carrots or potatoes. If you're eating with someone other than your cat, upgrade to sautéing.

- Cut your vegetables into thin slices. The thinner they are, the quicker they'll cook.
- Heat the pan before adding vegetables. The less time vegetables are exposed to heat, the fewer nutrients they'll lose.
- Stir constantly so the vegetables cook evenly.
- Do a taste test after a minute or two. You want cooked but still crisp.
- See the leftover liquid on the bottom of the skillet? Any nutrients that have leached out are still there. Pour the juice over your vegetables, add it to rice, sop it up with bread, or suck it through a straw. Just don't let it go down the drain.

PERCENTAGE OF AMERICANS WHOSE DIETS ARE MADE UP ALMOST ENTIRELY OF FAST FOOD: 14

Belly Up to the Bar

Is beer more or less fattening than wine and liquor?
—T. M., Eugene, Oregon

Neither. Whether it's in the form of beer, wine, or a slippery nipple, all alcohol is fat-free, says Carter, R.D. But hold up on the high fives: It's not calorie-free. In fact, after fat, alcohol has the highest caloric density of any food source (7 calories per gram)—that means one serving of beer (12 ounces), wine (6 ounces), or liquor (1.5 ounces) is worth between 105 and 150 calories, or about 54 jujubes.

To cut back on calories, opt for light beers; there's no such thing as light wine or Goldschlager. Light beers are less filling because they have less alcohol, which drops their calorie count by about 45. For a light beer that also tastes great, Paul Gatza, director of the Homebrewers Association, recommends Old Milwaukee Light, a two-time taste winner at the Great American Beer Festival Championships. Of course, if you really want to shave calories, stick to nonalcoholic brews, which float in at between 58 and 90 calories per 12 ounces. You won't be wearing lamp shades at your next party, but at least your pants will fit.

Waterlogged

I keep hearing that I need to drink eight glasses of water a day. I don't like water. (Doesn't anyone notice it has no taste?) Can I drink coffee or diet soda instead?
—S. R., Chattanooga, Tennessee

Absolutely. Some old-school nutritionists are too hung up on straight H_2O. Don't listen to them. Think "fluids," not specifically "water," says Mark Kantor, Ph.D., a professor of nutrition at the University of Maryland. But keep an eye on the calories that soft drinks and sports drinks deliver. They can quickly go to your gut.

Another point: A lot of nutritionists dis Diet Coke and coffee because caffeine is a diuretic. But don't worry about peeing yourself dry. The *Journal of the American College of Nutrition* reported a small study showing that when men drank caffeinated beverages, they were as well-hydrated as when they downed an equal amount of water.

PERCENTAGE OF AMERICANS
WHO REGULARLY DRINK BOTTLED WATER: 54

PERCENTAGE WHO BELIEVE THEIR TAP
WATER IS NOT AS SAFE AS IT SHOULD BE: 32

Popeye's Pasta

Does spinach pasta count as a vegetable?
—J.B., Grapevine, Texas

Sorry. There's hardly any spinach in spinach spaghetti. Look at the nutrition label on the pasta box. You probably won't see vitamin A listed, even though spinach is loaded with it. This is a sure sign that there's little spinach inside. Most spinach pasta is made of semolina and spinach powder or paste. Sure, it's green, but it's nowhere near a vegetable. Instead, try this idea: Stir a cup of thawed, drained, chopped spinach into your pasta sauce. A serving will give you 35 percent of your daily requirement of vitamin A, plus lutein and zeaxanthin, two nutrients known to protect vision.

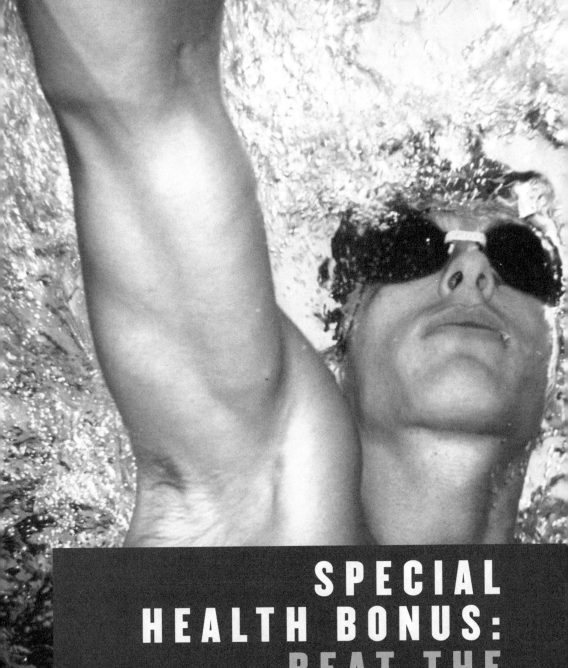

SPECIAL HEALTH BONUS: BEAT THE MEN KILLERS

Who Will Die First?

Will one of these guys be 6 feet under soon? Or will you?

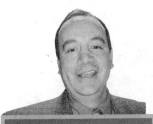

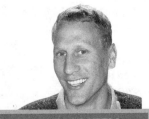

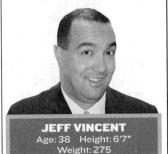

BOB SELL
Age: 37   Height: 5'11"
Weight: 195

BOB CASSAZELL
Age: 33   Height: 6'2"
Weight: 167

JEFF VINCENT
Age: 38   Height: 6'7"
Weight: 275

GREATEST RISK FACTOR
- Stress

VITAL STATISTICS
- Married 15 years, no kids
- Has borderline high cholesterol/blood pressure
- Gets a physical exam with stress test every 2 years
- Is a partner in a consulting firm
- Flies 125,000 miles per year
- Averages 4 to 5 hours of sleep per night during a 60-hour workweek
- Eats a moderately high fat diet
- Dinners range from a gourmet meal to cereal
- Exercises infrequently
- Drinks at an occasional party
- Smokes an occasional cigar

FAMILY HISTORY
- Heart disease on father's side (dad and grandmother died in early fifties)
- Longevity on mother's side (grandparents lived past 70)

BOB'S PREDICTION
- "I believe genetics plays an overwhelming role in determining our fate. Although my dad died young, his lifestyle brought that on. He continued to smoke and drink after his bypass. So I think you can discount genetics as one of my risks. I say Cassazell goes first."

GREATEST RISK FACTOR
- Genetics

VITAL STATISTICS
- Married with two kids, ages 3 years and 5 months
- Has normal cholesterol/blood pressure
- Sees a cardiologist annually with complete physical every 3 years
- Owns a construction company
- Works 6-day, 60-hour weeks
- Eats a relatively low-fat diet with minimal red and processed meats
- Has fruit for snacks
- Drinks 32 ounces of water daily
- Former college runner (4:04 mile); runs 15 miles per week
- Occasionally plays basketball
- Drinks four beers a week
- Never smokes

FAMILY HISTORY
- Brother died of a heart attack at 36
- Sister has heart disease
- Grandmother has a heart condition, and several of her brothers and sisters died of coronary failure in their forties

BOB'S PREDICTION
- "The person under the greatest stress is in the most trouble. Mine is high, but it's nowhere near Sell's. I believe stress contributed to my brother's death."

GREATEST RISK FACTOR
- Inactivity/diet

VITAL STATISTICS
- Divorced for 5 years; wife has custody of two kids
- Is 50 pounds overweight
- Has normal cholesterol/blood pressure
- Gets a complete physical every 2 years
- Is a financial information salesman
- Has relatively low stress
- Takes a daily multi-vitamin, and eats whatever
- Dinners range from a home-cooked steak to happy-hour buffet
- Usually does an hour of calisthenics 3 days a week, but that's only "to keep my stomach from protruding farther than my chest."
- Has a few beers during the week, but partial to scotch on weekends
- Smokes an occasional cigar

FAMILY HISTORY
- No known chronic diseases, but as an African-American, he's at higher risk for high blood pressure and prostate cancer

JEFF'S PREDICTION
- "I think the deadliest combination is stress and genetics. So I think I have a good shot at outliving both these guys."

And the Loser Is . . .
Bob Sell

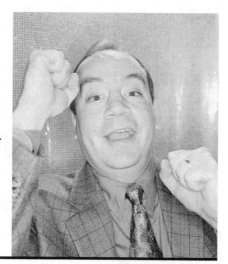

Ken Goldberg, M.D., founder of the Male Health Center in Dallas, helped us devise a scoring system that either awards or deducts points for specific traits and behaviors. The lower the point total, the greater the risk of premature death.

Check out the chart on the opposite page to see how Dr. Goldberg handicapped the competition—then figure out your own score to see where you stand.

HOW SELL IS BEATING THE OTHER GUYS TO THE GRAVE

"The odds of any of these guys dying in the next 5 years are very low," concludes Ken Goldberg, M.D., founder of the Male Health Center in Dallas, "but when you play this out over 10 or 15 years, some real problems emerge. I think it's a close race between Sell and Vincent as to who's going to do himself in first."

Although Cassazell has a frightening family health history, he has minimized most of his other risks. Participating in a comprehensive medical exam every few years ensures that any coronary artery disease that does develop will be caught early. And even though his job and family life are stressful, Dr. Goldberg says he shouldn't worry. Poor nutrition, lack of exercise, and excess weight are all more detrimental to longevity.

It's equally important for Vincent to continue having routine medical checkups. Being Black puts him at almost as high a genetic risk as Cassazell, even though Vincent's family history is relatively clean. Because he'll forever carry this health handicap, it's vital that he control what he can by exercising aerobically, eating smarter, and shedding fat.

And as for Sell, it's interesting to note that although he lost this match, of all our contestants, he controls his destiny the most. Since his good/bad family health history balances itself out, all of his remaining risks stem from his hectic lifestyle. If he can bring some sanity to this, there's hope for him yet.

"He's young enough that if he addresses his weight, diet, exercise, and stress problems," says Dr. Goldberg, "he could outlive us all. Preventive maintenance is the key to long life."

The Final Analysis

HEALTH FACTOR	POINT VALUE	SELL	CASSAZELL	VINCENT	YOU
PHYSICAL EXAM Preventive medicine is key.	Gets a physical at least every 3 years +2 Goes to a doctor only when there's a problem −2	+2	+2	+2	
MARITAL STATUS Statistics show that married men live longer.	Married +1 Single or divorced −1	+1	+1	−1	
FAMILY HISTORY Certain diseases are inherited.	Longevity runs in the family +2 One side of the family has longevity, the other dies young from disease 0 Strong family history of heart disease, diabetes, or cancer −2	0	−2	+2	
STRESS Chronic stress is a risk factor for high blood pressure and other problems.	Low stress +1 Moderate stress −1 High stress −2	−2	−1	+1	
DIET Good nutrition can slant the odds in your favor.	Healthy, low-fat diet +2 Unhealthy, high-fat diet −2	−2	+2	−2	
EXERCISE Aerobic exercise keeps your weight in check and reduces risk factors for heart disease and certain cancers.	Does aerobic exercise at least three times a week +2 Does some exercise but little or no aerobics −1 Exercises infrequently −2	−2	+2	−1	
CHOLESTEROL/ BLOOD PRESSURE High blood pressure and cholesterol readings could be cause for concern.	Normal readings +1 Borderline readings −1 High readings −2	−1	+1	+1	
TOBACCO Using no tobacco is best.	Never smokes +2 Smokes occasionally 0 Smokes daily −2	0	+2	0	
ALCOHOL Moderation is key.	Two or fewer drinks a day 0 More than two drinks a day −2	0	0	0	
WEIGHT Overweight raises your risk of diabetes, heart disease, and other threats.	At a healthy weight +2 Overweight −1 50+ pounds overweight −2	−1	+2	−2	
RACE African-Americans are at higher risk for high blood pressure, cancer, and other diseases. Latinos are at higher risk for diabetes.	Caucasian 0 African-American −1 Asian 0 Latino −1	0	0	−1	
TOTALS		−5	+9	−1	

▶ IF YOUR SCORE IS LESS THAN 0: You'd better make some serious lifestyle changes, or you're headed headed to an early grave.

▶ IF YOUR SCORE IS 0 TO 17: You may want to up your life insurance while you still can.

▶ IF YOUR SCORE IS 18 OR MORE: You'll live to a ripe old age.

MUST READS

A Ticking Time Bomb

He hasn't been trained in the latest technology. He isn't aware of the latest treatment. The tests he relies on will miss eight out of 10 cases. Yet the enemy he's fighting is heart disease, the leading killer of men. Who is he? He's your doctor

By Joe Kita

David Rubinson had a heart attack at age 39. But he blames himself for that. As a record producer and manager of such acts as Santana and the Pointer Sisters, he thought he was Superman. And eventually the late nights in the studio, the rich foods, and the extreme stress caught up with him. A poor lifestyle, combined with a family history of heart disease, became his kryptonite.

But he considers himself blameless for what happened next. In the ensuing decade, he transformed his life. He downsized his business, became a vegetarian, stopped smoking, started exercising, lost weight, and took up yoga. His total cholesterol plummeted from 380 to 210, he qualified for $2 million worth of new life insurance, he passed his treadmill stress tests, and his doctors gave him nothing but back pats. Then one night at dinner, almost 10 years to the day after his heart attack and just 12 hours after running 9½ miles across the Golden Gate Bridge, he felt a familiar dread.

"It wasn't real pain," he recalls. "It was more a sense of depletion, like somebody had pulled the plug and all the water was running out of the tub. Later, after I put everyone to bed, I went into my office at home and took a nitroglycerin tablet. And when it made me feel better, I knew I was in trouble. I woke my wife and told her we had to go to the hospital."

When doctors did an angiogram to assess the situation, Rubinson couldn't believe what he saw. "The grafts from my original bypass were completely dried up," he says. "They looked like black strings. I'd been running across that bridge on nothing. It's hard to describe what I felt. Rage, betrayal, terror. My son asked the doctors, 'How could this happen? My God, look at everything he's done!'"

So there was more surgery, five bypasses this time, and when Rubinson left the hospital, he was depressed and desperate. That's when he heard of a cardiologist named Robert Superko, M.D., who was perfecting a new type of blood analysis at a fledgling Bay area clinic. It identified 12 different sub-classes of cholesterol-carrying particles, plus other substances that influence heart disease. Dr. Superko claimed that total cholesterol and even levels of HDL and LDL were too general to be dependable predictors of cardiovascular trouble. In fact, he said, they were often misleading, creating a false sense of worry or security.

Rubinson had never heard this theory before, even though he'd been seeing some of the country's best cardiologists. So, with nothing to lose, he submitted a blood sample and, to his amazement, found an apparent explanation for his heart disease. "Dr. Superko showed me all these new numbers," he explains, "things like small, dense lipoprotein and homocysteine. Then he told me, 'You can diet and exercise all you want, but there are genetic factors at work here that must be managed in other ways.'"

With Dr. Superko's guidance, Rubinson continued his healthful lifestyle and started taking medication to thwart the most lethal of these new types of cholesterol. Now, almost 10 years after his second bypass surgery, Rubinson has all these new numbers within acceptable ranges and can claim, with confidence and authority this time, that his disease is under control.

"When I talk about Superko, tears come to my eyes," says Rubinson. "Because he saved me. Without this man, I'm gone."

Without realizing it, you may be in a situation similar to Rubinson's. You may think you're taking good care of your heart: exercising, eating right, and having your cholesterol checked. And your numbers may be good. Even your doctor may say you have nothing to worry about. But should you believe him?

- The landmark Framingham Heart Study, which has been tracking thousands of people since 1948, found that 80 percent of those who develop coronary disease had the same basic cholesterol numbers as those who didn't.
- At least 50 percent of arteriosclerosis (narrowing of the arteries) can't be explained by the standard risk factors (smoking, diet, lifestyle, high cholesterol). There are other agents at work that routine lab tests miss.
- For 25 percent of men with a family history of cardiovascular problems, the first sign of heart disease is sudden death.

Getting nervous?

You should be. Despite all the advances in heart disease treatment within the past decade (new drugs, surgeries, means of prevention), it remains the country's number-one killer. A staggering 60 million Americans (one in every five persons) has some form of it, and each year 725,000 men and women die of it—the equivalent of one victim every 44 seconds. And although science has arrested its growth, there's still been no sign of a precipitous drop-off.

Statistics like these contradict the impression most people develop at the doctor's office, where basic cholesterol numbers, treadmill stress tests, and lifestyle factors parade as ironclad predictors of risk and benchmarks for treatment. On its Web site, the American Heart Association (AHA) encourages people to think of high cholesterol as a "leading risk factor for heart disease . . . a vital sign, similar to blood pressure." It makes the following recommendations.

- Total cholesterol—below 200 milligrams per deciliter (mg/dl)
- HDL (good cholesterol)—above 40 mg/dl
- LDL (bad cholesterol)—below 130 mg/dl
- Triglycerides—below 150 mg/dl

These four components of cholesterol, the so-called basic panel, are the only ones the AHA mentions. When your blood test results fall within these guidelines, your doctor will probably conclude that you have nothing to worry about. Conversely, when your numbers exceed these boundaries, he'll recommend lifestyle changes and maybe even cholesterol-lowering drugs. But as we've seen, heart disease isn't so clear-cut. In fact, some impressive research refutes the dependability of these guidelines.

Total cholesterol. Drawing from a study of 360,000 men, researchers found that 24 percent of those who died of heart attacks had total cholesterol levels below 200. "Total cholesterol is really a very bad test," says Christie Ballantyne, M.D., director of the center for cardiovascular prevention at Methodist Hospital/Baylor College of Medicine in Houston. "If you're judging the health of your heart by it, you're way off."

HDL. According to data from the Framingham Study, the average HDL cholesterol of men with coronary artery disease was 43. That's slightly higher than what the guidelines say is protective.

LDL. Based on data from Framingham, the average LDL cholesterol of those having heart attacks was 150. The guidelines call that only "borderline high" risk.

Triglycerides. According to research from Framingham and other studies, keeping it below 150 appears to be the new consensus for safety. Until its 2002 guideline changes, the AHA had its threshold set at 200.

For these reasons and more, the basic cholesterol panel can predict coronary artery disease in only 20 percent of cases. "HDL, LDL, triglycerides—

THE AVERAGE GUY'S LDL CHOLESTEROL LEVEL: 140 MG/DL

WHAT IT SHOULD BE: LESS THEN 130 MG/DL

NUMBER OF MEN WITH LDL CHOLESTEROL HIGHER THAN 160 MG/DL: 1 IN 5

LDL CHOLESTEROL: HOW IT KILLS

A typical blood test gives you a general reading of your total low-density lipoprotein (bad cholesterol). But there are seven different types, some of which are more dangerous than others. Here's how they cause heart attacks.

I. From childhood onward, a high-fat diet and sedentary lifestyle increase the LDL in your bloodstream. The smallest, densest particles (IIIa and IIIb) are the most likely to burrow into artery walls and cause lesions.

2. Bigger, less dense LDL particles (I, IIa, IIb, IVa, and IVb) can add to the damage, over time calcifying into plaque.

3. One day, a piece of plaque breaks off and rides the bloodstream into your heart or wedges in a blood vessel, closing it off. Starved of oxygen, your heart muscle shuts down. If you're lucky, you reach the hospital in time.

that's the bare minimum," says Dr. Ballantyne. "And before you think you're safe, remember that ideally you want an LDL less than 100, an HDL over 45, and triglycerides less than 150. Unfortunately, most people don't fit nicely into these categories. Anyone in the gray zone needs more information." And that's where the new blood tests come in.

Small, dense lipoprotein. Fibrinogen. C-reactive protein. Homocysteine. Lipoprotein(a). HDL2b. These are just a few of the measures that appear on reports from the Berkeley HeartLab, an advanced cardiovascular diagnostics center in San Mateo, California, headed by Dr. Superko. These gauges are unfamiliar, for patients as well as many doctors, but they represent the cutting edge of heart disease prevention. Dr. Superko has published more than 100 scientific articles on the topic and is a fellow in the American College of Cardiology.

When asked why anyone needs such detailed blood work, especially when he often must pay $150 to $700 to get it, Dr. Superko points to two substances, the preponderance of which can dramatically increase your risk of coronary disease.

The first is small, dense lipoprotein, and it's the worst of the seven types of LDL cholesterol that can now be measured. It's dangerous because it's the likeliest of all the particles to worm its way into artery walls and plaques. This creates arterial lesions, contributes to the growth of existing ones, and may make plaque less stable and more susceptible to rupture. The combined results of three major studies found that small, dense lipoprotein conveys a threefold increase in cardiovascular risk.

The second substance is called lipoprotein(a), or Lp(a) for short. This is a bastard form of LDL that's so predictive of coronary disease that it's been called "heart attack cholesterol." Researchers at Oxford University in England found that among 5,400 people with heart disease, those with the highest levels had a 70 percent greater chance of having a heart attack.

As you'll learn in "Will He Live, or Will He Die?" on page 148, other rarely measured blood components can have similar dire consequences. Even though the mechanisms by which they all work are not fully understood, clinical evidence is mounting that they play influential roles in heart disease. How vital it is to know yours depends on your family history and the lifestyle you lead. But what's disturbing is that so few doctors are offering their patients this opportunity.

"It's a national scandal," says Thomas Yannios, M.D., associate director of critical care and nutritional support at Ellis Hospital in Schenectady, New York. "I'd estimate that only 5 percent of doctors in the United States are using these specialized blood tests. There's an incredible lack of understanding of this science on the part of the medical profession. It's exasperating to me because we now have the ability to look into a person's metabolic soul."

The Berkeley HeartLab isn't the only business of its kind. LipoMed in Raleigh, North Carolina, and Atherotech in Birmingham, Alabama, offer similar analyses, using different methodologies. One independent study, which utilized the Berkeley program, reduced the risk of future heart events by 43 percent over 4 years. And Atherotech claims it can raise a physician's ability to predict cardiovascular disease from 40 percent to 90 percent. These are bold promises the AHA is still considering, but some doctors are already convinced.

Dr. Yannios is one of them. After attending lectures on the subject at American College of Cardiology conferences, he started doing some anecdotal research. While making rounds in the intensive care ward at his hospital, he began asking patients about their cholesterol profiles.

"I was horrified to find so many who had been through the mill of cardiac specialists, and others who supposedly had zero risk, hospitalized with heart problems," he says. "Something big was being missed."

HOW TO GET THESE TESTS

If you have a family history of heart disease and/or basic cholesterol numbers that are suspicious, ask your doctor about these specialized tests. If he's unconvinced, call the Berkeley HeartLab at (800) 432-7889 for a referral. If the tests reveal a problem, your doctor may prescribe niacin. Take niacin only under a doctor's care; it can cause liver damage in the large doses that are necessary to be effective.

Dr. Yannios subsequently wrote a book called *The Heart Disease Breakthrough* in which he pulls together much of the supporting research for these specialized blood tests. In the book, he points out that this is neither flimsy science nor recent theory. The foundational research dates to the 1950s, when scientists at the University of California at Berkeley discovered multiple cholesterol-carrying particles. And what's more, the Framingham Study has for decades been citing connections between many of these components and heart disease: fibrinogen in 1987, homocysteine in 1990, and lipoprotein(a) in 1994. So why aren't more people, and especially more doctors, ordering these tests? There are a number of reasons.

The science is very complex. "Traditionally, biochemistry is one of the first subjects you take in medical school," explains Dr. Yannios, "and the cholesterol stuff is at the end. It's not a very glamorous topic, and that mentality gets carried on. A lot of doctors either don't want to or don't have the time to master this biochemistry because it seems so complex."

Cardiologists are mainly plumbers. When you develop a clog, they'll scour it out, but traditionally they haven't offered much advice on keeping your pipes clean. "Doctors tend to treat what they can see, not what is potential," says Dr. Yannios. "And when the issue becomes more complex, that reinforces the behavior."

Insurance may not pay for it. Although these tests are much cheaper than the bill for a bypass, health insurance plans don't typically reward prevention. Unless your provider is progressive or your cardiologist insists upon these tests, you probably won't have much luck with reimbursement.

The prescription is a vitamin. The antidote to many of these evil new particles is not a high-tech drug but a B vitamin called niacin. It reduces triglycerides and LDL cholesterol—including Lp(a) and small, dense lipoprotein—while it raises beneficial HDL. In fact, niacin can be more effective at treating these things than popular cholesterol-busting drugs, which tend to act more generally on total cholesterol and gross LDL. (Be careful, though. Niacin has serious side effects and should be taken only under a doctor's supervision.)

The point of all this is that doctors are so busy they often rely on drug company salesmen for information about new treatments. Because niacin has historically been the prescription when these new numbers are out of line, "there was never any fat wallet promoting it," says Dr. Yannios. In other words, unlike the commercial anti-cholesterol drugs, which generate $16 billion in annual global sales for pharmaceutical companies, there was never any business reason for anyone to educate doctors about these other blood components. That's changing, however. A company named Kos makes a timed-release prescription product called Niaspan, and Kos recently partnered with DuPont to promote it.

WILL HE LIVE, OR WILL HE DIE?

Our writer submits his own blood for analysis

By Joe Kita

In many ways, I'm the perfect lab rat for this. My father died of a heart attack at age 61, and I'm now 41. For the past 15 years, my total cholesterol has remained borderline high (210 to 240) and my LDL elevated (130 to 160) despite my losing weight, exercising, and eating a low-fat diet. In fact, with the results of every blood test, I grow more frustrated. All my lifestyle changes have apparently had little impact. Lately, I've been considering cholesterol-lowering drugs.

But physicians who have looked at my numbers have been reassuring. They point to my high HDL (55 to 75), low triglycerides (sub-100), and good HDL/LDL ratio (less than half average risk) and tell me I have nothing to worry about. But the cardiologist David Kann, M.D., who drew my blood at a small hospital in Carlisle, Pennsylvania, has learned not to make such assumptions. "Personally, I thought I had no risk of heart disease," Dr. Kann explains. "Then I sent my blood off and found there's a pretty good chance I could have a heart attack."

There is nothing special about the way blood is drawn for these tests. You fast for 12 hours, then roll up your sleeve for the usual needle prick. Afterward, the sample is packed with ice in an insulated container and shipped. Dr. Kann prefers the Berkeley HeartLab because he says it's very reliable. Ten days later, I have the results (and the bill, $695, not covered by my insurance). As you scan my report (the numbers in parentheses are my readings), I'll let the experts explain what we're seeing.

Apoprotein B (107 mg/dl): This is the protein cap that each LDL particle wears. By counting these, you get a precise measure of the LDL particles in the bloodstream, a truer indication of your genetic predisposition to heart disease. These particles may damage your arteries and cause blockages, so it helps to know how many you've got. I'm over the recommended limit of 100. Dr. Yannios calls it "a fin breaking the water."

Lipoprotein(a) (3 mg/dl): This "heart attack cholesterol" accumulates around arterial lesions and promotes clotting. Lp(a) alone can raise your risk of heart attack by as much as 70 percent. Furthermore, it does not respond to diet and exercise. Niacin is the best way to treat it. Dr. Superko recommends keeping Lp(a) below 20. Seeing mine so low is a relief.

Fibrinogen (324 mg/dl): This is a protein molecule that promotes clotting and also thickens the blood. The more there is, the greater

But in the meantime, doctors across the country continue dispensing basic cholesterol tests and writing prescriptions for anti-cholesterol drugs that may not target the patient's specific problem. Dr. Superko points out that even though people taking cholesterol-reducing medication experience a 25 percent reduction in cardiovascular events, "there are still an awful lot of people on them having heart attacks."

Bob Bakke is a classic example of this. Despite a strong family history of heart disease, he thought he had everything under control—just like Ruthe likelihood that your heart is struggling to pump sludge. High levels seem to correlate with cigarette smoking, obesity, inactivity, aging, and diabetes. Levels above 350 double the risk of coronary disease. Mine is approaching that, but still okay.

C-reactive protein (0.07 mg/dl): This substance is produced in the liver when arteries become inflamed. The more of it there is, the greater the chance that arterial plaque will rupture and cause a heart attack. Levels above 2.5 mg/dl convey a twofold to fourfold increase in risk and are capable of predicting first heart attacks 6 to 8 years in advance. Mine is practically nonexistent.

Homocysteine (11.6 micromoles per liter): This is an amino acid that promotes clotting. It appears to work in conjunction with fibrinogen and Lp(a). Levels above 14 can increase your risk of heart attack and stroke by two to four times. Fortunately, it's one of the easiest of the new blood components to control. Dr. Yannios says it responds well to folate and B vitamins. Mine is getting close to the ceiling, so it bears watching.

Insulin (4 micrograms per milliliter—mcg/ml): This is a hormone secreted by the pancreas to regulate blood sugar. Testing for insulin isn't new, but it's important. When combined with high triglycerides; low HDL; high fibrinogen; and high levels of small, dense lipoprotein, high insulin levels strongly predispose you to atherosclerosis. The goal is to keep this under 12 mcg/ml.

LDL IIIa and IIIb (15.6 percent): There are seven subclasses of LDL particles, with such catchy names as I, IIa, IIb, IIIa, IIIb, IVa, and IVb. Overall, LDL is bad cholesterol, but IIIa and IIIb are the most destructive types. These are the smallest, densest particles—the ones most likely to work their way into artery walls and form plaques. People with lots of small, dense lipoprotein are dubbed pattern B and have a threefold greater risk of developing heart disease. I'm a healthy pattern A, but it's only because my lifestyle changes have helped suppress these destructive molecules.

HDL2b (21 percent): There are five subclasses of HDL particles, labeled 2a, 2b, 3a, 3b, and 3c. Overall, HDL is good cholesterol, but 2b is the most beneficial. The more you have of it, the less likely you are to suffer a heart attack. Mine is bountiful.

So I'm safe for now. After 15 years, I can finally breathe easy. My diligence has paid off.

"Your genes want to do bad things," concludes Dr. Yannios, "but you've completely throttled them by making all the right lifestyle changes. Keep it up and you'll be around for a while."

binson—running 3 to 5 miles daily, eating a low-fat diet, keeping all his standard cholesterol numbers within recommended ranges. In fact just for extra insurance, he was taking one of the most popular cholesterol-busting drugs on the market (Mevacor) and had recently passed a cardiac stress test. Yes, life as a healthy, slim 44-year-old university research administrator in Chico, California, was good. Then, while running on a gym treadmill and chatting with his 14-year-old daughter, Bakke suddenly passed out. The treadmill flung him against the wall so hard, emergency personnel initially thought he had injured his neck. But later, in the hospital, it was discovered that three of his major coronary arteries were 90 percent blocked. Four days later, he had a quintuple bypass.

"It was devastating," he says. "Suddenly I didn't know whether I'd live or die."

With Dr. Superko's help, Bakke, now 52, has gotten his heart disease under control.

He takes 4 to 5 grams of niacin daily and has continued with his healthful lifestyle. A series of ultrasounds of his once-narrowed arteries has shown a 36 percent improvement in circulation. No, he's not going to be surprised again. And neither should you.

"These tests are a way to know for sure," Bakke says. "With the information available now, I believe you can actually beat this thing."

Are You Eating Yourself to Death?

Across America, a skyrocketing number of young men are being stricken with diabetes—a disease that could leave them blind, impotent, disabled, or dead. The scary part: You may have it and not even know it

By Christopher McDougall

Depending on your nerve, John Buse, M.D., Ph.D., is either the first or the last guy you want to see coming toward you in a shopping mall. His specialty: the ultimate gut check.

With a crew cut topping his stocky frame, the 43-year-old Dr. Buse has the air of an army recruiter as he stands by his information table, intently scanning the streaming crowd for men who need his help. "I can look at a guy once and say, 'Hey, you look like you've got diabetes,'" says Dr. Buse. The tip-off is the belly, that bulging sack of fat lolling over an unassuming shopper's belt. Fat, especially belly fat, has been linked to an increasingly common and lethal form of diabetes, a disease that dumps toxic levels of sugar into the bloodstream. Dr. Buse, who heads the diabetes center at the University of North Carolina, spots more and more men carrying that dangerous chunk of fat these days. But as he travels through his home state, offering warnings, most men don't want to hear it. "They wave their hands and say, 'Whoa, no thanks! I don't want to know.'"

Such persistent denial is one reason diabetes rates have been soaring over the past decade. What those hand wavers don't realize is that diabetes's newest victims are not the elderly or the virally infected, as in the past, but men just like them, and maybe you—guys in their twenties, thirties, and forties who

ARE YOU BECOMING A DIABETIC?

Full-blown diabetes is easy to spot: frequent, uncontrollable urges to urinate; virtually unquenchable thirst; numbness in your hands and feet. But the symptoms leading up to the full-blown disease are easier to ignore. And ignorance isn't bliss; it's amputation—or death. Here are the top silent alarms.

You feel sleepy right after a meal. If your body gets flooded with sugar it can't process, it'll stage a sort of rolling blackout. It will pull energy from other systems to marshal the resources needed to pump out the extra sugar.

Your vision has become a little blurry. When too much sugar crowds into your blood-stream, it can cause the lenses in your eyes to stretch, resulting in blurred vision. Also, watch for headaches after reading or doing paperwork.

Your blood pressure is higher than usual. It's hard to tell which comes first, the diabetes or the high blood pressure. But it seems that even slightly higher than normal blood pressure levels are related to insulin resistance.

Your breath constantly smells like nail polish remover. Without enough insulin to turn carbohydrates into energy, your liver will begin to break down fat for fuel. "Acetone breath" is one by-product of fat combustion.

otherwise appear to be in perfect health. What they also don't comprehend are the frightening consequences diabetes can have if it isn't treated. Impotence. Blindness. Heart attack. Stroke. Amputation. Death.

Nervous yet?

"I was one of those guys," says Greg Barsh, a burly 38-year-old attorney and avid downhill skier from suburban Philadelphia. Last year, Barsh had his blood tested only because his father, a physician, kept nagging him about his weight. Barsh wasn't worried. He had been a jock most of his life, and though he'd gained 40 pounds since finishing law school and getting married, he still exercised and felt great. "I was always full of energy, and I thought I was eating okay," Barsh says. "I wasn't into sweets, so I ate a lot of fruit and yogurt. I'd eat, like, 15 tangerines at a time."

Barsh was so blasé that before his blood test, he stopped at a lunch truck parked outside the clinic and snacked on fruit salad and an egg roll. "I was still wiping my lips when I entered the hospital," Barsh recalls. When the doctor told him the results, he nearly fell off the stool. "I lit that test up like a Christmas tree. A minute ago, I'm feeling like a million bucks, and now they're reading me a death sentence." A blood sugar level greater than 125 is considered diabetic; two different tests put Barsh's above 250.

"The doctor said I'd have a heart attack within 5 to 10 years," Barsh says quietly. He has no family link to diabetes; he isn't a member of a high-risk ethnic group; he hadn't become prone to diabetes through viral infection.

At 5 foot 10 and 220 pounds, Greg Barsh was just slowly, unknowingly eating himself to death. That egg roll was probably the last one he'll ever touch.

"The increase in diabetes among younger people has been astounding and truly alarming," says Dr. Buse. "Over the past decade, we've seen a 70 percent increase among people in their thirties." If you look at a graph of diabetes rates in men, you'll see a slope that's frighteningly alpine—since 1990, the climb has been fast and unrelenting.

In 2002, the Centers for Disease Control and Prevention (CDC) in Atlanta found 7.8 million American men with diabetes.

Even more chilling is the fact that one-third of those with diabetes—roughly 2 million men—have yet to be diagnosed and don't know they're dying. Many men don't want to know, as Dr. Buse learned from his come-to-God missions in the malls. Others may simply believe they have no reason to worry. Misled by misconceptions about sports drinks, nutritional supplements, fruit juices, and fat-free foods, they may feel fine and be convinced they're eating right. "There's so much misinformation about what's healthy," says Dr. Buse, "that thousands of people are killing themselves and don't have a clue."

LIFE IN THE FAT LANE

There's never been a worse time and place for self-inflicted eating ailments than 21st-century America. Culture, cuisine, and technology have combined to make our lives more sedentary, our food more plentiful, and our opportunities to eat more frequent. The fact that one pizza franchise has in-

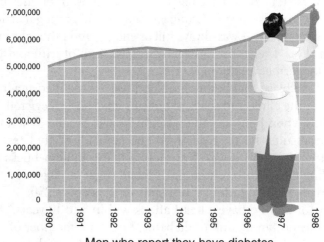

Men who report they have diabetes

YOUR NEEDLE-EXCHANGE PROGRAM

We'd like to report that a cure for diabetes is just around the corner. But we can't because it isn't. However, what is imminent is almost as good: a cure for a lifetime of insulin injections.

Cell replacement. PPL Therapeutics is working on converting immature cells, a.k.a. stem cells, into insulin-producing islet cells, which can be injected into diabetics. "Islet cells from organ donors can help type I diabetics get off insulin," says Robert Sherwin, M.D., president of the American Diabetes Association. "If stem cells can be converted into islet cells, we'll have enough to treat type 2 diabetics as well."

Gene therapy. Poking its head above all the human genome hype is a gene called SHIP2. Belgian researchers found that diabetic mice born without the SHIP2 gene were significantly more sensitive to insulin than those with the gene. "If we can turn SHIP2 off, we may be able to boost insulin sensitivity in type 2 diabetics," says

Stephane Schurmans, M.D., a coauthor of the study.

Inhalable insulin. Take a deep breath. Soon that's what it might feel like to give yourself insulin. When University of Vermont researchers gave type 2 diabetics powdered insulin to inhale, they discovered it was as effective as injectable insulin. "It may ultimately provide even better blood sugar control than injections," says William Cefalu, M.D., the study author. FDA testing is under way.

Alternative therapy. Deep in the Congo lies pseudomassaria, a fungus with the ability to lower blood sugar levels. "It activates receptors that make the insulin you have more effective," says Michael Pirrung, Ph.D., a Duke University chemist. Duke researchers have already found a way to reproduce the active compound in the lab. The next step: turn the compound into a pill.

vented a way to pack even more cheese into a pie by force filling the crust is all you need to know about America's *vive le fat* mentality.

Developers build suburbs without sidewalks, knowing that few of us bother to walk anywhere anymore. Our morning cup of joe is now likely to be a latte with a pint of milk. Our workweek has gotten longer, not only reducing exercise time but also screwing up our eating habits. Instead of regular, well-balanced meals, many of us wolf down fast food at our desks at odd times of day, using food as a way to stay awake or relieve the tedium of long hours behind the keyboard.

"Our lifestyle has changed dramatically over the past 100 years, but our genes haven't kept pace," says Mitchell Lazar, M.D., director of the University of Pennsylvania's diabetes center. Men were once hunter-gatherers, he explains, which meant they exhausted lots of calories in pursuit of food. Those humans with the "thrifty gene"—the capacity to store fat—were the ones who were able to survive the harsh, unpredictable search for food, and they passed on their low metabolisms to us.

But now that every street corner is well stocked with calories for sale, that fat-storage capability has become a liability. "It takes thousands of years for DNA to alter, but our food supply becomes more abundant by the year," Dr. Lazar explains. "Isn't it ironic? The low-metabolism adaptation, which allowed the human race to survive the lean years, is now contributing to this raging increase in diabetes."

Even "healthy" foods can be a problem when consumed in excess. We've convinced ourselves that if it's low fat and vitamin-packed, we have license to pig out. But as Barsh discovered, even tangerines contain calories, and 15 of them contain a lot of calories. And the calories you can't burn, you convert into fat cells that pad your gut a little more. You don't binge? You could still be piling on weight from eating healthful but extremely calorie-dense foods. "Juices are a big problem—16 ounces of juice equals five apples, and no one would think that eating five apples is less than gluttony," says Dr. Lazar. Same thing goes for those ubiquitous energy bars. "You can swallow 400 calories in 30 seconds," says Dr. Buse.

Another major misconception is that diabetes comes only from eating too much refined sugar, like the kind found in chocolate candy and ice cream. But it's more about a diet that's loaded with any high-carbohydrate foods that are easily converted into glucose—foods like bananas, orange juice, white bread, wine, and pasta. Fatty foods are also a problem, but for a different reason. Down one 20-ounce bottle of Coke and it will be processed and gone in an in-

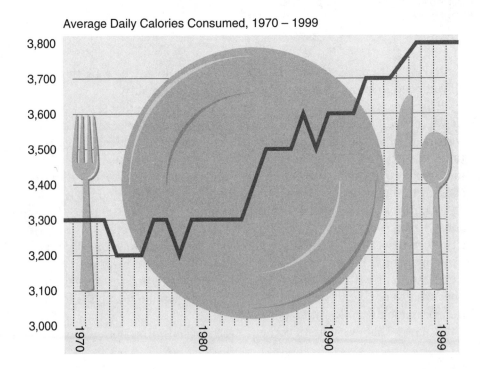

Average Daily Calories Consumed, 1970 – 1999

stant, but that chunk of fried mozzarella will keep oozing glucose into your arteries for quite a while. When you keep your blood sugar levels constantly elevated this way, you increase your risk of developing diabetes even if you aren't overweight.

Aggressive eating was certainly a problem for 26-year-old Neil Mowery. Last year Mowery, a former hockey player with the nose to prove it, was diagnosed with type 2 diabetes. "I was completely blown away when I found out," says Mowery. "I've always been thin, even when I was playing ice hockey in high school, so I'd lift weights five times a week and down 8,000 calories a day, trying to add muscle mass." But instead of helping him gain weight, the daily pasta binges flooded his bloodstream with glucose. "I'd make a family-size box of Tuna Helper and eat the whole thing myself, thinking it was good for me." Eventually, Mowery's body had had enough and hit him with chronic fatigue and sudden weight loss. When he finally went for testing, his blood sugar was 380.

HOW THINGS GO AWRY

Diabetes is actually an easy disease to understand. Basically, it's an interruption in the body's supply line of food. Here's how it works. Just about everything we eat is digested and turned into glucose, also called blood sugar. The glucose is then carried to the body's cells, where it's burned as fuel. One crucial element makes the entire process possible: insulin, a hormone secreted by the pancreas that allows glucose to penetrate the cell walls. "I like to think of insulin as the key that opens the door," explains Dr. Lazar. "You have all this glucose surging around in your blood. It wants to enter the muscles, but it needs to get through a receptor in the cell wall. The receptor is the lock; the insulin is the key. Once the insulin unlocks the receptor, the glucose can flow in."

Diabetes occurs when there's a breakdown in that glucose stream. It can happen two ways: First, the pancreas can malfunction and stop producing insulin. The cause is a virus that tricks your immune system into wiping out the cells that manufacture insulin. That's type 1 diabetes (formerly known as juvenile diabetes, when it was thought to show up only in children). In other cases, the pancreas produces plenty of insulin, but for some reason the insulin doesn't unlock the receptors, so the glucose can't flow in. That's type 2. It's the more common form, comprising 95 percent of all people with diabetes.

No one knows exactly how you develop type 2 diabetes, but Dr. Lazar's team at the University of Pennsylvania recently made an important discovery. In an animal study, they found that fat cells secrete a hormone called resistin. Resistin acts like rust in the lock, somehow jamming the works and preventing insulin from opening the receptors so glucose can surge into the cells. "The more fat cells there are, the more resistin there is and the greater the chance of diabetes," Dr. Lazar says. If Penn researchers are able to prove that this also happens in humans, they may be able to design a medicine that can counteract it.

Whether it's type 1 or type 2, the effects of diabetes are about the same: The body keeps converting food into glucose, but because the glucose can't enter the cells, it starts building up in the blood. Some is converted to fat; the rest turns toxic and throws off poisons that can destroy your heart, kidneys, and retinas. Your vision will get blurry, you'll have trouble breathing, and you'll get dehydrated as your body tries to urinate the sugar overload. You can drop into a coma, and you're very likely to die of a heart attack or stroke. Diabetes is the seventh leading cause of death in the United States, but it may take even more lives than the statistics show. "Eighty percent of diabetics will die of cardiovascular events," says Mark Schutta, M.D., the leader of a diabetes treatment team at the University of Pennsylvania Hospital. "But the heart at-

EVASIVE MANEUVERS

Getting diabetes is no accident; it's a head-on collision that we steer our lives straight into. Consider these five tips your defensive driving course.

Walk off your belly. The scientific name for your gut is *visceral fat*. And the scientific way to lose it? "Aerobic exercise, particularly walking, is one of the best ways to get rid of visceral fat," says Frank Hu, M.D., Ph.D., a Harvard University epidemiologist. In one study, Dr. Hu found that those who walked the fastest and longest had reductions in visceral fat that cut their risk of diabetes in half.

Eat the right carbs. Get to know the glycemic index, a measure of how quickly the carbohydrates in a particular food can be converted to glucose and released into the bloodstream. In a Harvard study, men who ate foods with the lowest indexes, like whole wheat bread, were 37 percent less likely to develop diabetes than those who ate high-index foods such as white rice. For a complete list of foods, go to www.glycemicindex.com.

Reach for a drink. Somewhere between blitzed and sober is a blood alcohol level that can help ward off diabetes. According to a study published in the *Archives of Internal Medicine*, light to moderate drinkers—three to six drinks a week—are 42 percent less likely to develop diabetes than those who drink more often than that or not at all. It's believed that alcohol may improve insulin sensitivity.

Take Pravastatin. Researchers at the University of Glasgow in Scotland analyzed the medical records of nearly 6,000 men and found that those taking the cholesterol-lowering drug Pravastatin had a 30 percent lower risk of diabetes than those not taking it. If you're already on a medication for your cholesterol, talk to your doctor about switching to Pravastatin.

Swallow 400 milligrams of E. In the alphabet soup of vitamins, E is the one that may prevent the big D. When Finnish researchers evaluated the diets of 944 men, they found that those with the highest vitamin E intake had a 22 percent lower risk of diabetes than men with the lowest intake. Vitamin E may also prevent the free radical damage that plays a role in the complications caused by diabetes.

tack is generally pegged as the cause of death, even though it was actually the diabetes that brought it on."

Meanwhile, as your blood is filling with rancid sugar, your glucose-deprived cells are starving. Up to 70 percent of diabetics suffer nerve damage, which can lead to amputations, blindness, and coma. While men and women develop the disease about equally, men suffer slightly harsher consequences: We're twice as likely as female diabetics to lose a foot or a leg (probably because men avoid the doctor and tend to be diagnosed later), and more than 20 percent of men with diabetes are left impotent—including 60 percent of those over the age of 50.

And in the case of type 2, the damage is largely self-inflicted. You can't do much to protect your pancreas and avoid type 1 diabetes, but as Greg Barsh and Neil Mowery learned the hard way, type 2 is primarily a matter of diet. Granted, some people face a higher risk than others—if you're over 45, for instance, or related to a diabetic, you're more vulnerable. Also, Blacks, Latinos, and Native Americans are more prone to diabetes than Caucasians. But for most diabetes sufferers, it's simply a matter of what they put into their mouths, combined with a genetic predisposition to store fat. That paunch Dr. Buse is so obsessed with? It's the first sign that sustainable fat is becoming dangerous. When it's spread around the body, fat is less damaging; but when it sags into the belly, look out.

"With obesity on the rise, we can expect diabetes rates to increase sharply," warns Jeffrey Koplan, M.D., director of the CDC. "If these dangerous trends continue at the current rates, the impact on our nation's health and medical costs in future years will be overwhelming."

LOOKS CAN BE DECEIVING

If you think of yourself as lean, don't feel smug just yet. You might be in for the same shock I got when I called Steven Heymsfield, M.D., an obesity expert at Columbia University College of Physicians and Surgeons. I'm a marathon runner and a big consumer of fish and vegetables, and though I've expanded to a 38-inch waist from my usual 36 (double lattes, Guinness Stout, and giant Nestlé's Crunch bars are weaknesses), I still run or lift weights five times a week. I could lose a little, sure, but I'm reasonably trim. Right?

"No, you're actually 1 pound overweight," Dr. Heymsfield told me. "At 6 feet 4 inches, you should weigh 172 pounds on the low end and 205 on the high end." My 206 pounds suddenly thrust me into a completely different social group, one I'd always felt a whole lot skinnier than. He tried to console me. "Don't worry. I see men in the clinic every day who are astounded to hear they're badly overweight." While I'm not in that extreme category, Dr. Heymsfield says we can no longer trust our own eyes when it comes to evaluating our bodies. How can we accurately gauge who's chubby and who's not when 59 percent of American men are overweight? You may be lean compared with more than half the men around you, yet still be way over your recommended weight.

The only true measure, believes Dr. Heymsfield, is the body mass index, or BMI. A BMI of 25 to 29 is overweight, while 30 and up is obese. So if you think you're trim, consider these numbers.

- At 5 foot 7 and 185 pounds, you have a BMI of 29—definitely overweight, and right on the border of obesity.
- If you're 6 feet and 185 pounds, your BMI is 25—overweight.
- At 5 foot 6 and 175 pounds, you have a BMI of 28, and only 11 pounds to go before crossing from chubby to obese. (You can calculate your exact BMI by dividing your weight in pounds by your height in inches. Then divide the result again by your height in inches and multiply that number by 703.)

Even tall, thin guys can be overweight; Dr. Heymsfield talks about "skinny fat" men who may look lean but actually have an unhealthy amount of fat layered over stringy muscle and bone. These men may have dangerously high glucose levels, which they never think to have checked because their deceptive body shape masks the problem. "The ironic thing is, they're probably being encouraged all the time to eat more!" says Dr. Heymsfield.

Athletes are also at risk. Diabetes specialists find that many men who work out regularly think a little sweat turns their bodies into all-purpose incinerators, capable of cleansing their systems of whatever fried, fermented, or honey-glazed calorie bombs they choose to swallow.

The truth: Exercise may prevent all that glucose from being turned into fat, but your blood sugar levels may still be too high. Take Les Strayhorn, a former Dallas Cowboys running back who's one of Dr. Buse's patients. "Les was 30 years old when he had to retire because of a knee injury," Dr. Buse says. "He goes back to graduate school, and after a few months he starts complaining of fatigue. He can't figure out why on earth he feels more tired now than when he was playing." Turns out Strayhorn's blood sugar measured 400. Without help, he might have lost a limb or worse.

"This guy subscribed to the American gospel of a football player's diet," Dr. Buse says. "His whole life, he'd been eating processed carbohydrates like pasta and bread, and drinking gallons of juice instead of eating fruit." When you add the straight sugar jolt from the maple syrup on his pancakes and the high-fructose corn syrup in his sports drinks, Strayhorn was swallowing a massive glucose infusion each day.

Another of Dr. Buse's patients, a middle school football player, made the

PERCENTAGE INCREASE
IN YOUR RISK OF DIABETES IF YOU
WATCH 20 OR MORE HOURS OF TV A WEEK: **73**

same mistakes. "This kid is 6 foot 4 and 250 pounds and was already being eyed by high school coaches," Dr. Buse says. "His brother is a scholarship player at college, and the two of them work out together in the summer, trying to beef him up." The training diet of the 13-year-old boy consisted of huge amounts of milk and processed carbs. At his team physical, the doctor diagnosed him with type 2 diabetes.

"He's lucky," says Dr. Buse. "I've seen people in their mid-twenties who've lost both legs and their eyesight because they caught it too late."

DEFEATING THE BIG D

Once diagnosed, diabetes is fairly simple to treat. The frontline sugar-lowering strategy is threefold: lose weight, exercise more frequently, and eat meals that won't dilute your blood with too much glucose. Often this is all the treatment needed.

If not, the next step is "diabetes pills." They come in three classes: those that stimulate the beta cells in your pancreas to release more insulin, those that make your body more sensitive to the insulin you already have, and those designed to slow the conversion of carbohydrates into glucose. While they're easy to take, diabetes pills aren't always effective and can have side effects; some patients have reported diarrhea, hypoglycemia (blood sugar that's too low), and even liver damage.

If the pills fail, or if your blood sugar is stratospheric right from the start, you'll have to resort to insulin shots. Most type 2 diabetics who need shots get by with just one injection a day, but some need as many as three.

Still, anyone who doubts he can not only control his diabetes but also lead a vigorous, healthy life just needs to consider Joe Largay. On the surface, you see an extremely fit 41-year-old with surfer-blond hair and a lean, almost bony face. What you don't see is the type 1 diabetes lurking underneath. In some ways, type 1 is even more difficult to manage than type 2, but Largay sees the disease as a life reformer rather than a handicap.

"There's an old saying: If you want to be healthy, contract a chronic disease," Largay says. Fifteen years ago, when he was a young competitive cyclist, Largay's normally reliable body began to develop odd problems. He was always thirsty, he was constantly urinating, and he was having more and more trouble recovering from his workouts. Doctors told him his pancreas had shut down. Largay had virtually no insulin circulating in his blood and an astounding blood sugar level of 600.

Many newly diagnosed diabetics refuse to accept the news, or they sink into depression. Largay had a different reaction. "Beating the disease was another goal to reach, another hill to go over," he says. For solidarity, he banded together with three other type 1 diabetics and formed a bike racing team. "We think of our diabetes as a positive force in our lives," Largay says. "It has made us keenly aware of our bodies and has almost never gotten in the way of performance." Last year Largay's team finished seventh out of 40 teams in a U.S. Cycling Federation 24-hour mountain bike relay.

"There is good news, but it's for people who catch their diabetes early," says Dr. Schutta. "Ninety percent of type 2 diabetics can be treated with pills. And if you catch it early enough, you can treat it with just diet and exercise."

Neil Mowery, the ex–hockey player, sticks to a diet rich in vegetables and lean proteins and manages to keep his blood sugar low. He still lifts weights five times a week, and he says he's never felt better in his life. Same with Greg Barsh: He lost 70 pounds in 6 months while still allowing himself the occasional platter of ribs or corned beef special. "It's easy," says Barsh. "I just look at my son and imagine him growing up without a father."

Barsh has also become a diabetes evangelist. "After hearing my story, the guy I fish with in Florida got so scared he's already lost 35 pounds," he says. "But don't get me wrong; I'm not the kind of guy who tries to turn people over to a healthy life—I went to grad school in New Orleans, for God's sake. It's just that sometimes you can use your own near-death experience to get people's heads out of the sand."

Not Just Your Father's Cancer

You're young, you're healthy, you don't think about prostate cancer. Neither did this guy

By Gil Gaul

This is how it begins: in the pale blue haze of an early November morning, the phone rings as I'm heading out the door to work. It's my family doctor, Tom Hanley, M.D., a good, caring soul in an increasingly brutalized profession. The results of my blood work are back, he says. The cholesterol looks good, but there is this one thing. My PSA is slightly elevated.

PSA . . . PSA . . . PSA . . . I rummage through my memory banks. Doesn't that have something to do with old men, cancer?

"It's probably nothing to worry about," Dr. Hanley says. "But I want you to see a urologist. You don't want to end up like Frank Zappa or Jimmy V."

"Sure," I say, a little dazed and on automatic pilot. "Let's set something up."

After he hangs up, I call my wife, Cathy, at her job. "What did Frank Zappa die of?" I ask.

It turns out Zappa died of prostate cancer in December 1993, just shy of his 53rd birthday. I wasn't paying attention at the time. Like most middle-age men, I had no reason to, or so I thought.

Survivor Story #1
NORMAN SCHWARZKOPF, GULF WAR HERO

"If you've been getting checkups on a regular basis and they find it early, then all it is, literally, is a temporary pain in the ass. So don't be an idiot—go in and get a checkup. None of us enjoy the digital rectal examination—or I should say *most* of us don't enjoy it—but if you've got half a brain in your head, you'll make a point of asking for one. You know, 31,000 men will die of prostate cancer this year . . . but no one should die of it. Because it's detectable and curable."

Jimmy Valvano, the hyperactive basketball coach at North Carolina State, died of cancer the same year. His case is more complicated. The source of Valvano's cancer was never identified. But some of the complications—severe back pain and a rapid spread of the cancer to his bones—resemble advanced forms of many cancers, including prostate.

It is the fall of 1999. I am 48 years old. A father. A husband. My back aches.

A week after Dr. Hanley's phone call, I find myself in the waiting room of a local urology practice, surrounded by shuffling old men and their wives, my head filled with voices and ghosts. I clutch a copy of my blood work in both hands like an immigrant holding his papers to the New World, the world of the ill.

The papers say my PSA—or prostate-specific antigen, which measures traces of cancer in the blood—is 5.4. That's a relatively low level, but still not good.

A doctor I have never met before, Michael R. Bernstein, tall, young, with a bemused smile, quizzes me on my voiding practices. How many times do I get up at night? How often do I go during the day? Any bothersome symptoms when I void? Do I ever have accidents?

Accidents?

Wet yourself.

Never, I reply. But I do go to the bathroom a lot. Then again, I always have gone to the bathroom a lot. I attribute this to a small bladder and multiple Diet Pepsis.

Dr. Bernstein nods. Later, he'll write:

The patient is a 48-year-old white male with a history of abnormal PSA. He has occasional nocturia; however, he denies any bothersome voiding symptoms. Specifically, he denies any frequency, urgency, or urinary incontinence.

Urologists are the plumbers of medicine. They ply their trade in dark, hard-to-get-to corners, clean out drains, patch holes. In the prostate exam, a doctor jams a finger up the rectum and roots around, checking the size of the prostate gland, whether it's tender or hard, and whether there are any telltale nodules hinting of cancer.

Dr. Bernstein reports that I seem fine, but he wants me to come back for a biopsy. Protocol, he says. You're probably fine.

It's difficult to say what I'm feeling. Fear. Confusion. A little anger on the side. I don't feel ill, other than the bad back that sent me to the doctor. Yet I may have cancer—prostate cancer. How can this be? I'm too young. I'm not ready. I want to go back and start over. But it doesn't work that way.

I struggle with this notion for days. Both of my parents died young, although not of cancer. As far as I know, there is no history of cancer in our genes. A thought flares that I am doomed, unlucky, that I won't live long enough to see our boys—now 19 and 14—become men. I feel guilty. How could I be so selfish? Isn't an illness, with all of its consuming needs and irrational fears, the ultimate expression of selfishness?

As usual, my wife comes to the rescue. I'm getting ahead of myself, Cathy says. She convinces me to have another PSA—a more sensitive version of the test, intended to distinguish prostate cancer from benign disease. She has been reading up on prostate cancer, and to me her logic is irrefutable. Why undergo an invasive biopsy when the first PSA might have been a false positive? My doctor resists at first, but he ultimately agrees to have the blood work done: My PSA is 3.7, down from 5.4. But the percentage of so-called free PSA, the more sensitive measure, is 23.5. In this instance, the higher the percentage of free PSA, the better. Mine is relatively high, but not high enough. Below 25 percent, biopsy is recommended.

THE WAIT

My biopsy is performed in early December, in the same urology office. A technician with a portable ultrasound machine sets up shop in the examining room. A different doctor, one who specializes in prostate biopsies, introduces himself. He asks me to slide back on the table, spread my legs. He holds an in-

Survivor Story #2
MICHAEL MILKEN, FOUNDER OF CAP CURE, A PROSTATE CANCER ORGANIZATION

"My good friend Steve Ross, head of Time-Warner, had just lost his battle with prostate cancer, so I decided to ask for a PSA test during a physical. 'You're too young,' my doctor said. 'Humor me,' I replied. A second PSA and a biopsy confirmed that cancer had spread beyond my prostate to the lymph nodes. I was given 12 to 18 months to live. After lying down for 24 hours to get over the shock, I moved into action to fight back against the disease."

Survivor Story #3
BOB DOLE, FORMER U.S. SENATOR

"The highlight for me was having the catheter taken out . . . and finding out I wasn't incontinent. They send you home with these pads and tell you you can get more at the drugstore. I think I took home 30 or 40, but I needed only three or four. I was lucky—some guys have to endure incontinence for years, or for the rest of their lives."

strument that looks vaguely like an electric hair curler, with a needle and a tiny camera.

Try to relax.

This sort of thing happens to women all the time, and we shrug off their complaints. I understand now. The cruelties of medicine, thrusting and probing in one's most sensitive corners. The abandonment of all sense of ownership of one's body. The pretenses to dignity.

The doctor informs me that he plans to take a half dozen or so samples, angling around the prostate, which is roughly the size of a walnut. I should feel a little jab, he says, but it shouldn't be very painful. Earlier, I was offered a Valium, but I turned it down. I want to have a clear head, to understand what they're doing to me.

I lose count after the first few samples. Having the instrument inserted into me isn't the problem. I barely feel it. But there is something I can only describe as an aftershock, which jars my insides and leaves me breathless each time a sample is taken. In the end, I'm holding my breath, anticipating each next shock, slightly nauseated. Finished, the doctor congratulates me on how well I did and sticks a dressing up my bum to collect leftover blood. I shuffle back out to the lobby, suddenly feeling very old.

Another week passes slowly by. Time seems to expand around this curve of uncertainty, lengthening my days. I wake up and want to curl back up in bed. Work—I'm a reporter—is suddenly hard. I find myself drifting, unfocused. I startle when the telephone rings, and barely hear what others say. My normal passion for research, details, complex issues, has vanished. I'm shutting down emotionally, looking for an escape hatch, a way up to air, light.

In a vacuum, the calculus of disease is exponential. Every ache and pain is magnified, takes on new meaning. I imagine the worst and then quickly talk myself out of it. All of my life, I've been healthy. A champion javelin thrower in high school. A scholarship athlete in college. Later, a sub-3-hour marathon runner. I've watched my weight, eaten lots of fruit, avoided McDonald's. That has to be worth something.

Illness took me by surprise. I wasn't prepared for it. For the first time in my life, I feel fragile. Vulnerable. Mortal.

At last, the results arrive.

Of a half dozen tissue samples, four are clean, one is characterized as suspicious, and one, taken from the right base of my prostate, is cancerous, with a diagnosis of adenocarcinoma, a malignant tumor in a secretory gland. The good news is that only 2 percent of the tissue in that sample is deemed cancerous. It's given a Gleason score—a classification of the grade of cancer—of six, an average grade. The higher the score and number of positive cores, the more likely the cancer has spread outside the prostate wall.

In truth, I'm one of the lucky ones. The PSA test appears to have picked up the cancer in its early stages, before it could spread into my lymph nodes— exactly the argument for using the test more routinely, especially with younger men, when there's still time to save their lives.

Still, I'm not off the hook. I have cancer.

PLAN OF ACTION

The next few weeks are spent doing more research, learning the vocabulary of cancer, consulting with doctors, having my biopsy slides read by other pathology experts to confirm the diagnosis.

I've already decided on surgery. It seems like the safest bet for someone my age with my diagnosis.

My wife and I make contact with many former prostate patients by phone or online. Some of what I read frightens me. It seems that only men with problems—especially men whose cancers have come back—write in. I'm not ready emotionally to handle bad news, and I back off. I need to maintain the illusion that everything is going to be fine.

One suggestion I embrace is to find a doctor and a hospital specializing in prostate cancer. With my HMO's blessing, I travel to Johns Hopkins for a consultation with Jacek Mostwin, M.D., a urologist experienced in prostate surgery. After studying my lab work and examining me, Dr. Mostwin reassures me that I have a small tumor and am an ideal candidate for treatment. He explains how the surgery—known as radical retropubic prostatectomy—works. An incision is made in the abdomen. The surgeon then cuts through the urethra and separates the prostate gland from all of the tissue, blood vessels, and nerves that are connected to it. The prostate—and hopefully the cancer—is removed, while the wafer-thin nerves that sit on either side of the prostate, and are essential for an erection, are preserved.

The complications include short-term incontinence and impotence. But most men my age with small tumors do fine, Dr. Mostwin says. By 3 months, patients are usually dry. By 6 months, they're starting to have spontaneous erections.

Right, I'm thinking. Let's cut the sucker out and get on with life. But Johns Hopkins is much in demand, a place where sheikhs and other luminaries come to have their prostates removed or bombarded with radiation. Dr. Mostwin alone has operated on nearly 1,000 men. He checks his handheld Palm and informs me that the earliest he can get me on his schedule is in 7 weeks. Seven weeks! That seems like forever to a man who has made up his mind.

GOING UNDER THE KNIFE

The weeks drag by. Logically, I know I'm going to be okay. But there are moments, especially when my back is aching, when I'm far less sure of myself. It's interesting how illness—or even the threat of illness—does that. I've always thought of myself as a strong person. Now I am full of doubts. I have trouble making decisions, hesitate, second-guess myself.

I have my surgery on March 27, 2000. Coming up from the anesthesia, I hear the doctors who are stapling me back up debating the merits of *Who Wants to Be a Millionaire. I don't think the questions are very smart.* Thud. *I don't know. Some of them are tricky.* Thud. *Tricky, sure. But that's not the same thing as smart.* Thud.

Guys, I want to shout, please, this is me you're stapling back together. Enough with the television talk. But I can't. I'm numb, mute, floating around the room like a cloud in a Magritte painting. Then one of the doctors announces the time: 54 minutes. That doesn't seem possible either.

In the waiting area, Dr. Mostwin informs Cathy that everything went smoothly (2 days later the pathology report confirms that the cancer was confined to the organ). He tells Cathy that I had the largest prostate he has ever seen for a man my age. Not inflamed or cancerous, just large. That's nice, I say back in my room. Do I get bonus points for a big prostate? Can I add them to my frequent-flier miles?

I'm up and shuffling the next day. The hall is crawling with guys just like me, some young, some old. We form a shambling group, attached to our IV poles, holding our catheter bags, slogging up and down the hall in slow mo-

AMONG 1,000 MEN SURVEYED, PERCENTAGE WHO WEREN'T SURE WHO (MEN, WOMEN, OR BOTH) HAS A PROSTATE: **32**

PERCENTAGE OF MEN SURVEYED WHO HAVE NEVER SPOKEN TO A DOCTOR ABOUT PROSTATE CANCER: **57**

PERCENTAGE WHO SAY THEY'VE NEVER HEARD OF THE PSA TEST, DESPITE THE FACT THAT IT'S THE BEST METHOD CURRENTLY AVAILABLE FOR EARLY DETECTION: **76**

Survivor Story #4
RICHARD PETTY, FORMER NASCAR CHAMPION

"You know what? Even though I've got 200 NASCAR Winston Cup Series wins and I won seven NASCAR series championships, none of it compares with going back to my doctor for my regular follow-up PSA test and getting the all-clear sign again."

tion. There are no passing lanes here. No testosterone-laden road rage. No frat-boy good cheer. Everyone obeys the speed limit and keeps to the right. Smiles are grim and tight.

LIFE AFTER SURGERY

I leave Hopkins on a beautiful spring day. The sky is Windex blue. The magnolias are blooming. I've gotten through the hardest part. Now to get on with life.

The first few weeks pass slowly and with their own peculiar rhythm. I get up, empty my catheter bag, eat a little, read the paper, rest, take short walks, rest, eat, sleep. For someone used to being so active, it's hard slamming on the brakes like this.

The catheter is the worst. It's uncomfortable, it's awkward, it gets in the way. Occasionally the line snags, sending a backwash of urine into my penis. That grabs my attention. The catheter bag is like a small dog that won't leave my side. I tape it to my calf when I need to walk. When it's hot and I'm in shorts, I carry it in a tote bag, as if I'm on my way back from the library.

About a month after my surgery, it's disclosed that Rudy Giuliani has prostate cancer and is considering whether to drop out of his Senate race against Hillary Clinton. Even if the mayor opts for surgery, the *New York Times* reports, he could be back on the campaign trail in 3 weeks. I'm a little more than 1 month out and can't imagine myself running to the bathroom, let alone for the Senate.

It seems that prostate cancer is taking on celebrity status. Wasn't that what Bob Dole had? There's a tendency to reduce it to a few sound bites: Oh, sure, it's bad. But they can yank it out and a few weeks or months later, you're back on your feet. What gets lost—as is true with other public diseases—is the array of subtleties that make the disease what it is: unpredictable, chronic, hard.

I leak heavily for 3 months and have to use three or four pads a day to stay dry. For the most part, it's more annoying than uncomfortable, more depressing than painful. Only once do I have an accident: I'm waiting to interview someone at city hall. I sit on a hard wooden bench in the hallway outside the office. Ten, maybe 15, minutes go by. When I get up, the rear of my pants is soaked; the bench is wet. Mortified, I slip my briefcase behind me, holding it there with two hands, and walk quickly back to the office, where I've stashed a spare pair of pants.

Four, 5, 6 months pass and I'm still leaking, especially when I do anything stressful, such as bend, lift, or walk quickly. I have to hire a lawn crew to cut the grass—in my twisted mind, a crushing defeat. Fall rolls around and I'm still dribbling. I'm reduced to using a leaf blower instead of a rake. Winter. Forget about shoveling snow. Spring, and the anniversary of my surgery, I'm still wearing one pad. I can tell Dr. Mostwin is a little disappointed when we talk. You're doing well, he reassures me, but it could take up to 2 years before you dry up.

Two years? This is news. Some men take longer, Dr. Mostwin says. You're doing well.

I try. Some days are hard. I sulk: Why me? But that only gets me so far. I remind myself that I'm not the only man leaking a year after surgery. I see the postings on the Internet. Besides, I could be a lot worse off. I could be leaking heavily, having accidents. I could still have cancer. To date, I've had three blood tests, the most recent on the anniversary of my surgery, and all have been negative.

RISING TO THE OCCASION

I am doing better on the potency issue. A little more than a month after surgery, I experience a tingling sensation similar to an orgasm. Whoa, what is that? I blurt. It's you, silly, Cathy says. Me? Really? My penis is slightly swollen, but hardly what I would call erect. Still, there's feeling. A good thing.

There's no delicate way around this. Prostate surgery changes everything. You aren't as hard. You aren't as large. It takes a little getting used to—and a sense of humor.

As the months pass, my erections grow, though I still haven't returned to where I was, and expect I never will. I would characterize my erections as serviceable—a flag at half-mast, versus a flag blowing stiffly in the breeze. I use something called a vacuum erectile device to get me going. I insert my penis into a plastic tube, and pump to create a vacuum; blood flows into my penis, resulting in an erection. I then slide a soft rubber ring around the base to hold the erection. It's not exactly spontaneous. But Cathy and I are happy enough. Besides allowing me to enjoy sex, the pump exercises the muscle and floods the traumatized nerves with blood, helping to rehabilitate them.

**PERCENTAGE OF PROSTATE
CANCER CASES MISSED BY TISSUE BIOPSY ALONE:** 14

TO BE SCREENED OR NOT TO BE

For years, prostate cancer was an old man's disease—an obstacle your aging dad had to deal with as he began collecting social security checks. But in the last dozen years, the face of the ailment has grown significantly younger.

Why? Credit more aggressive screening. Thanks to the development of the PSA blood test and heightened awareness, tumors are being identified—and treated—in younger men than ever before.

So this is a good thing, right? Identify cancer early and you have a better chance of beating it? Instinct might say yes, but the medical community remains split on the issue. While the American Cancer Society recommends that doctors offer prostate screenings beginning at age 50, other medical organizations, including the National Cancer Institute, oppose routine testing.

Their concern: So far, no study has proved that identifying prostate cancer early helps a patient live longer (most prostate tumors are slow growing and can take decades to make you ill). What's more, skeptics say, screening can be harmful as it leads many men to be treated for small, slow-growing tumors that would never have hurt them. Since treatment can cause impotence and temporary incontinence, the cure may end up being worse than the disease.

Advocates of screening admit that not every man who has a positive biopsy and gets his prostate removed would have had his life shortened by cancer. But, they argue, some would—and so the only way to protect yourself is to catch the disease early through screening.

Our take: While we understand screening's downside, we'd rather not gamble on prostate cancer. Follow the ACS guidelines and begin screening when you turn 50 (45 if you're African-American or have a family history). But talk to your doctor beforehand about what the results might mean and what your options will be.

Viagra, the ludicrously expensive little blue pill, also helps with erections, though it isn't perfect. I first try Viagra at around 7 months. It doesn't work very well for me; I am only slightly larger. Later on, I use Viagra in combination with the pump, and, other than a headache the next morning, it works like a charm. I'm bigger and able to hold the erection significantly longer. Next time, I use half a pill without the pump and it works fine—plus no headache.

One good side effect is that my orgasms are more intense than before. They seem to come in waves and last longer. Why this is, I can't say. I suspect it's the result of moving the nerve bundles during surgery. Whatever the explanation, I am thankful.

I can even see this becoming a fad. Men will have their prostates removed in order to enhance their sexual experience. It will be viewed as another form of cosmetic surgery. Today on Maury: Men without prostates and their lovers! Yeah, baby.

Some men writing on the prostate sites seem depressed by all the changes. I suspect they're men whose lives before surgery were intimately tied to having sex. The changes to their equipment are crushing. They're forced to adapt, reinvent themselves, redefine their sense of manhood.

Truth be told, it is pretty damn depressing. But what choice do you have? You can lose the cancer and suffer a little, or stick with the cancer and die. It's okay to mourn the loss of your true self. But it's also important to move ahead. I've opted to try to laugh. So I leak a little. Big deal. Oops. Okay, I'm not as big as before. Get over it.

Think of the upside: I've learned how to shop in the women's aisle of the supermarket. Ah, Kotex is on sale this week.

Okay, it's a joke.

Here's another: Around my house we've taken to referring to my prostate as the Prostate Formerly Known as Gil. It's a Prince thing. Maybe you have to be there.

The way I look at it, something bad happened to me. I can't explain it. I had no genetic history and lived a healthy life. For some reason, it was my turn. Now I have to deal with it. I have my life and some relatively minor inconveniences.

I don't think of myself as a survivor. I reserve that lofty term for men and women who have endured far more than a leaky valve and a limp penis.

Someday, maybe a few months from now, maybe a year, I'll be doing better than I am now. I can live with that.

Wake-Up Call

Last night, 10 million men fought for breath and lost their struggle for a good night's sleep. Today their jobs, maybe even their lives, are in jeopardy

By Donovan Webster

Each morning at 8 o'clock, they begin to arrive. As the doors open, a fresh human tide—mostly men—shuffles into the clinic of Steven Koenig, M.D., a pulmonologist specializing in sleep disorders at University of Virginia (UVA) medical center.

Some of the men are in Dr. Koenig's office at the request of their wives or bedmates. Others are here on referrals from their physicians. All of them share one thing: They have a potentially life-threatening health condition even they have trouble describing since it affects them only when they're deeply asleep. It's called sleep apnea, and it means that every night after they doze off, they go through regular periods in which they completely stop breathing.

Dr. Koenig, a tall, sandy-haired man in his forties with the firm but friendly manner of a seasoned airline pilot, is a national authority on sleep apnea. He leads me into an examination room where his first patient of the day, Jack, a 40-something man of average height and weight, is sitting. Jack's wife, Linda—thin and fit, her graying brown hair cut short—balances on a stool nearby. Jack, a hospital records administrator, is dressed comfortably in a navy blue wool sweater and khakis, and he appears barely awake. As he sits, his upper body weaves back and forth like a reed in a light breeze. He has shaggy gray hair, and his eyes—sunken deep inside dark circles—are three-quarters shut. He has what Dr. Koenig will later call "sleep drunkenness."

"Good morning," Dr. Koenig says. "So, how are you doing?"

Jack rouses a little. It takes him a moment to gain his composure. Apparently, he was conked out when we walked in.

"Ah . . . it's getting progressively worse since I saw you last summer," Jack says. His speech is slow and slurred. "Now I never fully wake up. It's like I've crossed below some threshold . . . and I'm always more asleep than awake. I fall asleep in elevators . . . wake up to find myself leaning against a wall, having missed my floor completely. I fight to stay awake at work. When I come home each night, I fall asleep. If nobody wakes me, I'll sleep until the next morning. . . . I sleep all weekend."

Linda is nodding.

"After you sleep a long time," Dr. Koenig asks, "do you wake up feeling alert and rested?"

Jack shakes his head. "No. Never."

Dr. Koenig pauses. "Have you fallen asleep while driving yet?"

Linda shivers. "Oh, God, please don't say *yet*."

In the cool antiseptic white of the examination room, Dr. Koenig looks soberly at Jack and Linda. "I'm afraid falling asleep while driving is next," he says. "I think, Jack, you're at the point where you shouldn't drive by yourself anymore."

CAN YOU REST EASY?

Sleep apnea can affect anyone, but men age 40 or older, with a neck size 17 inches or larger, are at particular risk. Here are six signs you may have the condition.

- You snore.

- You have high blood pressure.

- You experience night or morning headaches.

- You occasionally wake gasping for air.

- You fall asleep during the day.

- You sleep 8 or more hours and still feel sleepy.

If three or more of these symptoms apply to you, go to www.absm.org/Diplomates/listing.htm to find a doctor in your area who's board-certified in sleep medicine.

A KING-SIZE PROBLEM

Jack's case may be severe, but in a way he is lucky—and not just because he hasn't nodded off going 75 miles an hour on the interstate. It's estimated that at least 10 million men suffer from sleep apnea, but only 18 percent (Jack among them) have been diagnosed as having the condition. The rest? Perpetually tired guys who, at this very moment, are pushing through their days unaware that they're being suffocated at night.

"That's the biggest problem with this disease," says Daniel Loube, M.D., a sleep researcher and spokesman for the American Sleep Apnea Association. "Because you're sleeping when you exhibit symptoms, many people don't believe there's anything wrong. So it's hard to get them to a doctor."

Unlike snoring, which vibrates but doesn't close a sleeper's airway, sleep apnea is defined by the complete or near-complete cessation of respiration for a minimum of 10 seconds an episode. Depending on the severity of the apnea (a Greek word meaning "want of breath"), these miniasphyxiations can occur between 20 and 90 times an hour. When oxygen starvation becomes critical, sleepers briefly awaken with a snort and a second or two of air-starved choking. Unfortunately, these arousals are just long enough to prevent sufferers from getting the deep, restorative sleep they need, but too short for them to recall the following morning.

In the majority of cases, untreated sleep apnea manifests itself in lowered energy, compromised memory, depression, and sometimes headaches (which arise from the high levels of carbon dioxide in the bloodstream). Worse, it's estimated that as many as one-third of men with sleep apnea suffer from erectile dysfunction.

But it's not just the quality of a man's life that's affected. Research also indicates that untreated sleep apnea gives a person twice the risk of cardiac arrhythmias, four times the risk of congestive heart failure, and an eight-times-greater risk of stroke. "There are a lot of long-term health dangers," says Meir Kryger, M.D., a sleep specialist at the University of Manitoba. "That overnight behavior—deep sleeping and waking up with a jolt—places a lot of stress on your blood pressure, venous system, and heart muscle. That constant reactivation of your nervous system, well, it's just very hard on a body. Night after night, apnea takes its toll."

Of course, you can avoid all the cardiovascular consequences of sleep apnea and still end up dying of the condition. A recent Canadian study found that untreated sufferers of sleep apnea are three times more likely to have a car accident than those without the disorder. In fact, the link between sleep apnea and motor vehicle collisions is so strong that California legislators passed a law requiring doctors to give their local health officer the names of sleep apnea patients who nod off while driving. The health officer must then report the patients to the state department of motor vehicles for possible license suspension.

SLEEPWALKING

Bill, an otherwise healthy 50-year-old sales and marketing executive, began seeing Dr. Koenig 3 years ago. An umpire for youth and adult league baseball in his spare time, the 6-foot-2-inch, 185-pound father of three had been feeling his daytime consciousness slipping away.

"I'd be in meetings or behind the wheel of my car—especially in the afternoons—and I would be overcome with drowsiness," he says.

It was his wife's early-morning observations that finally convinced him to seek medical help. "I always thought, No, she's just sensitive," he recalls. "After all, she hears rain in the downspouts and it keeps her awake. But when she began to tell me I was stopping breathing . . ."

After a meeting to assess Bill's history and symptoms, Dr. Koenig referred him to the sleep study center at UVA medical center. Located just 5 minutes from Dr. Koenig's office, behind padded, soundproof double doors, the center is outfitted with banks of computers and four well-appointed bedrooms. In each there's a bed, comfortable chair, and television. In fact, except for the wires and plugs that hook into the control box by the bed, they look much like standard hotel rooms.

Once Bill had made himself comfortable in the bed, technicians began wiring him for observation. Sensors were taped around his skull for elec-

THREE NEW BED PARTNERS

The last big sleep apnea breakthrough came in 1979 with the invention of the CPAP machine. Here's what researchers have been doing for the past 23 years.

Vestibular-in-line Pressure System (VIPS). This strapless butterfly-shaped mouth-piece is designed to replace the CPAP's standard nasal mask. In a study at Western Pennsylvania Hospital in Pittsburgh, patients using VIPS reported none of the claustrophobia, air leaks, or nasal congestion felt by those wearing the nasal mask. "In preliminary tests it's been shown to be just as effective as the nasal mask," says Lewis Kline, M.D., one of the study authors. VIPS is available by prescription.

Hypoglossal nerve stimulation. Feel that stringy piece of flesh underneath your tongue? It's called the genioglossus muscle, and Johns Hopkins University researchers found that hitting it with painless zaps of electricity reduced apnea episodes by as much as 50 percent. "The stimulation moves the tongue forward and prevents it from blocking the throat," says Alan R. Schwartz, M.D., the lead researcher. A home unit is expected to be available within 5 years.

Serotonin antagonists. University of Illinois researchers are testing medications that will control a person's tongue and throat muscles at night so they don't relax and block the airway. So far serotonin antagonists, drugs that target the nerves that direct those muscles, look the most promising. Human trials are currently under way.

troencephalogram (EEG) brain wave monitoring and on his eyelids for electro-oculogram (EOG) readings, which measure the patient's levels of rapid eye movement (REM) sleep. He was also fitted with an electromyogram (EMG) sensor on his chin to measure muscle movement—a sign of how deep a level of sleep is being achieved—and small sensors above his upper lip to record mouth- and nose-breathing rates. Finally, a pulse oximeter was attached to his finger to record the amount of oxygen being exchanged with each breath.

Just minutes after the minimum 90 minutes of monitoring, technicians determined that Bill was having 32 apnea events an hour. They woke him with the results. "It didn't take them long," he says. "Or maybe they just didn't want me to die in their care."

"YOU'RE BLOCKING MY WINDPIPE"

Dr. Koenig diagnosed Bill as having obstructive sleep apnea, the most common form of the disorder, affecting 99 percent of sufferers. The other types are central sleep apnea, caused by neurological misfires between the brain and diaphragm, and mixed sleep apnea, a combination of obstructive and central.

Obstructive sleep apnea takes its name from the way it obstructs night-time breathing. Normally the throat muscles, tongue, tonsils, and uvula (the fleshy tissue hanging at the back of your throat) relax and sag slightly when you lie down. But if one or more of these parts are particularly loose and droopy, or if you have a small airway to begin with, airflow will be blocked when you're sleeping. This effect becomes exaggerated as you age and your body begins to lose muscle tone.

Smoking, drinking, and popping sleeping pills can also contribute to obstructive sleep apnea by further relaxing the tissue surrounding the airway. But the one vice that causes the most trouble is overeating. Being even 15 to 20 pounds overweight translates into more floppy flesh to block things up. "People aren't fat in just one place," says Dr. Kryger. "They have extra tissue inside and out, and that accumulated flesh can block a person's airway when he lies down to sleep." Overweight males are at particular risk, Dr. Kryger adds, because they tend to carry their weight higher—in their shoulders and necks—than females do. Researchers believe this is one reason sleep apnea affects twice as many men as women.

Naturally occurring growths or changes in the bony surfaces behind the jaw, nasal passages, or back of the throat also can block a sufferer's upper airway, by pressing on surrounding flesh. "Weight issues affect roughly 60 to 70 percent of all sleep apnea patients, but the rest aren't overweight," says Dr. Loube. "Really, anyone can develop this condition."

Even the complexities of brain chemistry (which affect how strong and regular a person's breathing is during sleep) may play a role. "In most cases, sleep apnea is probably the result of the complex relationship between a sleeper's breathing and the upper airway," says Safwan Badr, M.D., president of the American Sleep Apnea Association. "It's something we're still trying to understand. In fact, I tell my students that if they can determine the exact cause of sleep apnea, they have a high probability of shaking hands with the king of Sweden someday. It's worthy of a Nobel Prize."

BECOMING AN AIRHEAD

Every time you pull into a gas station to fill an underinflated tire, you're using a treatment for sleep apnea: compressed air. Continuous positive airway pressure (CPAP) is the fastest, most effective, and most widely prescribed remedy for the disorder. Costing about $500, a CPAP machine has two main parts: a small mask the patient wears over his nose, and a shoe-box-size "blower" that's connected to the mask by a tube. The blower sends a constant stream of slightly pressurized air into the nasal passages, filling the patient's upper airway like a splint and preventing the throat from collapsing during sleep. The CPAP machine has been shown to relieve the symptoms of sleep apnea in most patients who use it consistently. The trick? Convincing patients to use it consistently.

"Really, the CPAP machine is the best protocol for most forms of sleep apnea," says Dr. Koenig. "The issue is getting people to use it and keep using it. The machine and mask are just big and annoying enough that people don't like them." Imagine slipping under the covers each night with an elephant mask on your face and you'll get a good picture of the problem. According to a 1993 study at the University of Pennsylvania, only 46 percent of patients consistently complied with CPAP treatment for 4 or more hours.

Jack, the near zombie I met at Dr. Koenig's office, was a noncomplier. He had been using the CPAP machine only about 30 percent of the time. Bill gave up on it completely. "I remembered what Dr. Koenig had told me about trying to comply with the treatment, and I stuck with it for a few months," he says. "But the machine was uncomfortable, and it wasn't working."

As Bill found out, the other treatment options for sleep apnea are pretty limited. Aside from the obvious—refraining from drinking and smoking—the

SAVE YOUR BREATH

Not everyone finds the CPAP machine to be an elephantine torture device. Take James. When this 50-year-old man first visited Steven Koenig, M.D., an expert on sleep disorders at University of Virginia medical center, sleep apnea was pointing him in the direction of a heart attack or a concrete median. "This guy was having 82 ap-neic events, plus another 12 partial closures, an hour," Dr. Koenig says. James initially refused to use the CPAP machine. Then he had that heart attack and began to use it religiously. "Now I've got energy day and night. I sleep well. I just feel really good. The CPAP machine has become my friend."

main do-it-yourself fix is to lose weight. Even a 10 percent reduction can help some people with thick necks. Becoming a side or stomach sleeper also can help (sacking out flat on your back causes more flesh to hang down in the middle of your airway), as can a specially designed mouth guard. The purpose of a mouth guard, a.k.a. a mandibular advancement prosthesis, is to pull the wearer's jaw and tongue slightly forward in order to help open the airway.

Then there's surgery, a treatment choice even less popular than CPAP. The simplest procedure, a basic tonsillectomy, seems to benefit children but not adult sleep apnea sufferers. In another procedure, UPPP (short for uvulopalatopharyngoplasty), a surgeon removes the uvula, the tonsils, and part of the soft palate, opening up your throat like a Roto-Rooter opens your house's sewer lines. But for all the flesh that's being bored out, UPPP is effective only about half the time. The most drastic measure of all, a tracheostomy, is usually reserved for people with truly severe sleep apnea (fewer than 5 percent of sufferers). A surgeon cuts a hole in the patient's windpipe, then inserts a tube that can be uncapped at night, essentially bypassing the problems in the mouth and throat. The upside of the procedure is a 100 percent cure rate. The downside? You have a hole in your throat.

COPING UNTIL THERE'S A CURE

Bill went for a mouth guard. "I didn't need surgery. I just needed to be a little less tired some afternoons," he says.

Dr. Koenig also prescribed the stimulant Ritalin. In addition to its being widely used for attention deficit disorder, Ritalin is given to sleep apnea sufferers who still have daytime sleepiness even after receiving treatment. Ritalin's main drawback is that it can be addictive, which is why doctors prescribe the non-habit-forming stimulant Provigil when insurance will cover it. Bill's policy wouldn't.

"I resisted for months because I don't take drugs," Bill says. "But when I was still tired in the afternoons, still endangering myself behind the wheel, I decided to try it."

Bill takes the drug sparingly—just a half dose—and says he's functioning well again. "Between the oral appliance and the Ritalin, I'm safer from the danger of falling asleep while driving. Now my condition's livable."

As for Jack, he's going to give the CPAP machine another shot. He knows that he might get his waking life back if he can somehow tolerate hooking himself up to the device every evening. And if he can't? There's always surgery or a mouth guard or a combination approach that includes medication.

But there's still no single, convenient cure for sleep apnea. That's a while off, and, truthfully, it might never come. Still, that doesn't mean millions of men have to die of the disorder; doctors know what the enemy looks like and what it's capable of. And while that may not be enough for us to breathe easy, it should at least keep us alive.

KNOW THIS

Raising the Bar

A new government policy may require all hospital medications to carry grocery-style bar codes that could be scanned before being used. Bar codes could save some of the 100,000 patients a year who die as a result of medical errors.

Butt Out

Researchers in the United Kingdom are developing a new antismoking vaccine. The drug—called TA-NIC—prevents nicotine from reaching the brain. By eliminating the buzz that people get from lighting up, the scientists hope to make it easier for smokers to give up cigarettes for good.

In related news, a Mayo Clinic study found that men who quit smoking and took the antidepressant bupropion for an entire year were less likely to gain weight or start smoking again than men who took a placebo.

Surge Protector

A new drug called Covera-HS may eliminate the surges in blood pressure that make morning heart attacks so common. In a study of 357 people with high blood pressure, University of Connecticut researchers found that Covera-HS was 30 percent better than other medications at controlling morning blood pressure levels. "The chance of having a heart attack or stroke in the first few hours after getting up is two to three times greater than at virtually any other time of day," says William White, M.D., the study author. Controlling morning BP surges is one of the best ways to reduce your risk of having a heart attack, he says.

PERCENTAGE OF AMERICAN ADULTS WHO SMOKE CIGARETTES: 26

PERCENTAGE OF AMERICAN ADULTS WHO WANT TO TOTALLY BAN CIGARETTE SMOKING IN RESTAURANTS: 44

IN THE WORKPLACE: 38

Double-Duty Drug

The breast cancer drug tamoxifen may also reduce cholesterol levels in men. In clinical trials, English researchers found that men with heart disease who took the drug were 30 to 60 percent less likely to die as a result of their disease than men getting standard treatment. After 4 weeks, the men's cholesterol levels dropped significantly, while the average diameter of their blood vessels more than tripled. Tamoxifen appears to work by enhancing the elasticity of arteries and veins.

A Test Worth Taking

A highly effective new blood test—that's widely available only in the United Kingdom—may soon help doctors diagnose cancer in its earliest stages. In clinical trials, DR-70 was 84 percent effective at detecting more than a dozen different types of cancer. The test works by measuring levels of compounds that are released into the bloodstream as tumors grow and destroy surrounding tissue. Doctors in the United Kingdom recommend that anyone who is over age 40 or who has a family history of cancer get the test, which costs under $100. To find a U.S. doctor who can perform it, click on www.dr-70.co.uk.

Kick the Cancer, Keep Your Prostate

A new study in the journal *The Oncologist* suggests that a drug combination called a triple androgen blockade may be an even better treatment than surgery for prostate cancer. The drugs—which are typically used if prostate surgery fails—work by blocking production of testosterone, the hormone fuel that allows prostate cancer cells to grow. In a 13-month trial of 110 men with prostate cancer, androgen blockade therapy significantly lowered the men's levels of prostate-specific antigen (PSA) and kept them low throughout a 3-year follow-up. "Hormone therapy stops the growth of tumors, without the risk of surgical side effects such as impotence or incontinence," says Robert Leibowitz, M.D., the study author.

PERCENTAGE OF CANCER SURVIVORS
WHO SAY LIFE IS AS GOOD AS, OR
BETTER THAN, WHEN THEY WERE DIAGNOSED: 74

DOWN THE PIKE

Dead Man Walking

According to research from the University of Pittsburgh, it may soon be possible to bring people back to life after they've been nearly frozen. In experiments on animals, researchers found that by rapidly flushing blood vessels with a cold saline solution, they can chill a body to 50°F—stopping the heart from beating. "We can then revive the body after up to 2 hours of clinical death," says Peter Safar, M.D., the study author. In the future, victims of a car crash could be chilled at the scene and resuscitated once proper medical care was available.

Nix the Needles

Diabetics are one step closer to a pill that would take the place of insulin shots. Researchers at Purdue University have developed a tablet that connects to the lining of the small intestine, allowing insulin to be absorbed directly into the bloodstream. In addition to treating diabetes, the new insulin pill may be a treatment for heart disease. A University of Buffalo study found that insulin reduces inflammation within blood vessels, helping to reduce the risk of a heart attack. Research on the pill, which has yet to be named, is still under way.

Worth a Shot

You've been vaccinated against measles, mumps, and polio, and you may soon be able to get a vaccine against atherosclerosis, too. "Researchers are working to develop vaccines that block the buildup of arterial plaque and prevent rogue antibodies from damaging heart muscle," says Carl Alving, M.D., chief of the department of membrane biochemistry at Walter Reed Army Institute of Research. "There's even a vaccine in development that prevents HDL (good) cholesterol from being turned into LDL," he says. Dr. Alving expects the first of several heart disease vaccines to be available in less than 10 years.

Mend a Broken Heart

Damage to the heart after a heart attack may not be permanent after all. New York Medical College researchers have discovered that muscle cells in the heart appear to be capable of regeneration. They're now working on treatments to accelerate that natural healing process.

No Stitch, Less Time

During bypass surgery, doctors use a needle and thread to stitch a transplanted artery to the heart—redirecting bloodflow around a blockage. The procedure is risky and time-consuming since patients' hearts are stopped. But Swiss doctors have developed an alternative. Using a tiny stainless steel clip, surgeons can now fuse blood vessels together, eliminating the need for stitches. "The device cuts operating time in half and reduces the risk of complications," says Friedrich Eckstein, M.D., the lead researcher. The device should be available in the United States within 3 years.

Another procedure—a nonsurgical bypass—may also be widely available in 3 years. During a traditional bypass, a vein is removed from the leg and transplanted into the chest. Researchers at Massachusetts General Hospital have developed a new procedure in which doctors send a catheter from a patient's leg up to the heart to route the blood to an unclogged neighboring vein, says Alan Yeung, M.D., codeveloper of the new technique. Nonsurgical bypasses could help the 100,000 patients who aren't healthy enough to undergo traditional surgery.

Waging War on Cancer

Within just a few years, doctors may not have to remove a tumor-riddled organ or inject a person with chemicals to battle cancer. Researchers at Johns Hopkins Medical Institute say a new antitumor treatment called a "cancer grenade" may soon be able to kill cancerous cells without damaging the cells around them. To set off the grenade, doctors inject the cancerous cells with a gene from the germ that causes diphtheria. "Once the gene enters the cell, it initiates a self-destruct signal and kills the cell without damaging the nearby healthy tissue," says Ron Rodriguez, M.D., the lead researcher on the project.

EASIEST WAY TO CUT
YOUR HEART ATTACK RISK: **WALK 2 MILES A DAY**

WHAT'S THE DIFF?

Blood Vessel vs. Artery vs. Vein

A blood vessel is any one of five conduits that carry blood through the body. The biggest of these are arteries—which transport oxygen-rich blood away from the heart—and veins, which transport oxygen-depleted blood back to the heart.

Arteriosclerosis vs. Atherosclerosis

We have no proof, but we believe doctors coined these terms to prove they can pronounce words the rest of us can't. The next time a doc says "arteriosclerosis," call his bluff by saying, "Well, of course. That's a general term for 'hardening of the arteries.' Which form are you referring to?" He'll likely respond, "Atherosclerosis," which is the most common form, occurring when yellow plaques of cholesterol and other fats develop in your large and medium-size arteries.

Systolic vs. Diastolic

When a nurse straps a cuff around your arm in a doctor's office, she's not measuring your mighty biceps. She, of course, is taking your blood pressure. Specifically, she's measuring how high the pressure is when your heart contracts (systolic) and when it relaxes (diastolic). A normal reading is less than 130 mm Hg systolic and 85 mm Hg diastolic. (Hg is the chemical symbol for mercury, the liquid metal that was used to measure blood pressure until the advent of digital technology. Don't ask us why, but the name stuck.) A reading above 139 mm Hg systolic or 89 mm Hg diastolic indicates high blood pressure, and a reading below 96 mm Hg systolic and 61 mm Hg diastolic indicates low blood pressure. A reading of zero over zero indicates it's time to find a good undertaker.

PERCENTAGE OF ADULTS WITH HIGH BLOOD PRESSURE WHO DON'T TREAT IT CORRECTLY: 73

TAKE ACTION

When it comes to beating the top diseases that kill men, prevention really *is* the best medicine. From simple tips you can use right away to new hassle-free tests that stop these killers in their tracks, the following strategies will help you bypass a bypass, dodge diabetes, and much more.

1. Tell 'em where it hurts. You're having a heart attack, but don't tell that to a 911 operator. "If you say you're having a heart attack, it's only going to slow things down because we have to ask why you think you're having one," says Dale Dotson, spokesman for American Ambulance in Fresno, California. Instead, immediately give the address you're calling from and then describe your symptoms. According to Dotson, "chest pains" is the phrase to remember.

2. Cuff up while you work out. Your blood pressure levels will be higher than when you're sitting still, but according to a new study, this reading may be a better indicator of your overall health. When you're exercising, a healthy BP can go above 120/80 but shouldn't top 200/80, says Kerry Stewart, M.D., the study author. Your doctor can measure your exercising BP during a cardiac stress test. Or, for a slightly less accurate reading, gauge your own BP, using a battery-powered tester while riding a stationary bike.

3. Drop your BP. It used to be that a "high-normal" blood pressure reading rarely raised your doctor's eyebrows. That's changed. A new study using data from the benchmark Framingham Heart Study shows that people with high-normal BPs had a $1\frac{1}{2}$- to $2\frac{1}{2}$-times-greater risk of heart attack or stroke in 10 years than those with optimal BPs. "High-normal" means a systolic pressure (first number) between 130 and 139, and/or a diastolic number between 85 and 89. If you're high-normal, see your doctor and do this.

Say when. In research at Tulane University, heavy drinkers (that's three or more drinks a day) who cut their intake in half trimmed 2 or 3 points off both BP measures. That's enough to lower the chance of developing high blood pressure by nearly 20 percent, says Jiang He, M.D., Ph.D., a coauthor of the study.

Pick your tunes. You like Korn? Crank it up; it'll soothe you. Patients awaiting surgery dropped their BPs back to normal when allowed to choose the music played. Karen Allen, Ph.D., the lead study author, says it was having control and a choice that mattered, not the type of music.

Hang with your main squeeze. When you're with your spouse, blood pressure often drops by 1 to 1.5 points, compared with other social situations.

It may be the predictability that does it, says Brooks B. Gump, Ph.D., the lead researcher.

4. Check your neck. If strokes run in your family, consider having an MRI to check the carotid arteries in your neck. A recent University of Washington study of 49 men with severe atherosclerosis found that magnetic resonance imaging may be able to detect dangerous clogging in the neck that can trigger a stroke. So far, this is the most effective method found for detecting unstable plaque within the arteries in the neck, says Chun Yuan, Ph.D., the study author. Plaque deposits can significantly increase your risk of stroke—but early detection allows doctors to put you on medications that whittle down deposits and reduce the risk that a large blockage will come loose and cause a stroke.

5. Get help kicking butts. If you can't quit smoking, even with nicotine patches and gum, it's possible your body may produce a faulty liver enzyme, called CYP2A6. The enzyme feeds your addiction by breaking down nicotine so quickly that you need to light up again within hours to avoid withdrawal symptoms. Instead of going cold turkey, you may be helped by a drug called methoxsalen, which blocks production of CYP2A6. "When patients take methoxsalen, blood nicotine levels stay higher longer, and smokers light up fewer cigarettes," says Edward Sellers, M.D., Ph.D., who discovered the new use for the drug.

6. Outsmart smog. City dwellers, beware. Breathing dirty air can drastically increase your risk of heart disease. Harvard researchers monitored the heart function of 40 healthy middle-age men. They then tracked the men's exposure to airborne pollution, including soot, smog, and ash. "The more particles the men inhaled, the harder it was for their hearts to adjust to different types of activity," says David C. Christiani, M.D., the study author. To protect yourself: Keep windows closed on high-pollution days; exercise outdoors in the early morning, when pollution levels are lowest; and recirculate cool air in your car, rather than open the vents.

7. Spend more time in bed. According to a University of Chicago study, getting too little sleep can increase your risk of becoming diabetic. "Getting less than 6½ hours of sleep a night impairs the body's ability to use insulin by 40 percent," says Bryce Mander, a researcher who analyzed the study data. Insulin resistance is one of the primary symptoms leading to the development of diabetes.

AMOUNT OF TIME THE AVERAGE GUY WAITS TO GO TO AN EMERGENCY ROOM AFTER FEELING CHEST PAIN: **2 HOURS, 12 MINUTES**

TIME IT TAKES A HEART ATTACK TO DO IRREPARABLE DAMAGE: **1 HOUR**

8. Have your pancake and eat it, too. In the past, you needed to avoid eating for at least 8 hours before doctors could test your blood for diabetes. But now researchers at the Durham VA Medical Center have found that a simple blood test called hemoglobin A1c can detect diabetes without requiring a patient to fast beforehand. "The test was designed to monitor diabetes treatment, but it can also spot the disease in up to 75 percent of cases in which people haven't previously been diagnosed as diabetic," says David Edelman, M.D., the study author. Men who are overweight, have a family history of diabetes, or are chronically tired should consider undergoing the test.

9. Get your colon checked—without pain or discomfort. If the thought of having a tube shoved through your colon gives you pause, there's a new, widely available alternative worth considering. The procedure—called a virtual colonoscopy (or CT scan)—is as simple, and pain-free, as getting x-rayed. In clinical trials, researchers found that CT scans could detect more than 90 percent of the large polyps found during traditional colonoscopies.

10. Don't fall off the low-fat wagon. According to a study from Australia, even a single fatty meal can cause temporary damage to your heart. Physicians at the Baker Medical Research Institute in Melbourne gave a high-fat meal to one group of volunteers and a lower-fat, "control" meal to a second group. Three hours later, the doctors measured the change in elasticity of all the subjects' arteries. (We don't even want to know how.) "After just a single meal, the arteries of the patients who'd eaten the most fat were 25 percent stiffer than those of the patients who'd eaten the leaner meal," says Paul Nestel, M.D., the study author. And research shows that stiff blood vessels are one of the primary causes of both heart attack and stroke.

11. Avoid mixing a multi with certain meds. Antioxidant supplements and cholesterol-lowering medications are great on their own, but they don't mix. Researchers at the University of Washington compared three groups of patients: one group taking a cholesterol-lowering medication (simvastatin with niacin); one taking antioxidants, including vitamins C and E; and one taking both. Their finding: Antioxidants appear to alter the effectiveness of cholesterol-lowering drugs, preventing "good," HDL cholesterol from increasing.

12. Add this to your pre-op checklist. Previous studies have shown that herbal supplements may increase the risks of surgery. But now a study in the *Journal of the American Medical Association* has established some firm guidelines on the subject. The recommendations: Avoid ginseng, St. John's wort, and garlic supplements a week before surgery because all three products increase your risk of complications. You should also stop taking stimulants like ephedra, kava kava, or ginkgo at least 36 hours before surgery. "A third of patients undergoing surgery continue taking herbs without telling their doctors, which can lead to serious conditions such as internal bleeding," says Jonathan Moss, M.D., the study author.

ANY QUESTIONS?

Sneak Attack

What is a "silent" heart attack, and how would I know if I were having one?
—E. S., Ooltewah, Tennessee

You wouldn't know; that's why they call it silent. This type of heart attack can be detected only after it occurs, normally during a routine EKG, according to Richard Stein, M.D., of Lenox Hill Hospital in New York. "A patient's electrocardiogram shows that the heart has been damaged," says Dr. Stein, "but the patient cannot recount any symptoms of a heart attack. He was never sick, he never had chest pains, and he was never short of breath." Silent heart attacks are more likely to occur in elderly people and diabetics. If you have high cholesterol, if you smoke, or if you have other risk factors for heart disease, the best way to monitor your heart's condition is to have routine EKGs. Dr. Stein recommends them for all men over 50.

Weekend Worrier

I have no more than one or two cigarettes on weekends when I'm drinking beer with my friends. But I don't smoke at all on other days. Can this little bit really hurt me?
—F. A., Capitola, California

If you're looking for assurances, you won't find them here. "There's no established safe level for smoking," says Corinne Husten, M.D., of the Centers for Disease Control and Prevention in Atlanta. That's the government's line. We'll be more realistic: Of course smoking two butts a week isn't as bad for you as smoking a pack a day. But the truth is, there's no telling how the 4,000 chemicals in cigarette smoke will affect the unique biology of your lungs. You're taking the worst of risks—one without any known odds. But here's a sobering fact backed up by decades of research: "Over 90 percent of people who start smoking (even intermittently) go on to become daily smokers," says Dr. Husten, who adds that how many years you smoke may be a more important factor in determining risk of lung cancer than how many cigarettes you smoke.

THE NUMBER OF YEARS HAVING NEVER SMOKED ADDS TO YOUR LIFE: 1.3

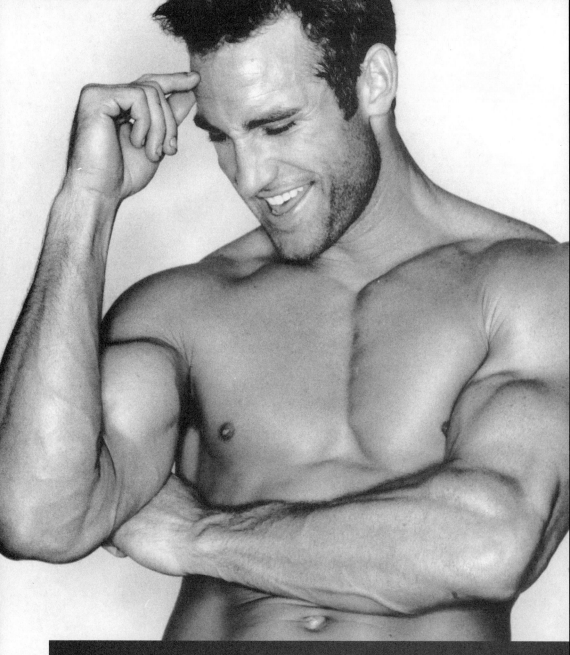

PART FOUR
BULLET-PROOF
YOUR BRAIN

GAME SHOW

Who Will Crack First?

Will stress get the best of one of these guys? Or you?

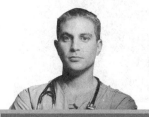

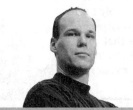

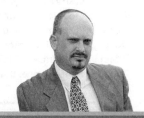

SCOTT BRAUNSTEIN
Age: 27   E.R. Doc Who Works
100-Hour Weeks

WARREN OSMOND
Age: 34   Bored Bingo Caller
Whose Wife Recently Left Him

MARK PEPER
Age: 38   Once Depressed Dad
Who's Had A Year of Mourning

WHY HE'S AT RISK

- Braunstein is a medical resident in two of his hospital's departments. He averages 4 hours of sleep but sometimes works 36 hours straight. A study of E.R. physicians found that about 25 percent felt burned-out and planned to leave the field within 5 years. Braunstein is only in the second year of a 6-year residency.

- He was jolted by his grandfather's recent death; mourning can turn into depression.

- His young age puts him at risk because he has less stability in his life.

- Religion, which can raise coping skills, isn't a priority for him.

WHAT PROTECTS HIM

- Though it's stressful, Braunstein likes his job.

- He's close to his family, and relationships are protective.

- He joined a 24-hour gym, and his 3 A.M. workouts keep his mind fit, as well as his body.

SCOTT'S PREDICTION

- "I may be under a lot of stress, but there's a light at the end of my tunnel. I have a promising career ahead."

WHY HE'S AT RISK

- Osmond is caught in a dead-end job that brings him little satisfaction. Bingo calling ("B-22!") is surprisingly demanding (he hasn't taken a vacation in 4 years), and he occasionally gets threats from sore losers.

- His wife of 3 years, who had a son from another marriage, recently left him. Although his doctor suggested he take antidepressants, he's been coping without them.

- Osmond doesn't go to church, and he has a temper. So drop that cane, blue-hair!

WHAT PROTECTS HIM

- Osmond has supportive friends and family, which could keep him from having a crisis.

- Although he's unhappy with his job, he's thankful for the security. The unemployed are twice as likely to experience anxiety and three times as likely to feel depressed.

- Osmond works out 5 days a week, which helps him relax.

WARREN'S PREDICTION

- "The doctor will lose it. His schedule is too crazy to keep up with for long."

WHY HE'S AT RISK

- Peper had 13 friends die recently, and the losses prompted him to evaluate and question his life.

- He has a family history of depression and was taking antidepressants until February; depression recurs in 50 percent of cases.

- After 13 years of marriage and two children, he's getting divorced. While he sees the split as a blessing, it's still a stressful time that makes his life even more unstable.

WHAT PROTECTS HIM

- He attends church, is surrounded by supportive friends, and likes his job. He works for a health care provider, which he finds challenging but not overly stressful; job satisfaction is a major protective factor.

- He feels less depressed since leaving his wife.

- He works out regularly, which helps manage depression.

MARK'S PREDICTION

- "My depression is under control. I think the bingo guy is on the verge of breaking down. If I had his job, I wouldn't last another day."

And the Winner Is . . .
Warren Osmond

We asked Ralph Swindle, Ph.D., a research scientist and psychology professor at Indiana University at Bloomington, to help us develop a test to determine how likely these men are to snap. The scorecard on the opposite page rates the major factors that could affect your chance of losing it. Play along. The lower your score, the greater your risk.

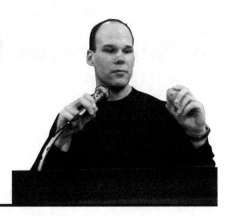

FINAL ANALYSIS

Creating balance is a key to maintaining control. It's not just men who are overwhelmed who break down. Men who don't have enough sources of fulfillment are just as likely to face mental health difficulties.

Crises don't just happen during midlife, either. "Younger men face more life instability, and the twenties are a key risk period for the start of psychiatric problems," says Ralph Swindle, Ph.D., a research scientist and psychology professor at Indiana University at Bloomington. "If a man gets into his forties without major problems, he may never develop them."

Since Osmond is unhappy with so many parts of his life, he is most at risk. Swindle says Osmond should see a doctor and should work on setting specific goals—like making a career change. Taking these steps will give him a sense of purpose and control over his life, which is vitally important.

Braunstein is managing his schedule, but Swindle is concerned about how long Braunstein can cope with working in two departments, and says he should focus on one. Lack of sleep is also a concern. If he's too tired at work and makes a mistake, the ramifications could be serious. He needs to make relaxing a priority and take time to grieve for his grandfather.

Although Peper has a history of depression, he's already come through the worst of it. The thought of having a relapse haunts him, so it's important that he maintain stability. The deaths are beyond his control, but had he not allowed himself to grieve, the stress could have aggravated his condition. And though separation is stressful, Swindle says Peper's unhappy marriage could have been more damaging. He's starting over, and that's one good way to improve your state of mind.

THE IMPLOSION INDEX

RISK FACTOR	POINT VALUE	SCOTT	WARREN	MARK	YOU
HISTORY OF DEPRESSION					
Depression commonly recurs and tends to run in families.	Been diagnosed? −3		−3	−3	
	Family history? −1			−1	
	No history? +3	+3			
TRAUMAS					
Divorce, separation, or death of someone close could trigger a breakdown.	Recent trauma? −2	−2	−2	−2	
	No recent trauma? +2				
WORKPLACE STRESS					
Dealing with a stressful work environment increases odds of burning out.	Extremely stressful job? −2	−2			
	Moderately stressful job? −1		−1		
	Fairly stress-free job? +2			+2	
JOB SECURITY					
Losing a job could trigger a breakdown.	Recent unemployment? −2				
	A mistake could get you fired? −1	−1			
	High job security? +2		+2	+2	
JOB SATISFACTION					
Hating your job is mentally taxing and affects other areas of your life.	Low job satisfaction? −2		−2		
	Average job satisfaction? 0				
	High job satisfaction? +2	+2		+2	
RELATIONSHIPS					
Having people to go to for support is protective.	Don't have supportive friends, family, or spouse? −2				
	Have supportive friends, family, or spouse? +2	+2	+2	+2	
RELIGIOUS FAITH					
Religion aids in stress management and lends a greater sense of purpose in life.	Not very religious? −2	−2	−2		
	Moderately religious? +1				
	Very religious? +2			+2	
ATTITUDE					
Having a pessimistic view of life increases your risk.	Pessimistic about life? −2		−2		
	Optimistic about life? +2	+2		+2	
PHYSICAL HEALTH					
Staying in good physical health helps you cope with problems and maintain good mental health.	Eat poorly, don't exercise? −1				
	Sleep-deprived? −1	−1			
	Overuse alcohol? −1				
	Exercise, eat healthfully? +1	+1	+1	+1	
	Sleep regularly? +1		+1	+1	
AGE					
Younger men typically have less stability in their lives than older men.	Under 30? −1	−1			
	30 to 40? 0		0	0	
	Over 40? +1				
TEMPER					
Angry and aggressive people get less support.	Sometimes blow up? −1		−1		
	Calm temperament? +1	+1		+1	
TOTALS		+2	−7	+9	

▶ **IF YOUR SCORE IS 5 OR MORE:** You're probably whistling as you read this. We're envious.

▶ **IF YOUR SCORE IS 1 TO 4:** You're stabler than most, but there are aspects of your life that trouble you. Face them while they're still manageable.

▶ **IF YOUR SCORE IS 0 OR LESS:** You're dissatisfied with your life, and it's time you made some changes. You know what's needed. Follow your instincts.

MUST READS

Stressed to Kill

New research shows that high levels of the hormone cortisol may be as bad as high cholesterol

By Hugh O'Neill

We struggle with one stay-well discipline—stress control. The most celebrated de-stressers—yoga, deep breathing, rose-petal baths—aren't exactly in our guy wheelhouse. But further, stress is a tough enemy to imagine. Cholesterol, you can actually picture gunking up your pipes. Stress is a guerrilla fighter, hard to center in the crosshairs.

If, like us, you need a bad guy to target, consider aiming at a stress hormone called cortisol. There's evidence linking chronically high levels of the stuff—usually caused by stress—to a passel of problems, including obesity, muscle loss, diabetes, heart disease, memory fade, depression, and prostate cancer.

"Over the long term, elevated cortisol may be as detrimental to overall health as elevated cholesterol or elevated blood sugar," says Shawn Talbott, Ph.D., a nutritional biochemist and author of *The Cortisol Connection*.

The case against cortisol is still taking shape. When a substance is associated with illnesses, it can be tricky to sort out chicken–egg questions. But for putting a face on stress control, cortisol will serve nicely as a motivating enemy to post on the locker room wall. Time to kick a little cortisol butt.

THE STRESS RESPONSE, STARRING CORTISOL

When you're in an acutely stressful situation, your adrenal glands release several hormones. Some make your blood surge toward your muscles. You'll

PERCENTAGE OF AMERICANS WHO SAY THEIR TOP REASON FOR CHANGING JOBS IS TO HAVE A LESS STRESSFUL POSITION: 14

PERCENTAGE OF WORKERS WHO SAY THAT RUDE COLLEAGUES OR CLIENTS LEAVE THEM STRESSED: 34

have fuel to throw a punch or to run away like a scared rabbit. Cortisol's particular job is to make sure your blood is high-octane fuel. It signals glucose, amino acids, and fatty acids to flood out of your tissues and into circulation.

Like most substances in our bodies, cortisol plays a gazillion roles in keeping us well. Many medicines are even derived from it. And everything's just peachy if, once you've escaped from the cops, your cortisol level returns to its pre-emergency baseline. But cortisol turns from staunch defender into bad news if your levels remain too high for too long.

For most of us, this is traceable not to real emergencies but to our chronically worried minds. Simply by our fretting, our brains stimulate the hormonal stress response that nature engineered only for actual, physical threats.

"If the body is constantly mobilizing energy," says Robert Sapolsky, Ph.D., a professor of biology and neurology at Stanford University, "it never stores it, and this increases the risk of a number of metabolic diseases."

Obesity. A study done at Yale University found that people with higher stress-induced cortisol levels ate more than people with lower levels—and ate more sweets, too. What's more, if your cortisol stays elevated, it eventually encourages your body to store fat, says Talbott. And guess where it stores the stuff. According to a new study of 50 overweight middle-aged men in Sweden, cortisol stimulates a fat-gathering enzyme that gravitates toward the abdomen more than to any other place in the body.

THREE MENTAL STRESS BUSTERS

We asked Robert Sapolsky, Ph.D., a professor of biology and neurology at Stanford University, for stress-control tips that didn't include the lotus position.

1. Take the wheel. A sense of control over some of the stressors in your life helps. "If you blast a volunteer randomly with a noise, his stress hormones rise," says Sapolsky. "But if you give him a button and tell him that pressing it will decrease the likelihood of the noise, there's a smaller stress response to the same sound." Getting organized, even in small ways, may help you feel more like the captain of your ship.

2. Make a plan. "People manage stress more effectively if they can believe that things are improving," according to Sapolsky. So make sure you always have something you're looking forward to. Help your wife understand why she should tease you saucily with a promise of the Lady of the Manor and the Gamekeeper on Friday night. Hope makes stress manageable.

3. Get spiritual. Remember the simple wisdom of Simone Weil: Any undivided attention is prayer. If we can stop the tumble in our heads and every day briefly commend our complete attention to something—a 10-foot putt, a 10-penny nail, or a 10-year-old child—we may acquire the serenity many find in formal faith.

Diabetes. High insulin and cortisol are often found together. Though it's not yet clear which comes first, Talbott believes that over time, high cortisol levels "may make your body less responsive to insulin, impairing its ability to manage glucose." This is a formula for adult-onset type 2 diabetes.

A recent study found that people with the most stressful life events were 64 percent more likely than others to have developed diabetes without knowing it.

Dumber brains. When researchers at the Washington University in St. Louis School of Medicine artificially raised people's cortisol levels, they found that after 4 days, 14 out of 15 showed declines in their ability to remember material that was read to them. Their memory improved once cortisol levels returned to normal.

Prostate cancer. Researchers at Stanford University studied a relatively rare form of prostate cancer that's resistant to hormone therapy and noticed that cortisol actually promoted its growth.

PLAYING DEFENSE

It's tough to limit your stress. Bosses hate it when you ask them to stop being egotistical tyrants. But even if you can't cut your stress, these damage-control steps may either reduce the level of cortisol coursing through your body or minimize its effect on you.

Grab a bagel, but hold the lox. Or eat any other starchy food that's low in protein when you start feeling stressed. When Dutch researchers exposed stress-prone people to tense situations, those on a high-carbohydrate, low-protein diet had a 14 percent lower cortisol response than those going protein heavy and carbohydrate light. According to Rob Markus, Ph.D., one of the study authors, the extra carbohydrates increased the production of serotonin, a natural stress reducer.

Skip Letterman. A University of Chicago study, published in the journal *Sleep*, showed that men who slept only 4 hours had cortisol levels 37 percent higher than men who got a full 8 hours of shut-eye; the men who stayed

PERCENTAGE BY WHICH TAKING A SINGLE WEEK OFF FROM WORK CAN DECREASE YOUR OVERALL RISK OF HEART ATTACK AND STROKE: MORE THAN 20

PERCENTAGE OF AMERICAN WORKERS WHO BELIEVE THEY HAVE TOO MUCH WORK TO GO ON VACATION: 33

PERCENTAGE WHO ARE AFRAID THEIR JOB WOULDN'T BE THERE WHEN THEY GOT BACK: 11

IS YOUR CORTISOL TOO HIGH?

You can have your cortisol tested through a blood draw at a doctor's office. There are also new home salivary tests on the market. You spit into a small vial in the morning and at midnight and mail back the goods for the results (www.bodybalance.com).

We had two of our editors—Mike Zimmerman (two small kids, new house) and Adam Campbell (way calmer)—take both tests. The blood tests had them both in the normal range for midday cortisol levels. (Zim was 17 percent higher—thanks, kids.) On the home test, Campbell was in the okay range for both readings, but Zimmerman's nighttime level was high. (So we gave Campbell half of Zim's work.)

Cortisol not only varies greatly throughout the day—meaning you have to measure it at different times—it also rises quickly in response to even simple stress (like not finding a copy of *Men's Health* in the clinic waiting room). For those reasons, doctors we spoke with said the tests aren't particularly accurate or even necessary. "Unlike with cholesterol, how you feel can be a good predictor [of cortisol]," says Shawn Talbott, Ph.D., a nutritional biochemist and author of *The Cortisol Connection*. "If you're harried and frantic and worried a lot, it's a good bet your cortisol is too high."

awake the whole night had levels 45 percent higher. Sleep specialists suggest that you strive for 8 hours per night.

Stop tossing and turning. How well you sleep matters, too. Another University of Chicago study showed that men who got plenty of deep sleep—the quality stuff without all the dreaming and rapid eye movement—secreted almost 65 percent more human growth hormone (HGH) than men who were short on good slumber. You want more HGH to help prevent the loss of muscle mass caused by cortisol.

Remember C, as in "crisis." If you're in a stressful time of life—wondering why the jury has been out so long, perhaps—load up on vitamin C. "For managing stress," Talbott says, "you probably top out the benefit with a daily intake of 1,000 milligrams (mg), divided into small doses throughout the day."

Don't have that last drink. Booze dehydrates you. Your body thinks there's a water shortage emergency, which bumps up your cortisol. How much alcohol is too much? Most of the smart money says three drinks a day.

Stop the Panic

These are anxious times, characterized by a nervous uptick of depression, anxiety disorders, panic attacks. The causes aren't going away soon, but you don't have to live with the symptoms

By Mike Zimmerman

I know what death feels like.

I knew it that day I was slumped over the hood of my car at a Jersey rest stop—my heart thrumming like a speedbag, my body soaked and shaking, my lips and fingers numb—and I still know it now. No peace. No tunnels. No bright lights. Just that knowledge, waiting for my heart to stop pounding, to stop period.

As the ambulance approached, the situation grew surreal. My extremities mutated into petrified claws. I held up those twisted, frozen fingers, asking, *What the hell is happening to me?* But I couldn't speak. My mouth had stiffened to a straw hole—Sylvester after Tweety feeds him some alum. Stroke? Heart attack? Aneurysm? I was collecting them all.

Despite my condition, the EMTs didn't seem the least impressed. They shoved tubes up my nose. Breathe slowly, concentrate, they said.

When my gurney wheels hit the tiles at Morristown Memorial, I could finally breathe normally. My hands and feet were my own once again. I could move my mouth even though I didn't feel like saying much.

Two hours later, as I shuffled through the sliding doors and back to reality a free and "healthy" man, I must have looked like Marty Feldman after a lightning strike. The doctor on duty told me that I'd hyperventilated from a combination of hangover, fatigue, and caffeine. Not unusual. The paralysis in my face and hands came from severe overbreathing. But now I was fine, he said. What he didn't tell me was that I'd had a panic attack.

I'd just coughed up initiation dues for a club that is more extensive than I'd ever imagined. And membership is on the rise: In a *Men's Health* magazine Web poll, 20 percent of those who responded listed anxiety/panic attacks as an adverse health effect of the September 11 tragedies. "Anxiety has soared," says Sandra Ceren, Ph.D., a clinical psychologist in California. "That's a big problem for people prone to panic attacks."

No one wants to join this club. But roughly 2.4 million people in any given year are thrust into membership by a buildup of stress, anxiety, uncertainty, and in the end, ignorance. For perspective, imagine the combined populations of Boston, Denver, San Francisco, and Washington, D.C., simultaneously freaking out.

Who in the world doesn't have stress? We're constantly pounded with information from all sides: Do this at work, don't do this at home, eat this, don't drink that, and—oh, yeah—watch CNN three times a day to make sure you're up-to-date on the latest domestic security risks. No wonder panic attacks have gone mainstream.

Tony Soprano gets them in grand style. And maybe you've used the term as a synonym for a total stress-out. But was it a panic attack? Maybe so . . .

PARALYZED BY FEAR

The American Psychiatric Association defines a panic attack as intense terror that strikes for no apparent reason, usually peaking in 10 minutes, with at least four of the following symptoms: racing pulse or heart palpitations, hyperventilation, choking sensations, sweating, trembling, chest pain, nausea, dizziness, numbness and tingling in the body, chills or hot flashes, a sense of unreality, and—most intensely—a fear of losing control, going insane, or dying.

This is not the garden variety "I have a presentation in the morning" anxiety. This is a full-body reaction as powerful and crippling as an orgasm. But instead of ooh-la-la pleasure, you get oh-my-God terror that can break deodorant in seconds.

Panic disorder develops when several attacks lead to a chronic fear of future attacks. Which can in itself trigger another attack—a vicious circle that spins even when the person knows exactly what's happening to him.

But here's a little-known fact: Panic disorder is not just severely debilitating. It's severely treatable. And even more compelling? For some people, it's severely self-treatable. I'm living proof. If you know the basics—why panic attacks happen, and that they won't hurt you—you can deflate them, prevent them, and eventually defeat them. And you can do it without taking a single pill.

WHAT TRIGGERS THE TERROR

Panic erupts when your body's fight-or-flight mechanism trips, causing an adrenaline dump that goads you into action. Grizzly bear in your beer cooler? Fight. Dentist with a drill? Flight. Panic attacks happen when the mechanism is triggered without any real threat.

"The brain is wired for survival and doesn't discriminate," says Bert Anderson, Ph.D., creator of the Healing Panic Recovery program, which has helped hundreds of people beat panic disorder. "It doesn't think out whether a situation is dangerous or not."

PERCENTAGE OF AMERICANS WHO HAVE LOST 5 OR MORE DAYS IN THE PAST MONTH DUE TO MENTAL HEALTH PROBLEMS: 8

So what pulls the trigger? You do. And you may not even know it. Epic life changes are usually a factor: a loved one's death, a divorce, bigger job responsibilities, moving. Chemicals don't help: Hangover, caffeine, nicotine, and the illegal stuff all contribute. Then there are the everyday stresses: the constant threat of another terrorist attack, fatigue, anticipating a drive on the freeway, an airline flight, a speech. Maybe you misinterpret sensations in your body: chest cramps, head rushes, gas. The resulting anxiety activates fight-or-flight, which sends you down the road to panic. In a dragster.

The biggest problem? It's different for everyone. There can be hundreds of combinations of symptoms. "The 'right' answer will come from the last person you talked to," says Anderson.

Sounds good, you might say, but everyone has anxiety, fear, and potential triggers. Why don't we all have panic attacks? There's no easy answer.

Here's what we do know: how many people suffer panic attacks each year. That panic disorder sometimes runs in families. That women get panic attacks more than men. That the attacks usually flare for the first time between late adolescence and your mid-thirties. That they rarely begin in people over 45. Other than that, no one can predict who will have panic attacks, how many they'll suffer, or how severe they'll be.

CHOKED BY A WEED

The seeds were planted in me about 5 years ago. I was running on a hot, muggy day when a gurgling sensation gripped my heart, as if bubbles were popping inside. An arrhythmia. It freaked me out, but I continued running. A week later, the bubbles popped again, but with the added bonus of pain—like a barbecue fork right into my heart. A split second. But frightening beyond anything I was willing to tolerate. Off to the doctor I went.

The diagnosis: gas. Ha! I didn't believe it for a second. Something had to be wrong with my heart. To check, they gave me the usual battery of tests (EKG, echocardiogram, and more). Same verdict. There was nothing wrong with me . . . physically.

Above the neck, I was a mess. Exercise—what was best for me—had become the source of something truly frightening. So I stopped running. What if the doctors missed something? What if I really did have a heart problem? What if I keeled over in the middle of a run? Or in midtown Manhattan as I was walking to work?

See? This is what invades your mind: tiny seeds. A noxious weed germinates that you cannot control, cannot hack back, and cannot ignore.

That's when the attacks started, usually while I was commuting to work. Brief at first—a couple of minutes, tops. I would listen to my heart, obsessed with every beat, knowing one day it must stop. If I detected anything strange—even imaginary—the adrenaline gushed like a heavy metal power chord. Then, one hungover Sunday, the Big One hit, the one you just read about that landed me in the E.R. I'd spent a weekend of bacchanalian bliss at my best friend's place: golf, beer, bad jokes. Two hours into the drive home, my mind was a ball of static. Sweat dripped inside my shirt. My nerves hummed as if an electric razor were mashed into the back of my neck. Then I found that rest stop, where every cardiac terror finally boiled over.

Later that night, when I came to my senses, the anxiety was replaced by anger. I needed to know, once and for all, what these attacks were. So I started reading. And thinking. And, eventually, healing. I'd endured the attacks for months, and I'd had enough. Some people endure them for years, even decades.

The question is, how much will you take before you seek help?

HELP IS ON ITS WAY

For a long time, getting help for panic attacks was kind of like getting Internet service: at first, nothing. Then it got better, and better, and better still. When I landed in that emergency room 5 years ago, I wasn't diagnosed with panic disorder—the term never came up. I had to discover it on my own. This kind of nondiagnosis once was common. "The situation was really bad 10 years ago," says Frank Wilhelm, Ph.D., of Stanford University. "It has improved a lot since then. Panic disorder is now recognized quite well by general physicians."

"The doctor is doing what he is trained to do, simply that," says Anderson. In other words, hear the complaint, examine the patient, assess the problem, prescribe a remedy. "The remedy," he says, "depends on the doctor's level of sophistication."

Which means your best first step is a trip to the ol' primary—armed with insightful questions about your treatment options.

Experts now point to breathing as an important part of any treatment. Many panic sufferers hyperventilate without knowing it. Prerequisites do not include paper bags and gasping. It's simply "subtle overbreathing," as Curtis Hsia, Ph.D., of the Center for Anxiety and Related Disorders at Boston University, calls it. Rather than use your diaphragm (insert birth-control joke here) to take full, normal breaths, you use your shoulders and chest to take short, quick breaths. This skewed breathing decreases the carbon dioxide in your blood, inhibiting your body's ability to transfer oxygen from the bloodstream to the organs—particularly the brain.

"A starving brain does not serve the senses very well," Anderson says, and that contributes to fear at the onset of panic.

Thankfully, research has increased. In an ongoing study that published preliminary results last year, Wilhelm—one of the nation's leading experts in respiratory assessment of anxiety—found that changing dysfunctional breathing patterns decreased the frequency and severity of panic attacks in all subjects. The treatment was simple: Teach people about hyperventilation, how to be aware of it, how to control it, and how to retrain their breathing at home.

But Wilhelm cautions, "Breathing awareness and training is one important pathway to control of panic, but not the only one."

FACE YOUR DEMONS

Cognitive behavioral therapy, or CBT, has emerged as a powerful uppercut in the fight against panic. CBT forces you to face your panic triggers so you learn that anxiety won't hurt you.

"Patients reach the point where if they are starting to have a panic attack, they can say, 'Oh, I know what this is; it's no big deal,'" says Hsia.

When a patient begins formal CBT, provoking an attack is often part of the therapy. If it doesn't occur naturally, some patients actually have to induce panic, breathing improperly and allowing their worst fears to consume them—on purpose, repeatedly. Sound fun? It's a vital first swing of the hammer that will eventually break the disorder. Patients need to see—the hard way—that panic is just a conditioned response, nothing harmful. As

THE ANTI-PANIC PLAN

"The good news is that anxiety disorders are treatable," says Jerilyn Ross, president of the Anxiety Disorders Association of America. Where to start:

See your doctor. Get a diagnosis. Panic symptoms can mimic serious health conditions, such as heart attack.

Be an educated patient. Ask specific questions about your doctor's recommendations. If he prescribes drugs, what are the side effects? How long will you be on them? Any alternatives? If he refers you to a specialist, is this person qualified to administer cognitive behavioral therapy (CBT, a proven weapon in the fight against panic disorder)? If not, what can they offer? If you're not getting answers, seek a second opinion.

Discuss treatment options. Your doctor may prescribe medication to help control the attacks, or refer you to a specialist, or both. When directed toward CBT, remember that successful treatment requires a willing patient. The more motivated the patient, the more effective the CBT.

Expect results. Length of treatment is variable: Severity of the disorder, dedication of the patient, and the presence of other health issues all affect progress. But, whether it's drugs or CBT, "you should begin to see results in 6 weeks," says Ross. "If not, reevaluate your treatment."

Other Places to Find Help and Referrals

National Institute of Mental Health (NIMH), www.nimh.nih.gov, (888) 826-9438 or (800) 647-2642

Anxiety Disorders Association of America (AADA), www.adaa.org, (301) 231-9350

Center for Anxiety and Related Disorders, Boston University, www.bu.edu/ anxiety, (617) 353-9610

DON'T PANIC, LITERALLY

When you feel an attack coming on, stay calm and focused. Understand that there is nothing physically wrong with you. Breathe normally. Don't fight the feeling. Let it happen. It will not hurt you. If possible, find a quiet place to calm down. Tell yourself, "This is no big deal. I know what this is. I can handle it." Remember: It will pass.

therapy progresses, patients go out into the world, accompanied by their therapists (and eventually on their own), to face repeatedly whatever situations trigger their panic.

"Prolonged exposure to the feared situation is the best treatment," says Wilhelm. "Anxiety is not dangerous, only very uncomfortable. Being able to accept it is an important part of overcoming it."

"What we want is for patients to be able to go anywhere and do anything," says Hsia. "So they can say, 'Even though I have these feelings, they won't kill me.' As they get used to the feelings, the feelings start to decrease."

There is a shortage of therapists qualified to administer CBT for panic, but they are out there. The program Hsia is involved with, at the Center for Anxiety and Related Disorders in Boston, has sessions that last 8 days or 13 weeks. Other programs vary, but patients should make sure they're getting formal CBT. (For referral information, see "The Anti-Panic Plan," at left.

A lot of doctors will simply write prescriptions. Antidepressants and other medications are definitely effective against panic disorder, especially in the early stages of treatment. But you may not need those drugs as much as you—or your doctor—believe.

"In the short term, medication is as effective as CBT," says Hsia. Long term, however, instead of learning that panic attacks won't hurt them, medicated patients learn deep down that they have a condition that is so serious they need a pill to control it. And when a panic attack hits? "They don't know what to do next, other than go back to the doctor for more medication," he says.

Wilhelm agrees. "Physicians are encouraged by the pharmaceutical industry to prescribe medication for this condition, which can be treated as effectively by CBT."

The bottom line: Ask your doctor. For this panicker's money, I don't want to be on anything that alters my day-to-day mood. Plus, some medications—the benzodiazepines, like Xanax—can be addictive. Then there's cost. And making sure you dose on time. Hey, if there were no alternative, I'd be the first one in line at CVS. But there are alternatives—good, sensible, effective alternatives that, to this untrained eye, make medication look a little medieval.

POWER OVER PANIC

Know how I beat panic? I stared it down. I studied the mechanism until I could see the little man behind the curtain. Then it wasn't so scary. When my condition was at its peak—as my "heart condition" delusions persisted—my doctor said something so casually brilliant, he basically cured me then and there: "When you have these attacks, other than the anxiety and palpitations, how do you feel?"

"Um . . . I feel fine."

"Then there's nothing wrong with you."

He was talking about my heart—not my panic disorder—but the shroud lifted. I stopped worrying about my chest, and I started listening to my gut, literally: The "bubbles and fork" struck when my digestive system surged to life. I finally heard what my body had been telling me all along. (Cue Cheech Marin: "It's just gas, man.")

Shortly thereafter, my panic attacks all but evaporated—without drugs or CBT.

Are they gone completely? The full-blown attacks, yes. The anxiety, no. I don't think there's anyone—Martha Stewart included—who can banish all anxiety from his or her life. Long drives by myself are still no fun at all since my rest stop incident. But when that ball of static starts to crackle in my brain, I simply breathe like a normal human should, and let it pass.

Living with panic isn't really living. It breeds with cousins in the anxiety disorder family: depression, agoraphobia, general anxiety disorder. What's worse, research has shown that panic's long-term pounding on your system might exacerbate any heart conditions you already have. Which means it's time to have an intelligent conversation with your doctor. Make sure you're physically healthy. Then ask about panic disorder. Ask about CBT versus drugs. Be curious. Be aggressive. The faster you get help, the faster you can reestablish a toehold in everyday life. "If you say, 'I want to get over this no matter what,' then you're going to do well," says Hsia.

But first you must believe that panic attacks by themselves won't hurt you. Believe that they are treatable. Believe that you'll do some of the best treatment on your own. And believe, above all, that this terror must end. For if you believe it, it will.

Happiness in a Pill?

The TV commercials for antidepressant pills seem to be describing exactly how you feel. Before you swallow what they're selling, here are 10 things to know

By Jeff Stevenson

Feeling anxious about the layoff rumors? Maybe you're bumming over a breakup and contemplating popping a few of your friend's Prozac. Or perhaps you're thinking of asking your doctor for samples of Zoloft or Paxil just to see if they'll make you feel better, as the TV commercials suggest.

"Folks come in all the time and say, 'I want to be on that pill for social anxiety (referring to Paxil)," says Shelley Nuss, M.D., assistant professor of medicine and psychiatry at the West Virginia University School of Medicine. "They'll list all the symptoms they heard on the commercial or read in the ad and say, 'They're talking about me!'"

Antidepressants, including Paxil with its antianxiety effect, are becoming like penicillin for our emotions. Each year, nearly 19 million Americans battle depression (6.4 million are men), and, over 10 years, the share of those who use medication for it has climbed to nearly 79 percent. The rise can be attributed in part to the direct-to-consumer advertising blitz for antidepressant drugs on television and in magazines.

These drugs are so commonplace that people forget antidepressants are potent, mind-altering medications. And it's likely they're not even aware of the potential for serious withdrawal symptoms that can occur if they stop taking the medicine because they've either let the prescription run out or simply forgotten their daily dose. Those common mistakes can put them in a world of hurt. (See "Higher Anxiety," on page 203.)

"If you're on antiseizure medication and you stop quickly, you can seize. . . . Suddenly stop taking beta-blockers, you can die of a heart attack. Antidepressants are no different from other classes of medication in this regard," says Jerrold Rosenbaum, M.D., a professor of psychiatry at Harvard Medical School.

PERCENTAGE OF AMERICANS WHO HAVE TALKED TO THEIR DOCTORS ABOUT PRESCRIPTION DRUGS THEY'VE SEEN ADVERTISED: 30

OF THOSE, THE PERCENTAGE WHOSE DOCTORS WROTE THEM A PRESCRIPTION FOR THE DRUG: 44

If you're planning to try an antidepressant medication, there are some important things you should know—things your doctor may not tell you.

1. Be certain there's really something wrong with you. Given the trying times we're living in, a certain level of anxiety and melancholy is normal. Don't make the mistake of believing you should be happy all the time or, even worse, that a pill can provide that.

"Some doctors are probably reaching for these medications prematurely," says Dr. Rosenbaum. "Sometimes patients might benefit more from counseling or even a watch-and-wait attitude."

2. Understand what the medications do. Paxil, Zoloft, Luvox, Celexa, and Prozac belong to a class of drugs called SSRIs—selective serotonin reuptake inhibitors. Some experts believe that depression and anxiety disorders are caused in part by a glitch in the brain's level of serotonin, a neurotransmitter responsible for ferrying messages between brain cells. It's kind of like a fleet of postal trucks: If there aren't enough trucks or the drivers don't have the correct addresses, then delivery is spotty. SSRIs smooth out the exchange of information in the brain by making more serotonin available—more trucks going in the right direction.

While SSRIs were originally approved to fight depression, their field of treatment has been steadily broadening. Paxil, for example, is the seventh most widely prescribed drug in the world, ostensibly because it has received additional FDA approval for treating panic, obsessive-compulsive, generalized-anxiety, social-anxiety, and post-traumatic-stress disorders. As a result, Glaxo-SmithKline makes almost $7 million from Paxil every day, or $2.4 billion annually.

3. Don't give an SSRI to your kids. Prozac, Zoloft, Paxil, and Celexa are not approved to treat depression in people under 18, yet physicians routinely prescribe them to kids. "Prozac is a very powerful mind-altering drug, and our children are popping it like candy," says Ann Blake Tracy, Ph.D., director of the International Coalition for Drug Awareness (www.drugawareness.org).

4. Get your SSRI from a psychiatrist. "Approximately three-quarters of all antidepressants are prescribed by primary care physicians, rather than psychiatrists," points out Robert Golden, M.D., chairman of the psychiatry department at the University of North Carolina. "Although most are skilled at treating straightforward cases of depression, some do not take the time to properly evaluate, educate, and monitor the patients to whom they prescribe these drugs."

5. Be patient. Your doctor should start you on the lowest effective dose possible. Keep in mind that it typically takes 2 to 4 weeks for the medication to build up in your system and become effective.

6. Take your medication at the right time. Some SSRIs, such as Zoloft and Prozac, have a stimulating effect and may be better taken with breakfast so

HIGHER ANXIETY

Ross Trimmer's joints ached so much, he couldn't sleep at night. "I felt so angry, I had trouble distinguishing dreams from reality. I thought I was going nuts."

Jeff Williamson* felt electric shocks in his head. "Zip, zip, zip—every 15 seconds; they were so strong they made my eyes squinch."

While their symptoms were different, these men had one thing in common: They had stopped taking Paxil.

Stop Signs

"Abrupt discontinuation can cause [these] difficulties," says Jerrold Rosenbaum, M.D., a professor of psychiatry at Harvard Medical School. "Every medicine that the body adapts to should be tapered when discontinued."

Trimmer and Williamson contend that their doctors never told them this. And what they experienced is apparently not unique. A number of class action lawsuits have been filed against GlaxoSmithKline, Paxil's manufacturer, on behalf of patients who allegedly became ill after they stopped taking the drug. And last year the Food and Drug Administration required Glaxo to strengthen its warnings about potential side effects of stopping the medication.

Paxil's Not Alone

Paxil isn't the only SSRI that can trigger withdrawal. Patients have had similar reactions with Zoloft, Luvox, Celexa, and Prozac.

In a study at Boston's Massachusetts General Hospital, 242 patients who had been taking one of the three most popular antidepressants for 4 to 24 months had their medication secretly replaced by a placebo. Sixty-six percent of those on Paxil, 60 percent of those on Zoloft, and 14 percent of those on Prozac reported new symptoms after discontinuing the drug. Many of the symptoms were thought to stem from the rapid removal of drug treatment.

One reason for this, explains Dr. Rosenbaum, the lead researcher, is the half-life of these drugs—the length of time it typically takes the body to halve the drug's concentration in the bloodstream once treatment has been discontinued. For Paxil, this is about 20 hours, for Zoloft approximately 24 hours, and for Prozac about 3 days. The faster these drugs exit the system, the more likely they are to cause problems. The World Health Organization (WHO) reportedly ranks Paxil as the toughest SSRI to quit.

Too Quick to Quit

Alan Metz, M.D., vice president of neuroscience at GlaxoSmithKline, insists, "There is no good scientific data to prove that Paxil, because of its half-life, is uniquely susceptible." He points out that the WHO information is based on "spontaneous report" data, which is less reliable than clinical trials.

"There's very good data to suggest that the length of time one should take an SSRI is 6 to 12 months," says Dr. Metz. "Unfortunately, in the real world the average duration a patient stays on an antidepressant is about 9 weeks. There's a good chance that people are stopping the medication too early and that the symptoms of their depression are returning."

* Not his real name

they don't interfere with sleep. Paxil, by contrast, may have a sedating effect on some people, in which case it's best taken at night. Ask your doctor when you should take yours.

7. Include exercise as part of recovery. Doctors often fail to inform their patients that exercise is a natural antidepressant. When Dr. Nuss prescribes an SSRI, she also prescribes 30 minutes of daily aerobic exercise. "In most cases, 5 percent of the improvement that results stems from the drug and 95 percent from the increased activity," she says. "Exercise is the real wonder drug."

8. Know the potential side effects. Each drug can affect a person differently. But the more common side effects shared by SSRIs include dizziness, nausea, dry mouth, sweating, constipation, insomnia, chills, and abnormal vision. SSRIs also are notorious for diminishing your sex drive. (Some antidepressants function differently in the brain and trigger fewer sexual side effects; talk to your doctor.)

9. Never stop cold turkey. Cutting off treatment abruptly, even after being on an SSRI for just a few weeks, can trigger serious side effects, including dizziness, vomiting, joint pain, irritability, and confusion—and worse. But you can avoid problems by tapering off your medication. The best way to exit an SSRI is first to determine that it's no longer necessary for your well-being. You do this by checking with your doctor. Then, if he concurs, he'll tell you how to reduce the dosage gradually over a period of weeks.

10. You won't become "addicted." SSRIs don't create junkies. "These drugs are not addicting in the way that cocaine or alcohol or heroin is addicting," says Dr. Golden. "We don't see a need to escalate the dose, we don't see misuse of the medication, and we don't see people devoting their lives to getting larger supplies because they crave the effects."

Dr. Nuss agrees. However, she suggests that there might be another type of attachment at work between the pill and the popper. "My patients with major depression tell me it's the most horrible feeling imaginable, like they're in a dark hole with no hope of escaping," she explains. "I'll generally treat them with an SSRI for 6 to 9 months. Afterward, many say they never want to stop . . . because they can't fathom ever going back to that dark place."

PERCENTAGE OF PHARMACISTS WHO HAVE USED A MIND-ALTERING DRUG WITHOUT A DOCTOR'S PRESCRIPTION: 40

Sleep Better Tonight

How to snooze like a baby—no matter what your age

By Neal Thompson

In the crib, you had it made. Fuss a little and you got a breast in your mouth. And when you weren't suckling, you were comatose—up to 18 hours a day. Now? You sleep like a man—lousy. By the time you reach 20, that 18 hours is slashed to 6. And as you age, the number shrinks even further.

Here's why. Inside every brain lurks the suprachias-matic nucleus, or "internal clock." It knocks you out and wakes you up. At birth it's set for maximum crib time, but as you get older, the clock shifts your metabolism and hormones in ways that deprive you of deep, dead-to-the-world sleep. Add that to age-specific wake-up calls—alcohol when you're 20, kids when you're 30, your bladder when you're 50—and your bed becomes bedlam. And that puts you in line for any number of daylight nightmares, including high blood pressure, decreased resistance to invading microbes, a compromised bodily repair and maintenance system, and the tendency to fall asleep while the boss is talking, rather than safely back at your desk. That's why we came up with decade-by-decade strategies for dealing with life's worst sleep saboteurs.

Read 'em and yawn.

YOUR TWENTIES

Six hours and 54 minutes. That's the amount of shut-eye the National Sleep Foundation says you're getting. It's also 2 hours and 6 minutes shy of the 9 hours—not 8—the experts say your body needs. "We need more sleep from puberty through age 25 than at any other time in our lives, except when we're newborns," says James Maas, Ph.D., a Cornell University sleep researcher.

The Four-Step Fix

1. Be in bed by 9:30 every night. In no time you'll want to kill yourself, but at least you'll be well-rested for the job. The alternative: **Take every other night off.** If you go out on Mondays, Wednesdays, and Fridays, then turn in an hour early on Tuesdays and Thursdays. "While this is far from optimal, it will help pay off your sleep debt before it becomes so large that you feel tempted to try to make it all up on the weekend," says Michael Vitiello, Ph.D., a professor of behavioral sciences at the University of Washington.

2. On barhopping nights, order your last drink 3 hours before you call it quits. According to Vitiello, this should give your body time to process the booze before you (a) crash (on the drive home) or (b) crash (in bed). If your blood is clear of alcohol, you'll sleep more soundly. Or, if the damage is already done, **make**

the last call a double virgin screwdriver. Fructose, one of the sugars in OJ, can speed up the metabolism of alcohol by as much as 25 percent.

3. Each night at around 11, your internal clock shifts you into slumber mode by secreting the hormone melatonin. And that's a good thing, unless you need to fall asleep earlier. MIT researchers have found that **taking 0.3 milligrams of a melatonin supplement can help you fall asleep faster** (if you can't find the right dosage, pick up easy-to-break scored pills). Swallow one of these sleeping beauties a half-hour before you want to nod off into oblivion.

4. If you follow tips 1 through 3 and still feel like sleeping in on the weekends, don't. Your internal alarm clock will fight you all the way. Instead, **force yourself up at your normal waking time** and your inner clock will thank you with a deeper, longer sleep the next night. Awake but dragging? Hang on until noon. Japanese researchers found that sleep-deprived subjects who took a 15-minute nap right after eating lunch were less groggy and more alert for the rest of the day than the bleary-eyed control group.

YOUR THIRTIES AND FORTIES

You're probably getting a little more sleep than last decade, but still not enough. Worse, according to a recent study published in the *Journal of the American Medical Association (JAMA)*, men in their thirties and forties get 82 percent less deep, "slow-wave" sleep than men in their late teens and early twenties. Slow-wave sleep is the phase in which your body receives the serious R & R it needs to rebuild itself.

The Four-Step Fix

1. Before you go to bed, **pop some vitamin B$_5$** (pantothenic acid). According to Ron Klatz, M.D., president of the American Academy of Anti-Aging Medicine, this is your antidote to too much cortisol, the stress hormone that surges in middle-aged men. If that doesn't help, ask your doctor about taking some Bayer with your B; aspirin may also help lower cortisol production.

2. Until you get your cortisol under control, it will limit your deepest sleep so you'll spend the night teetering on the edge of consciousness. **Buy stuff to**

PERCENTAGE OF AMERICANS WHO SUFFER FROM INSOMNIA AT LEAST A FEW NIGHTS A WEEK: 58

PERCENTAGE WHO SAY THEY HAVE INSOMNIA ALMOST EVERY NIGHT: 35

PERCENTAGE WHO FREQUENTLY WAKE UP EARLY AND CAN'T FALL BACK ASLEEP: 24

HOW TO SWALLOW SOME SLEEP

For the occasional sleep emergency, avoid over-the-counter sleep remedies. They contain antihistamines that can linger in your body for 8 hours or more, leaving you groggy in the morning. Ask your doctor for a prescription instead. He could set you up with such old standbys as Valium or Dalmane, but the newcomers Ambien and Sonata are better choices. "The older sleeping pills suppress slow-wave, or deep, sleep. The newer medications don't," says Timothy Roehrs, Ph.D., of the Sleep Disorders and Research Center at the Henry Ford Hospital in Detroit.

• **If you can't fall asleep,** go with Sonata; it starts working in 15 to 30 minutes and leaves your bloodstream in about an hour. If tossing and turning is the problem, Ambien is the way to go. It sticks around three times as long as Sonata, but there's no morning hangover. Just remember that both drugs are only temporary fixes. "These have been tested only for short-term use, up to 5 weeks," says Roehrs. "The long-term effects just aren't known."

• **If you've been losing sleep for 2 weeks** (worrying about that embezzlement scheme), then a sleeping pill may be a good idea. But if a month goes by and you're still sleepless, you may have a more complicated problem. See your doctor in the morning.

screen out the distractions: specifically, MSA Safety Works foam earplugs, a SleepMate white-noise generator, and Roc Lon blackout drapes. You'll be less accessible than God.

3. Kids waking you up? Order a copy of *Solve Your Child's Sleep Problems* by Richard Ferber, M.D. It's knocked out generations of wakeful tots. If the problem is an older child, **take the TV out of his bedroom.** A study at Brown University showed a link between easy access to the tube and increased sleep disturbances.

4. **Go for a brisk six-block walk.** According to University of Arizona researchers, that's the amount of exercise that's best at reducing sleep disruptions in men. (A regular workout program came in a close second.) Just do it in the late afternoon, like when you get off work. This will cause your body temperature to drop a few hours later, making you drowsy right before bedtime.

YOUR FIFTIES AND BEYOND

Here's when it all comes apart. In the previously mentioned *JAMA* study, the researchers found that after men turn 50, they get 28 minutes less sleep with each decade that passes. "By the time men reach their fifties and sixties, they have almost no deep sleep," says Sonia Ancoli-Israel, Ph.D., director of the Sleep Disorders Clinic at the VA Medical Center in San Diego. A man in his fifties has nighttime cortisol levels 12 times higher than when he was in his thirties. Nearly one in 25 also has sleep apnea—a condition that interrupts normal breathing. And then there's the expanding-prostate problem: A swollen gland may prevent you from fully emptying your bladder, which means you'll make approximately 7,422 nightly trips to the toilet.

The Four-Step Fix

1. **Grab some vitamin B$_5$, and wash it down with Gatorade about half an hour before bedtime.** British researchers have found that athletes who down a high-carbohydrate drink have a lower exercise-induced cortisol spike than those who don't.

2. Get checked for sleep apnea. If it's just plain old snoring, **ask your doctor about injection snoreplasty.** During this 15-minute procedure, a doctor will stiffen your soft palate—the fleshy area above your uvula that causes snoring—with an injection of sodium tetradecyl sulfate. Cost: $35, which is cheap compared with a divorce settlement. Results last about a year.

3. **Check your medications.** A study published in the *European Journal of Clinical Pharmacology* found that beta-blockers, a common treatment for high blood pressure, decreased melatonin production by 80 to 90 percent. Carvedilol is the only beta-blocker that didn't affect melatonin levels. Another culprit may be Prozac and similar drugs, which can lead to as much as a 30 percent increase in awakenings. Contemplate a switch to Paxil; it may actually help you fall asleep faster.

4. If you're peeing three or more times a night, consult a urologist. Odds are that your prostate is enlarged, a common problem for older men. Before you try drugs or surgery, **consider taking saw palmetto.** In a *JAMA* review of 18 studies, saw palmetto reduced the incidence of nocturia—the nighttime urge to urinate—by 25 percent. Look for ProstActive by Nature's Way; it's the most clinically studied brand of saw palmetto available.

KNOW THIS

Think Better outside the Box

It's time to tell the boss that your work space, that miserable cubicle he sneeringly calls an office, is making you sick—and hurting his company. A study in the *Journal of Applied Psychology* found that people who work in cubicles have higher levels of stress hormones than those who work in offices with doors. More important (to your bottom-line boss) is another study showing that, compared with cubicles, open offices encourage productivity and increase morale. A team-oriented workplace without dividers enables workers to read one another's body language and gauge when to interrupt, says the study author, Frank Becker, Ph.D., of Cornell University.

Boot the Beast

Dogs and cats can be con artists, swindling prime nocturnal real estate on your bed. And if you're letting your dogs get away with it, they're probably stealing your sleep as well. John Shepard, M.D., medical director at the Mayo Clinic Sleep Disorders Center, found that 22 percent of the center's patients let their pets sleep on the bed, and 53 percent of those patients said their sleep was disrupted to some extent. Dr. Shepard believes that rate may be much higher—think of all that shifting, growling, and dream running going on next to you. So you miss the quality sleep your body needs to restore itself. We say kick out the canine. If you want to lose sleep with a bedmate, lose it the right way.

Supplement Scare

The German government is considering banning the sale of kava kava, an over-the-counter herbal supplement that reportedly helps treat insomnia and anxiety. The pills have been linked to more than 20 cases of liver damage in Germany. In the United States, food supplements, including kava kava, are not regulated by the Food and Drug Administration.

Head Case

After measuring the noggins of 2,000 people, University of Washington researchers found that men with both a gene linked to Alzheimer's and a small head (less than 21 inches around, measured around the crown, or a hat size of 6¾ or smaller) are up to 14 times more likely to develop Alzheimer's than men with an average-size cranium (22 inches or larger).

The best defense against the disease? Keep using your head.

People who stay mentally active throughout their lives are three times less likely to develop Alzheimer's disease than people who gradually give up mental activities as they get older, according to a separate study from Case Western Reserve University in Cleveland. "Staying active keeps neurons in your brain strong and makes them more resistant to the age-related degeneration that appears to trigger Alzheimer's," says Robert Friedland, Ph.D., the study author.

Stop Alzheimer's, Stat!

Cholesterol-lowering medications called statins may also reduce the incidence of Alzheimer's disease. In animal studies, the drugs simvastatin and lovastatin significantly reduced levels of a brain compound called amyloid, which is commonly associated with the development of Alzheimer's.

Smart Sauce

Moderate drinkers do better on IQ tests than nondrinkers. According to Japanese research, small amounts of alcohol improve bloodflow to the brain, enhancing memory and mental function.

Blue Matter

Tufts University researchers have found that anthocyanins—the chemicals that make blueberries blue—boost the ability of brain cells to send and receive signals from other cells. So toss some blueberries on your cereal and wise up.

DOWN THE PIKE

Can You Sit Still for This?

There may soon be a test for attention deficit disorder. Researchers in Boston are working to develop a procedure to detect chemicals in the brain that may signify the presence of the condition.

Mind Reader

A diagnostic test for Alzheimer's disease is also in the works. Researchers in California have developed a procedure that detects small lesions in the brain—one of the first symptoms of the disorder. Early testing may allow doctors to treat patients with the disease before it progresses to a more serious stage.

DOES IT WORK?

Herbal Cure-All

Ginseng—which is given credit for solving everything from depression to credit card debt—has suffered a couple of setbacks. In an Oregon State University study, 60 days of ginseng supplements did not improve the mood of 83 college students any better than a sugar pill did. And the journal *Nutrition Reviews* looked at recent studies and found "no compelling evidence" that the root extract helped physical function or energy level—caffeine works better, the journal said. "The jury is still out" on ginseng's purported effect on sexual performance and stress busting, says David Grotto, R.D., the director of nutrition education at the Block Medical Center in Evanston, Illinois.

Music for the Mind

The "Mozart effect" refers to the boost in spatial reasoning power caused by listening to a Mozart piano sonata. But the positive effects appear to be exclusive to Wolfgang's tunes. The latest confirmation, from the University of California at Irvine, shows that Mozart's music offers a significantly bigger boost than Beethoven's "Für Elise" or 1930s piano music. Take that, Ludwig van.

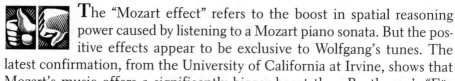

WHAT'S THE DIFF?

Psychiatrist vs. Psychologist

A psychiatrist is an M.D. who will listen to your problems and can write prescriptions. A psychologist usually is a Ph.D. and will listen to your problems but can't get you drugs.

Dementia vs. Alzheimer's Disease

Dementia is a catchall term for many different disorders that make you lose your marbles. True dementias, such as those caused by folic acid deficiency (which is reversible) or Parkinson's disease (which isn't), result from physical damage to the brain. The brain fog that sometimes accompanies depression and other mental disorders is known as pseudodementia.

Alzheimer's disease—the real thing, not "Now, where did I leave those keys?"—is the most common true dementia, accounting for up to 70 percent of senility in senior citizens.

TAKE ACTION

In today's computer age, we not only expect our PCs to boot up faster, offer a gazillion applications, and hold more memory—we expect the same from our brains. Well, consider this your guide to getting the most from that hard drive situated between your shoulders. These strategies will prevent any short circuits caused by stress or fatigue, not to mention they'll boost your brain-power, keep depression at bay, and help you stay sharp. Download away. . . .

1. Order Indian. A California study found that curcumin—a compound found in the Indian spice turmeric—may slow down or prevent the progression of Alzheimer's disease. "Curcumin is a powerful anti-inflammatory agent," says Greg Cole, M.D., the study author. The spice is so powerful, in fact, that Dr. Cole believes it may be responsible for the low incidence of Alzheimer's in India. Don't like food that burns? Curcumin is also available as a supplement.

2. Make like the Sailor Man. According to a new study, Popeye's favorite greens may help keep your brain younger and more active. Researchers at the University of South Florida recently found that rats who were given spinach supplements learned certain behaviors more quickly than rats that didn't get the supplements. The reason: Spinach contains high levels of vitamins C and E, along with several antioxidants known to protect cells from free radical damage, says Paula Bickford, Ph.D., the study author. Scientists have long suspected that free radical damage to cells increases the risks of developing Alzheimer's and Parkinson's diseases.

3. Wise up. So you missed the Ivy League by a few hundred SAT points. Make the most of your gray matter by heeding the latest advice of these brain researchers.

Gum up the works. British researchers found that chewing gum boosted heart rate and helped with short-term recall. Why? Either the faster heart rate delivers more oxygen and glucose to the brain, or saliva triggers a surge of insulin, stimulating learning and memory receptors, says Andrew Scholey, Ph.D., a researcher at the University of Northumbria.

Play mind games. Puzzles extend your dendrites, the antennae of your brain's neurons. Here are two easy teasers for your brain's right (artistic) and left (logical) sides, from *The Memory Bible* by Gary Small, M.D.

- Right brain: Arrange five toothpicks into the numeral 5. Then, without breaking any, rearrange them into the number 16.

- Left brain: Find the proverb in this string of vowel-less letters: RLL NGSTN GTH RSN MSS.

See page 216 for the answers.

4. Skip the bad news. Call them ill-informed, but people who turn off the news because it's too much of a downer could be staving off depression. Research found that a bad-news broadcast could trigger anxiety and depression in otherwise cheerful people. It's not the news itself that we worry about. Watching thousands starving in Somalia can trigger personal worries—anxiety about anything from a minor work crisis to a sick relative.

5. Fill up on fiber. People who frequently eat high-fiber foods have a more positive outlook on life and are less likely to have symptoms of depression than people who eat less fiber, according to a new U.K. study. Researchers are still working to determine the cause of the link.

6. Keep your edge when you're exhausted. Robert Montgomery, M.D., Ph.D., a transplant surgeon at Johns Hopkins Hospital, sometimes faces 12 hours of surgery followed by a day of seeing patients, teaching students, and catching up on office work. Here's how he copes.

Keep moving. "The challenge comes after I leave the operating room—then I feel like crashing, even though I'm not finished with work. I only do the things that require me to be on my feet. If I have to be in my office, I'll stand. I won't work at the computer. I'll do things involving human interaction that keep me engaged. And I take the stairs."

Shower. "It's worth 2 hours of sleep."

Catnap. "I won't nap for longer than 30 minutes, preferably only 15. And you can't get too comfortable, or you'll sleep too deeply and wake up feeling like you're drunk. I'll sit and put my head on my desk. A Barcalounger is death."

Play some tunes. "Surgery is like a dance, and music helps me get into a rhythm. I'll pick stuff that's both soothing and upbeat and play it loud, someone like Susan Tedeschi, Bruce Springsteen, Natalie Merchant, or one of my favorites, Barry White."

Lighten things up. "I'll go into a routine where I tease and joke and do a little Barry White impression—'Your sweetness is my weakness.' It keeps things lighthearted, and laughing raises your energy level."

7. Pop a pep pill. Another way to stay sharp on little sleep: Swallow some NADH, a coenzyme that may increase mental alertness and concentration.

PERCENTAGE OF MEN WHO RATE THEIR MENTAL HEALTH AS EXCELLENT OR GOOD: 89

PERCENTAGE OF WOMEN WHO DO: 82

In one New York–Presbyterian Hospital study, researchers tested 25 sleep-deprived people after the group had taken 20 milligrams of NADH and then again after they'd taken a placebo.

"When the people took NADH, they performed significantly better overall on a set of mental tests using a measure of speed and accuracy," says Margaret Moline, Ph.D., one of the study researchers. Look for supplements that say "ENADA" on the label; they contain the same NADH formulation used in studies.

8. Bypass the buffet. Ben Franklin once said, "A full Belly makes a dull Brain." He was right. The gastric acid your stomach uses to digest a protein-heavy meal forms bicarbonate, which alters your blood pH and indeed causes "dullness in the brain," says Philip Miner, M.D., medical director of the Oklahoma Foundation for Digestive Research. The best meal for a controlled release of energy throughout the afternoon: chicken on whole wheat with a piece of fruit and some juice.

9. Leave stress at work. The ultimate stress monster is a jaw-jutting, red-faced marine drill instructor. But after screaming at maggots all day, he has to leave his finger-pointing persona on the post. Gunnery Sergeant Rick Williams, the chief instructor at the Marine Corps's Drill Instructor School at Parris Island, South Carolina, told us how he chills out, after we asked. Politely. Sir!

- Williams ends each workday by mapping tomorrow's plan of attack. "That way I'm not doing it on the drive home from work, or at the dinner table, or in bed at 2 A.M.," he says. "I've got things wired tightly before I walk out the rear hatch."
- At 1631 (4:31 P.M.), Williams removes his "Smokey Bear" campaign hat and dons a ball-cap–style "soft cover" worn by all marines regardless of rank. "When I do that, I'm telling myself that that part of my day is done. It's over. Then I let it all go," he says. The next step: 5 to 15 minutes of thinking about anything but recruit training.
- Drill instructors (DIs) are known for screaming bloody hell and demanding perfection. But Williams reminds his students that being a Marine Corps DI is just a job. "It's a very important job, but a job nonetheless," he says. "When you realize that, it's easier to give yourself a break."
- Williams takes a nightly walk with his wife. Every DI needs to relax. "We don't like to admit it, but even marines are human," he says. "If you play the role every minute of every day, you'll burn out."
- "My wife and my kids are not recruits," Williams says. "They don't want to see Gunnery Sergeant Williams when I come home. They want to see Dad and husband. I want that, too."

10. Stop the juggling act. Multitasking is overrated, a new study suggests. Your brain's gear shifting takes time, and even a simple task can take up to 50 percent longer when you're distracted by other jobs, says one study coauthor, David Meyer, Ph.D., of the University of Michigan. Here are some tips for keeping focused on one job at a time.

Use an **L**-*shaped desk.* Designate one side for right-now work, the other for later-on work. "The **L** shape prevents you from being distracted by other projects right in front of you and saves time in sorting things out," says Stephanie Denton, president of the National Association of Professional Organizers.

Use vertical file holders on your desk. Papers scattered across your desk will keep screaming for attention. File them away—but not in a cabinet, where you might forget about them.

Take a cyber vacation. Use the "out of office" reply on your e-mail while you put your nose to the grindstone for a couple of hours.

Intercept the paper storm. Hang a plastic wall pocket on your door so incoming papers won't interrupt your concentration.

Create a schedule and stick to it. Work expands or contracts to fit the time allotted; you'll amp up your concentration if you're aware that time is running out, Denton says.

ANSWERS TO BRAIN TEASERS ON PAGES 213 AND 214: Make Roman numeral XVI; A rolling stone gathers no moss.

NUMBER OF MENTAL TASKS AMONG WHICH THE AVERAGE MAN IS CAPABLE OF DIVIDING HIS ATTENTION: 4

A N Y   Q U E S T I O N S ?

You Snooze, You Lose

Why does taking a nap make me feel worse than if I get no sleep at all?

—R. V., Birmingham, Alabama

If you doze through the full 60 minutes of *60 Minutes*, you're sleeping too long. The ideal nap length is 20 to 40 minutes, says Richard Rosenberg, Ph.D., director of the sleep disorders center at Evanston Northwestern Healthcare in Illinois. Any longer and your brain slacks off into REM sleep, a deep state of sleep and the one during which most dream activity occurs. Get suddenly rousted, and you may find yourself spouting vestiges of that dream with Cameron Diaz covered in Smuckers—bad during a board meeting. At best, you'll be left feeling groggy and discombobulated. At worst, your boss will start calling you Lady Marmalade.

To keep your snoozes short, find a private spot for a siesta and do what Salvador Dali did: Before dozing off, he would place a metal plate on the floor and hold a spoon in his hand. As he lapsed into REM sleep, his muscles would relax, and he'd drop the spoon on the plate and awake refreshed. Of course, those newfangled alarm clocks work, too.

"I'd Like to Make a Deposit"

I've got a crazy week at work coming up, plus a bunch of social events. Can I "store up" sleep by getting extra the week before?

—B. L., Dallas

Sorry, your body's not a bank account. If you're overdrawn on sleep, you can't just pluck it out of savings. In your case, the best bet is to improve the quality of the sleep you do get, so you won't end up with your nose in your salad on Thursday, says Jon Magee, Ph.D., director of the Sleep Disorder Center at Research Medical Center in Kansas City, Missouri. Do this for a few days before and during your crazy week.

- Squeeze 15 minutes of exercise into your day. Walking is fine. It'll enhance the quality of your sleep.

- Don't drink beverages with caffeine after 3 P.M., and avoid heavy foods after 7. Caffeine, of course, is a stimulant, but it also can trigger heartburn, indigestion, and acid reflux from a big meal.
- Stick to just two alcoholic beverages. Any more and your body will spend the night metabolizing alcohol, which interferes with quality sleep.
- Finally, if you are dead tired by Friday, try this strategy to prepare for important work. Drink two cups of coffee and immediately take a 20- to 25-minute combat nap. You'll be able to nap, says Magee, because it generally takes about 25 minutes for caffeine to reach your bloodstream. When you wake up, the combination of caffeine and rest will create an "alerting effect" that will last about 2 hours, he says.

Help for Hibernators

Every winter, all I want to do is stay holed up at home, eating, sleeping and writing angry letters to the phone company. Is there anything I can do about this?

—T. K., Lincoln, Montana

Some degree of unwillingness to face those dark, cold mornings is normal (along with the temptation to brighten your days with meatball sandwiches). But if you notice significant changes—you experience feelings of hopelessness and guilt, your sleep and eating patterns shift, you lose interest in watching hockey brawls—you may have seasonal affective disorder (SAD). This type of depression results from the waning daylight of the fall and winter, says Brian Doyle, M.D., clinical professor of psychiatry and family and community medicine at Georgetown University School of Medicine. Depression isn't something you can diagnose yourself, says Dr. Doyle, so see a psychiatrist if you suspect you have SAD. It's a common condition, especially in northern latitudes, and can usually be treated by spending time in front of an electric light box, which gives off light that's calibrated to mimic the natural light of the spring and summer. (Watching more TV won't have the same effect—sorry.) "Most people with SAD find that using these boxes for half an hour every morning makes a huge difference in how they feel," Dr. Doyle says. So can avoiding alcohol and picking up the pace of your exercise program.

PERCENTAGE OF THE WORKFORCE THAT
REGULARLY WORKS MORE THAN 40 HOURS A WEEK: 33

PERCENTAGE THAT WORKS
MORE THAN 50 HOURS: ABOUT 20

PART FIVE
SAVE YOUR SICK DAYS

Who Will Fight Off a Cold First?
One of these three snifflers—or you?

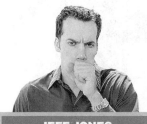

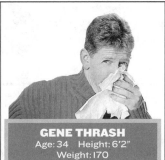

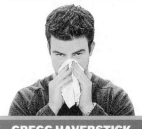

JEFF JONES
Age: 26   Height: 6'0"
Weight: 175

GENE THRASH
Age: 34   Height: 6'2"
Weight: 170

GREGG HAVERSTICK
Age: 25   Height: 5'9"
Weight: 165

STRATEGY
- Natural remedies. At the first symptom of a cold, Jones will pop vitamin C, echinacea, and zinc lozenges—natural supplements that he believes lessen cold symptoms.
- He'll work and exercise as usual.

POSSIBLE RISKS
- He's a business consultant who works under deadline 10 to 12 hours a day and travels frequently. Chronic stress can suppress the immune system because the body diverts energy to more immediate crises.
- Some nights he gets less than 4 hours of sleep, which may run down his body's defenses.

POSSIBLE DEFENSES
- Jones exercises at least three times a week and eats a healthful diet. Fresh fruits and vegetables fuel the body's defenses. Moderate exercise doesn't appear to help or hinder a cold once you have one.

JEFF'S PREDICTION
- "My friends call me Dr. Jones for a reason. My immune system is solid, so when the cold strikes, I'll be ready."

STRATEGY
- Take it easy and tough it out. No medication or herbal remedies.
- He'll take a break from his usual heavy exercise routine, go to bed early, eat chicken noodle soup, and drink lots of hot tea. Mother would be very pleased.

POSSIBLE RISKS
- Thrash is a high school teacher with a long workday, lots of stress, and plenty of exposure to sick students—three factors that might make him more susceptible to catching colds in the first place.
- He doesn't take any medications or remedies to lessen cold symptoms.

POSSIBLE DEFENSES
- Normally, he relaxes with lots of hard-core cycling, kayaking, and weight training. When sick, he'll take time off, which might be a good idea. Intense exercise may suppress the immune system during an infection.

GENE'S PREDICTION
- "I'll feel better in no time. The body recovers by itself, and I'm strong from all the exercise I normally do."

STRATEGY
- Over-the-counter medicine. Haverstick will take cold-and-sinus tablets with ibuprofen, but probably not until the symptoms get bad—a couple of days into the illness.

POSSIBLE RISKS
- He's a businessman who occasionally works late under deadline and entertains clients.
- In a typical week, Haverstick will have three dinner meetings scheduled, and he isn't likely to cancel one on account of a cold. He anticipates having at least three alcoholic drinks at each of these dinners.

POSSIBLE DEFENSES
- Overall, he regards his life as relaxed.
- He exercises several times a week, eats a balanced diet, and takes a daily multivitamin.
- He averages about 7½ hours of sleep per night.

GREGG'S PREDICTION
- "Nothing slows me down. I'm a healthy guy who never stays sick for long."

And the Winner Is . . .
Gregg Haverstick

Jack Gwaltney, M.D., head of epidemiology and virology at the University of Virginia School of Medicine, helped us devise the test on the opposite page to gauge which guy would stop sneezing first. Take it yourself to find out how you'll fare.

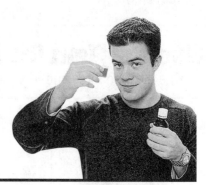

HOW HE BEAT THE BUG

Haverstick will be a step ahead of the other contestants because he plans to take medication that has been proven to work, says Jack Gwaltney, M.D., head of epidemiology and virology at the University of Virginia School of Medicine. "Thrash isn't treating it at all, and Jones is taking remedies that are less effective, if they work at all."

However, Haverstick will have the best relief if he takes a more effective combination of drugs, and takes them sooner. "He should take a first-generation antihistamine and a nonsteroidal anti-inflammatory drug such as ibuprofen," Dr. Gwaltney says. Look for the antihistamines chlorpheniramine, which is in Chlor-Trimeton, or clemastine. These drugs may cause drowsiness, but nonsedating antihistamines aren't effective in treating colds. Taking an antihistamine and ibuprofen every 12 hours reduces mucus by 30 to 40 percent and sneezing by 70 percent, according to Dr. Gwaltney's studies.

Jones swears by his natural remedies. However, Dr. Gwaltney says large doses of vitamin C help dry up mucus in the nose, but not as effectively as antihistamines, and vitamin C will not benefit other symptoms, such as sore throat and cough.

There's no valid reasoning behind Thrash's method. Although a cold is usually self-limited, which means it'll go away on its own, it could develop into a more serious problem, such as sinusitis. Also, why not feel better if you can? Thrash is wise to curtail his exercise and get extra rest. And although the soup and tea won't cure the cold, both will keep him hydrated, which is also a good idea.

As for alcohol? "I wouldn't recommend downing five or six beers when you have a cold," says Dr. Gwaltney.

COLD FACTS: How Do You Compare?

FACTOR	POINT VALUE	JEFF	GENE	GREGG	YOU
TREATMENT A cold should be treated at the very first symptoms.	Ignore? −2		−2		
	Wait a day or two? −1			−1	
	Treat immediately? +1	+1			
MEDICINE First-generation antihistamines and nonsteroidal anti-inflammatories work best to treat most cold symptoms. An oral decongestant may also be helpful if needed.	Don't take medication? −1	−1	−1		
	Take a first-generation antihistamine? +2				
	Take ibuprofen? +2			+2	
	Take decongestants? +1			+1	
	Take another pain reliever? +1				
OTHER REMEDIES Vitamin C has a mild effect on a cold, by drying up mucus in the nose. Most scientific studies have failed to show a useful treatment effect for echinacea or zinc.	Take zinc lozenges? 0	0			
	Take echinacea? 0	0			
	Take no natural remedies? 0		0	0	
	Take extra vitamin C? +1	+1			
SLEEP Adequate sleep is important for your body's overall ability to function well, particularly during an illness.	Sleep less than 7 hours a night? −1	−1			
	Sleep 7 hours or more? +1		+1	+1	
STRESS Psychological stress may make it more difficult to fight a cold.	Very stressed? −1	−1	−1		
	Recent stressful event? −1				
	Not stressed? 0			0	
EXERCISE Moderate exercise during a cold appears to be neither harmful nor helpful. Heavy exercise should be avoided.	Heavy exercise during a cold? −1				
	Moderate or no exercise during a cold? 0	0	0	0	
DIET A healthful diet may help keep the body's defenses strong.	Healthful diet? +1	+1	+1	+1	
	Low calorie intake? −1				
	Recent drastic weight loss? −1				
ALCOHOL Heavy drinking could lead to dehydration and cause further suppression of immune function.	More than a few drinks a day during a cold? −1			−1	
	Avoid alcohol during a cold? +1	+1	+1		
SMOKING Cigarette smoking is likely to worsen cold symptoms.	Smoker? −1				
	Nonsmoker? 0	0	0	0	
AGE Immune function decreases with age, so it may take your body longer to fight off an infection.	65 or over? −1				
	Under 65? 0	0	0	0	
TOTALS		+1	−1	+3	

▶ **IF YOUR SCORE IS +2 OR MORE:** You'll be feeling better in no time.

▶ **IF YOUR SCORE IS −1 TO +1:** You'll be stuck with this cold for the average length of time.

▶ **IF YOUR SCORE IS −2 OR LESS:** Get a few more boxes of Kleenex.

MUST READS

Put Out the Fire

Feel like somebody stuck a blowtorch down your throat? You may be one of the millions of men who suffer from acid reflux problems. Here's your fire extinguisher

By Bill Gottlieb

Tomato sauce almost wrecked Jim Donaldson's life.

Donaldson—a 42-year-old corporate VP—has a wife who used to make the same dinner every Wednesday night: spaghetti with homemade tomato sauce. Delicious, acidic tomato sauce. And every Wednesday after dinner, Jim staged a scene from the little-known Verdi opera *Bruciore di Stomaco*. He belched. He bloated. He burned. When he went to sleep, the acid rolled from gut to gullet like a swell in the Atlantic during a nor'easter.

Soon Jim's symptoms showed up every night; restless nights made him oversleep. He became so irritable his boss nearly canned him, so he finally saw a doctor, who told him he had the same problem that 60 million other Americans had. The diagnosis was gastroesophageal reflux disease, or GERD.

GERD is the foul-sounding acronym for all the symptoms of acid reflux disease—a bio-blenderized mixture of hydrochloric acid, bile salts, digestive enzymes, and liquefied food that travels north instead of south, repeatedly seeping out of the stomach and into the esophagus. It's what produces familiar frat-house symptoms like bloating, burping, heartburn, trench mouth, and nausea. And for about 10 percent of men—mostly the 40-plus crowd—years of acid reflux trigger weird cellular changes that may become esophageal cancer.

Thankfully, most causes of GERD are linked to things you eat or stuff you do, which means you can control the problem yourself. Take Jim. He beat it by cutting down on acid-triggering foods, stopping his after-dinner snack habit, and regularly popping an acid-blocking drug. So whether your acid-spitting monster is life-threatening or life-bothering, easy solutions and new medical treatments can help stop the burning.

THE DINNER OPTIONS

Hold the pepperoni. Fat triggers a hormone that relaxes the lower esophageal sphincter (LES). That sphincter is important not only because it's a great punch line in *SNL* skits but also because it's the valve that stops acid from flowing back into your esophagus. When the LES relaxes, acid can creep into your throat, says Steven Peikin, M.D., head of the division of gastroenterology and liver disease at the Cooper Hospital/University Medical Center in New Jersey. Fatty foods also delay digestion, giving acid more time to do its dirty work. Go for 30 percent of calories or less from fat at any meal.

Chew gum. Saliva contains a natural bicarbonate that neutralizes stomach acid, helping to clear it from the esophagus, says Donald Castell, M.D., a professor of medicine at the MCP Hahnemann University School of Medicine in Philadelphia. Like Charles Barkley, gum chewers generate a lot of saliva.

Put an ice cube in your coffee. Hot beverages aren't dangerous only to your crotch. They can also damage the tissues of the esophagus, which makes the tube more vulnerable to acid, says Roy Orlando, M.D., chief of gastroenterology at Tulane University's health sciences center in New Orleans. Studies show that people with heartburn prefer their drinks hotter than people who don't have the disease, so you'll consciously have to cool your drinks. Example: Some fast-food restaurants serve coffee at 176°F, but the safe level for reflux sufferers is 120°F to 130°F. No thermometer on your money clip? If it's too hot to put a finger in, it's too hot to drink.

THE ANTI-ACID PIZZA

Doctors will tell you that a pepperoni pizza is just about the worst food an acid reflux sufferer can eat. This recipe from *Men's Health* magazine's Chef Vinny is an alternative that'll give you twice the spice and half the pain. The mango chunks contain an enzyme that improves digestion, and the ginger and mint can help calm a queasy stomach. The black beans? Well, they're one of the few bean varieties that won't add gas to an already shaky situation.

Buy This

• I can (IO ounces) Pillsbury Refrigerated All Ready Pizza Crust

• I can (15 ounces) mango chunks, drained

• 7 ounces black beans (from a can), drained

• I teaspoon minced ginger (from a jar)

• 2 tablespoons shredded fresh mint

• I½ cups shredded light mozzarella cheese

Do This

Spray a baking sheet with cooking spray. Unroll the dough and press it into a thin crust. Bake the crust at 425°F for 7 minutes or until it begins to brown, then remove from the oven. Mix together the mango chunks, black beans, ginger, and mint. Top the crust with the cheese, then layer it with the bean mixture. Bake at 425°F for 6 minutes or until the cheese is slightly melted. Makes 5 slices.

Per slice: 260 calories, 17 grams (g) protein, 39 g carbohydrates, 4 g fat, 3 g fiber

Skip after-dinner mints. At the table, limit your GERD-triggering foods, such as tomatoes, citrus juice, calcium, carbonated drinks, and salt. And no after-dinner mints or chocolates: They'll keep your LES relaxed and trigger the burn.

THE AFTER-DINNER OPTIONS

Loosen up. Most men don't suffer from heartburn during the day. That's because gravity helps keep acid out of your esophagus. The trouble comes after dinner—when you're lying on the couch, in bed, or next to the bar stool. After dinner, loosen your belt or slip into sweats. Relieving the pressure on your gut can keep the acid from squirting up into your esophagus, says Dr. Castell.

Sleep on your left side. Quick anatomy lesson: The stomach is on your left side, and the esophagus enters it from the right. When you lie on your left side, the esophagus is higher than your stomach, so stomach contents pool away from the organ, says Dr. Castell. You roll over more than an SUV? Put a pillow behind your back. And don't eat within 3 hours of bedtime.

Prop yourself up. If you elevate the head of your bed 6 inches, acid will be less likely to flow into your esophagus.

THE MEDICAL OPTIONS

Try an OTC remedy. Dr. Peikin recommends Pepcid Complete, which combines an antacid (to make stomach contents less acidic) and an H_2 blocker (to cut down on acid production). Using antacids more than twice a week? See a doctor.

Get a prescription. If OTCs aren't effective, your doctor may suggest taking an H_2 blocker, like nonprescription Zantac or Tagamet HB, to control the symptoms. Or he may prescribe a proton pump inhibitor (PPI), like Prevacid or Prilosec, to both control reflux and heal a damaged esophagus.

Clean out your medicine cabinet. Heart, blood pressure, and asthma medications can cause reflux, while aspirin and ibuprofen can worsen an inflamed esophagus. Ask your doctor if there are any medications you can ditch.

Take the test. If you're older than 50 and you've had heartburn for at least 5 years, you're probably going to need an endoscopy. A doctor will insert a very slender tube with a tiny video camera through your nose into your esophagus. The thin tube is so unobtrusive you won't need sedation for the 15-minute procedure. (Really. We saw Dr. Benton do it once on *ER*.) The doctor wants to detect or rule out the presence of chronic inflammation of the esophagus (esophagitis), an esophageal ulcer, or esophageal cancer.

Consider surgery. Surgery is usually reserved for people who don't want to stay on acid-controlling drugs for the rest of their lives. A procedure called laparoscopic Nissen undoplication will put you in the hospital overnight and back to work in a week. Too busy for that? The FDA recently approved two outpatient GERD procedures that tighten the lower esophageal sphincter (insert audience laugh track here).

The Best Drugs for the Job

Thousands of over-the-counter remedies are vying for a spot in your medicine cabinet. But only a handful provide the ingredients you need

By Ted Spiker

I'm itching—in a place I'd rather not mention. Not to my doctor, not to my wife, and certainly not to anyone who's about to shake my hand.

I'd much rather stand in the anti-itch aisle of the drugstore, scan the products anonymously, and clear this whole thing up tonight. So I'll try a hydrocortisone cream. But maybe benzocaine would be better. Or perhaps diphenhydramine, or propylene glycol, or aloe barbadensis, or oatmeal. Oatmeal?

Uh, I'll take the one in the green box.

Surely you've had a nagging ailment and rushed to a drugstore for relief, only to be baffled by the selection of remedies. And you do what anyone would do when faced with a multiple-choice exam he hasn't studied for: You guess. I guessed wrong. Five bucks bought me the tactile equivalent of a jellyfish in my underwear. And I'm still scratching.

See the problem? The best medicines are worthless if we never find them. So we turned to the experts who actually know what the heck is in the roughly 100,000 nonprescription products sold in the United States. When we said, "Sore throat," they said, "Suck on this." When it came to "Unmentionable itch," they didn't hesitate: "Avoid the green box." And so on, until we had it all. Picking the right medicine is still a test, but at least now you have the answer key.

ALLERGIES (SNEEZING, WATERING EYES)

First, get her cat off your lap, then pop an allergy medicine that contains the antihistamine chlorpheniramine. It'll help dry up your watery eyes and stop the sneezing without making you drowsy. If staying conscious isn't an issue, go with diphenhydramine; it's the most effective ingredient for relieving allergy symptoms. "But chemically, it creates the highest degree of drowsiness," says Paul Doering, a national OTC expert at the University of Florida.

Brand to look for: Chlor-Trimeton Allergy 4-Hour Tablets, or generic

What the package doesn't tell you: If you also have an allergy-induced headache, take a separate painkiller (whatever you'd normally take for head pain), rather than an allergy medication that comes with a pain reliever in it. "You want to be able to have the flexibility to take a little more or less painkiller within the label guidelines," says Doering.

ATHLETE'S FOOT AND JOCK ITCH

Annihilate the itch with a product containing terbinafine. Australian researchers found that 85 percent of people using terbinafine had their athlete's foot clear up in 1 week, compared with only 56 percent of those using the antifungal agent clotrimazole. If the infection lingers for longer than 3 weeks, ask your doctor about the more powerful, oral form of terbinafine.

Brand to look for: Lamisil AT

What the package doesn't tell you: Lamisil AT is the only product that currently contains terbinafine, but man, is it pricey. Go with the 1-ounce spray bottle ($9); you'll get more uses out of it than you will with the 0.85-ounce cream ($13).

YOU WON'T NEED A DOCTOR'S NOTE

There's no explosion and flash of light when the FDA makes a prescription drug available over the counter. It's still the same drug. The big difference is the dosage and that you'll now have instant access to a medicine that may be more powerful than anything else in the aisle. But don't get too excited; the switch to OTC doesn't happen often since safety concerns are the reason most drugs are prescription in the first place.

Here's a list of possible OTC candidates, courtesy of Donna Edenhart, a spokeswoman for the Consumer Healthcare Products Association.

Prilosec. It's the best-selling prescription heartburn medication, thanks to the proton pump inhibitor (PPI) omeprazole. PPIs do the same trick of stopping acid flow as H$_2$ blockers, only better. In fact, some research has shown that omeprazole relieves the symptoms of acid reflux more effectively than other prescription ingredients.

Cholesterol-lowering statins. Even though FDA officials turned down Merck's request to switch lovastatin to OTC, it's likely that Merck and other drug companies will try again. According to Edenhart, the companies now know what the FDA's concerns are and are probably working to address them.

Allegra and Claritin. Even the least-sedating OTC antihistamines can cause a little drowsiness. Not Claritin and Allegra; they're the only nonsedating antihistamines available. However, Paul Doering, a national expert on OTCs at the University of Florida, says that anecdotal evidence shows this may come at a price of slightly decreased effectiveness.

Appetite suppressants. Doering says any drugs that appeal to vanity may work their way into OTC status. (Rogaine used to be prescription.) Some appetite-suppressing drugs—like Adipex, Bontril, and Meridia—fall into this category, but the stimulating effects of their ingredients—phentermine, phendimetrazine, and sibutramine—raise safety concerns that may keep them in the pharmacy.

CANKER SORES

While you're waiting for these painful mouth ulcers to heal, numb out with a gel that contains 2-octyl-cyanoacrylate. "It's effective because it seals off the nerve endings that trigger the pain," says Nicholas Popovich, Ph.D., a professor at the University of Illinois at Chicago college of pharmacy. While oral pain relievers that contain benzocaine can also deaden the pain, they've been known to cause allergic reactions.

Brand to look for: Colgate Orabase Soothe-N-Seal

What the package doesn't tell you: Canker sores can take 14 days to disappear, but if yours hasn't healed by then or begins oozing, see your doctor to rule out a more serious infection or mouth cancer.

CONSTIPATION

Leave the Ex-Lax for the practical jokes. Stimulant laxatives not only clear out today's waste; they go so far up your intestinal tract that they clear out tomorrow's waste, too. As a result, you won't have the urge to go tomorrow, so you may mistakenly think you're still constipated and need another laxative, says Steven Pray, Ph.D., a professor of nonprescription products and devices at Southwestern Oklahoma State University. The remedy that works: a stool softener that uses docusate, an ingredient that helps more of the water in your bowels mix with the solid stuff, making it easier for you to pass.

Brand to look for: Phillips Liqui-Gels

What the package doesn't tell you: If the docusate isn't budging things, drink something hot 30 minutes before you normally take a seat; this should help stimulate your colon into action.

COUGH (DRY, HACKING)

There are two ingredients that can suppress a cough: codeine and dextromethorphan hydrobromide. Codeine (available without a prescription in many states) is more effective, but potentially addictive. So stick with dextromethorphan—20 milligrams every 4 hours. "A dose of dextromethorphan should take effect within a half hour, no matter what form it comes in," says Peter Casano, M.D., an otolaryngologist at the University of Mississippi. As for cough drops, their active ingredient, menthol, has a mild effect on pain—it's not a cough suppressant.

Brand to look for: Robitussin Maximum Strength Cough

What the package doesn't tell you: If you have chest congestion, dextromethorphan will work against your body's attempts to cough up the phlegm. Use a product that contains both dextromethorphan and guaifenesin (see page 230) only when you're chest is congested and your cough is keeping you awake.

COUGH (WITH PHLEGM)

Skip the cough suppressant and pick up a cough assistant, otherwise known as an expectorant. Guaifenesin, the only OTC expectorant, helps to thin out and loosen up the mass of mucus lodged inside your lungs, making it easier to, er, dislodge. "You can take as much as 400 milligrams every 4 hours," says Dr. Casano. Once the phlegm's gone, the cough should disappear, too.

Brand to look for: Robitussin (expectorant), or generic

What the package doesn't tell you: Drink as much water as you can handle in between doses of guaifenesin. The extra fluid will help the medicine thin out your chest congestion even further.

CUTS AND SCRAPES

Unless your gash is so huge it requires a shoelace tourniquet, treat it with an ointment that contains the topical antibiotics polymyxin and bacitracin. "Antibiotic ointment kills bacteria that may interfere with the cell growth necessary for wound healing," says Scott Plantz, M.D., an emergency medicine physician and cofounder of eMedicine.com. Dr. Plantz recommends applying fresh ointment up to three times daily; this will keep the wound from scabbing, which in turn will help it heal from the inside out and prevent scarring.

Brand to look for: Polysporin ointment, or generic

What the package doesn't tell you: Don't fall into the trap of thinking that those "triple-antibiotic" ointments must be better than the double-antibiotic preparations. Not only do polymyxin and bacitracin contain all of the germ-fighting firepower you need, but the extra antibiotic, neomycin, can sometimes cause allergic reactions.

DANDRUFF

Women aren't the only ones who get yeast infections—the blizzard conditions on your head are a sign your scalp has one right now. "It's believed that decreasing the quantity of yeast on your skin will diminish the reaction," says John Romano, M.D., a professor of dermatology at Cornell Medical Center in New York City. Since yeast is really just a type of fungus, Dr. Romano recommends that you lather your pate with a dandruff shampoo fortified with ketoconazole. "Ketoconazole is an effective antifungal against this organism."

Brand to look for: Nizoral A-D antidandruff shampoo

What the package doesn't tell you: Try preshampooing with honey, a natural antifungal. In a study published in the *European Journal of Medical Research*, dandruff sufferers who washed their scalps with honey (diluted with warm water) daily had no more flakes or itching after 5 weeks.

DIARRHEA

It's called the runs because an infection is forcing water to run out the nearest available exit. The antidiarrheal ingredient loperamide helps put the brakes on your bowels long enough for your body to absorb excess water. In one University of Texas Health Center study, loperamide cleared up diarrhea about 5 hours faster than attapulgite, the antidiarrheal ingredient in Kaopec- tate. In addition to being more effective than other antiexplosives, loperamide doesn't have their side effects, such as constipation.

Brand to look for: Imodium A-D, or generic

What the package doesn't tell you: Stop drinking soda until the medicine really kicks in. "You're mainly taking in sugared, flavored water, which further dilutes what few electrolytes you still have," says Pray.

FEVER

If your body is slow-roasting at 102°F, take 500 milligrams of aceta- minophen; it should cool things down by 2 or 3 degrees. It's also easier on the stomach than aspirin, ibuprofen, and naproxen and has less of a chance of in- teracting with other cold and flu medications. That said, if the acetaminophen hasn't budged the thermometer after about 4 hours, try a 200-milligram dose of ibuprofen. "Since people respond better to some medications than to others, switching types on the second dose may increase your chance of bringing the fever down," says Pray. Still no relief from the heat? See your doctor.

Brand to look for: Tylenol Extra Strength, or generic

What the package doesn't tell you: A University of Maryland study found that acetaminophen and aspirin might actually lengthen the duration of the flu by a day or two. Researchers are still investigating, but in the meantime, if you think your fever is flu-induced, try lowering it with ibuprofen and naproxen exclusively.

GAS

Next time you feel the need to "share," reach for an antigas product that lists simethicone as its main ingredient. While it won't eliminate the air bub- bles trapped inside you, it will speed up your body's processing of them— without any side effects. "Simethicone is a safe and benign ingredient, compared with the charcoal in other OTC drugs, which may reduce the ab- sorption of some antibiotics and antidepressants, and may also cause in- testinal obstruction and dehydration," says Eli Ehrenpreis, M.D., a gastroenterologist and author of *Clinician's Handbook of Prescription Drugs*. Take 750 milligrams daily until your flatulence has blown over.

Brand to look for: Gas-X Extra Strength tablets

What the package doesn't tell you: You may have to do more than just avoid beans and other legumes to short-circuit a gas attack. Foods that are high in pure carbohydrate sugar, like candy and chocolate, can also cause you to detonate. "Bacteria that feed on these carbohydrates form 80 to 90 percent of rectal gas," says James A. Surrell, M.D., a colon and rectal surgeon with the Ferguson Clinic in Grand Rapids, Michigan.

GENERAL PAIN

Advil, Motrin—they're both code for ibuprofen, the best OTC medication for pain associated with swelling and inflammation (think minor arthritis, muscle sprains, minor surgical procedures). According to a recent study published in the *Journal of Rheumatology*, osteoarthritis sufferers preferred ibuprofen over acetaminophen two to one. Start with 200 milligrams four times a day, and if that doesn't help, you can go up to 400 milligrams.

Brand to look for: Advil, or generic

What the package doesn't tell you: You can find even faster pain relief by using the new Advil Liqui-Gel capsules, which contain dissolved ibuprofen. According to a study published in the journal *Clinical Drug Investigation*, Liqui-Gel capsules were absorbed 58 percent more quickly into men's bloodstreams than standard tablets.

HEADACHE

What worked the last time? If it was acetaminophen, go with that. Ibuprofen? Pop some. "The effectiveness of a pain reliever in treating a headache varies from person to person, and it's a matter of trying different ones to see which works best," says Pray. If they all seem equally ineffective, try a pain reliever that also contains caffeine (like some variations of Excedrin), or just wash it down with a cup of coffee or a big glass of iced tea. In a study published in the journal *Clinical Pharmacology and Therapeutics*, 80 percent of headache sufferers who took ibuprofen and caffeine reported significant pain relief, compared with 67 percent who took ibuprofen alone.

Brand to look for: Excedrin Extra Strength

What the package doesn't tell you: If the pounding is particularly bad, talk to your doctor about taking a 600-milligram magnesium supplement daily. Research shows that keeping blood levels of this mineral high may reduce the frequency of migraines.

HEARTBURN

Douse the flames with an H_2 blocker. Whether it's Pepcid, Zantac, or Tagamet, all H_2 blockers are about equally effective at reducing your stomach's acid production, says David Brooks, M.D., a gastroenterologic surgeon at Brigham and Women's Hospital in Boston. The one drawback: You'll need to take a separate antacid to neutralize the existing juice that's sitting

SHOULD YOU TAKE A MULTISYMPTOM OTC?

Drugs that treat four or five different symptoms are the multitools of medicine: They jam all your survival essentials into one neat package. But unlike your trusty Leatherman, a multi-symptom drug can't be used just one part at a time. Got a wicked cough and sinus congestion but no fever? Tough—you're taking 500 milligrams of acetaminophen whether you like it or not. And what happens when the cough clears up but your nose is still stuffed? Oh, well.

"If you don't need the ingredient to treat the symptom, you also don't need the side effect that comes with it," says Steven Pray, Ph.D., a professor of nonprescription products and devices at Southwestern Oklahoma State University. Sure, separate medicines cost more and mean more stuff to swallow, but that's the price of being sick.

around in your stomach. The only brand that combines an acid-reducing ingredient and an antacid in one tablet is Pepcid Complete.

Brand to look for: Pepcid Complete

What the package doesn't tell you: H_2 blockers may not completely stop your stomach's acid production, in which case you may need a Gaviscon chaser. It's an antacid that also contains alginic acid, a substance that forms a marshmallow-tasting mixture that floats on top of the stomach acid. So when that acid backs up, you taste marshmallow, not DieHard.

THE BIG "H"

Not a hangnail, hemorrhoids. If you have the pain and itch of swollen blood vessels "back there," buy a tube of 1 percent hydrocortisone cream. "Hydrocortisone depresses the response of the cells that cause inflammation, rendering them relatively inactive but not killing them," says Benjamin Krevsky, M.D., a gastroenterologist at Temple University.

Brand to look for: Preparation H, or generic

What the package doesn't tell you: If there's any bleeding at all, or if you're still itching after a week of hydrocortisone treatment, see your doctor immediately: You may be suffering from an anal fissure, rectal cancer, or anal herpes.

ITCHY RASHES AND BUG BITES

After fine-grit sandpaper, the most powerful itch reliever is an anesthetic that contains 20 percent benzocaine. It starts working within 3 minutes of application and lasts for 3 to 4 hours. (If you're allergic to benzocaine, try a spray with 2 percent lidocaine or 1 percent pramoxine.)

Brand to look for: Maximum Strength Lanacane, or generic

What the package doesn't tell you: Before you spray on the benzocaine, rub in some 1 percent hydrocortisone cream. "The cortisone takes the swelling out to relieve pressure on the skin's itch receptors," says Pray.

MOTION SICKNESS

Once your stomach starts somersaulting, there's no stopping it. So plan ahead, and swallow an OTC medicine that contains meclizine before motion sickness strikes. Meclizine won't cause as much drowsiness as Dramamine can, and may even work better than scopolamine, a prescription motion sickness drug. In one NASA study, people who took meclizine reported fewer motion sickness symptoms than those who used scopolamine.

Brand to look for: Bonine or Dramamine Less-Drowsy tablets

What the package doesn't tell you: If you still feel drowsy, skip the meds and slip on a ReliefBand. This watchlike device gives off electrical signals that interfere with the nerves that cause nausea. Sounds like bunk, but it works—the FDA has approved the ReliefBand for the treatment of nausea. "It's the most effective defense on the market," says Brent Blue, M.D., an aviation medicine expert.

NASAL CONGESTION

Swallow now, spray later. According to Dr. Casano, the best way to clear out clogged nasal passages is to take a pseudoephedrine capsule in the morning and give yourself a blast of oxymetazoline or propylhexedrine nasal spray at night. You won't have to worry about being kept awake by pseudoephedrine's stimulant side effect, and you can use the decongestant nasal spray for 5 days straight (instead of the usual 3) without suffering from rebound congestion.

Brand to look for: Sudafed 12-hour and Afrin nasal spray, or generic

What the package doesn't tell you: Take a 12-hour timed-release pseudoephedrine capsule instead of the 4-hour tablet. When you first take the tablets, there's a spike in the release of the medication that's followed by a quick drop, says Dr. Casano.

RED, ITCHY EYES

Stop rubbing them long enough to find eyedrops that contain either tetrahydrozoline or naphazoline. According to Patricia Williams, Ph.D., director of the Thomas R. Lee center for ocular pharmacology at Eastern Virginia Medical School, both ingredients constrict the dilated blood vessels back to normal size. "They're equally effective, so you can make your choice by price," says Williams. Just don't use the eyedrops for more than 2 or 3 days, or your eyes will become redder than before.

Brand to look for: Visine, Clear Eyes, or generic

What the package doesn't tell you: Even if the instructions say to put two drops in each eye, use only one. "Your eye physically can't hold two drops. 'Two drops' only sells more drugs," says Williams. And once you put that drop in, keep your eye shut for about 3 minutes; this will give it time to absorb the medicine.

SORE THROAT

In the world of sore throat lozenges, there is no Mariano Rivera, no reliever that blows away the competition. However, according to Pray, lozenges containing dyclonine are better than anything else warming up in your medicine cabinet, for two reasons: They're less likely to cause an allergic reaction, and they won't offend your taste buds, an important consideration in an OTC medicine you're sucking, not swallowing. Look for lozenges that pack 3 milligrams of dyclonine, the maximum amount available.

Brand to look for: Sucrets Maximum Strength lozenges

What the package doesn't tell you: Take 200 milligrams of ibuprofen, too. "While a lozenge will anesthetize the area when it dissolves, an internal analgesic like ibuprofen will reduce the swelling that's triggering the pain," says Pray.

SUNBURN

Cover your red lobster shell with 20 percent benzocaine cream; it'll numb even the worst burns. Allergic to the stuff? Use a moisturizing lotion that lists mineral oil as the main ingredient. It will replenish the moisture the sun baked out, and can help relieve the sensation that hundreds of needles are pricking your skin, says Popovich. And if you're considering using aloe vera, too, think again. "Aloe is unproven and can cause allergic reactions in some people," says Pray.

Brand to look for: Maximum Strength Lanacane, or generic

What the package doesn't tell you: Once you're well-oiled, take 200 milligrams of ibuprofen to relieve the pain from the inside out.

Bad to Your Bones?

As you read this, your bones are becoming shorter, thinner, and more brittle. Do you know how to stop the decline?

By Ted Spiker

A broken bone is a badge of honor. It shows the world that you're a man who takes risks, a man who plays the game to win, a man who doesn't pass out at the sight of a protruding ulna.

It also shows that you may be one of the more than 2 million men suffering from osteoporosis, a bone-deteriorating disease that, over time, increases your risk of breaks and fractures, worsens your already poor posture, and shaves inches off your height. We know what you're thinking. Only postmenopausal women get osteoporosis. But that's a myth.

"Under the right circumstances, any man of almost any age can be affected," says Eric Orwoll, M.D., an osteoporosis researcher at Oregon Health Sciences University. It's "circumstances" like exercising too little, drinking too much, and smoking (at all) that make a guy more likely to snap in his thirties and almost certainly shrink in his fifties.

Fortunately, this article is Rust-Oleum for your bones. We've pulled together five stay-intact strategies that, if applied regularly, will fortify your frame against osteoporosis. Your skeleton has stood up for you all these years; now it's time to return the favor.

I. MILK IT

Doctors tell women to consume about 1,000 milligrams (mg) of calcium a day to help maintain their bone density. Pretty good advice for men, too, except for one thing: You have a prostate. In a recent Harvard University study, men who took in more than 600 mg of calcium a day had a 32 percent higher risk of prostate cancer than those who got less than 150 mg. "High intakes of calcium tend to suppress 1,25 dihydroxyvitamin D_3, a substance that helps protect against prostate cancer," says June Chan, Sc.D., a urological epidemiologist at the University of California at San Francisco.

How to stay rock solid: Shoot for 1,000 mg of calcium and 400 international units of vitamin D daily. "The extra vitamin D will enhance the absorption of calcium and maintain your levels of dihydroxyvitamin D," says Jing Ma, M.D., Ph.D., a professor of medicine at Harvard Medical School. Low-fat dairy products fortified with D are your best sources of calcium, but if you need a supplement, stick with calcium citrate; it's absorbed better than calcium carbonate.

WHEN THE CREAK RISES

Diagnosed with osteoporosis? New drugs can beat it before it breaks you.

Fosamax: The only FDA-approved osteoporosis drug for men, Fosamax slows the rate at which old bone is broken down. In an Oregon Health Sciences University study, men who took Fosamax had a 7 percent increase in bone density, compared with 2 percent in the control group. The men taking Fosamax also ended up with an 80 percent lower risk of spinal fractures.

Supplemental testosterone: Some men need a little extra help to boost testosterone. To see if you're one of them, have your blood levels measured. If they come in lower than 280 nanograms per deciliter, ask your doctor about testosterone shots or the patch. While the patch is the most effective delivery system, you may not like where you have to stick it (on your scrotum). If that's the case, go with monthly injections.

Parathyroid hormone: Unlike most other treatments, which only stop bone loss, parathyroid hormone injections actually help form new bone. Columbia University researchers found that men given parathyroid injections had nearly a 14 percent increase in bone density after 18 months. Parathyroid hormone should be available soon.

WATCH YOUR BACK

You've never broken a bone in your life, but you suddenly feel inexplicable back pain. It could be your body's osteoporosis alarm. "Any height loss or a back pain caused by something minor like coughing is a sign that you may have fractured a vertebra due to osteoporosis," says Lynn Chard-Petrinjak, of the National Osteoporosis Foundation. Ask your doctor to check you out with dual energy x-ray absorptiometry (DEXA), a low-radiation test that measures bone density. You'll have to pick up the $200 tab since most insurance plans won't cover DEXA, but it's worth it; even if your skeleton is sound, the results will serve as a baseline for future exams.

2. DEFY GRAVITY

Swimming and cycling do great things for your heart, your waist, and the Lycra industry, but little for your bones. When your skeleton is being held up by water or pedals and a seat, it doesn't have to work against gravity to support your body. And, just like muscles, bones need to lift weight in order to grow, says Gordon Strewler, M.D., an osteoporosis expert at Harvard Medical School. "When stress is placed on the skeleton, it remodels itself to increase its strength."

How to stay rock solid: Move metal. According to Tufts University researchers, the greatest increases in bone density have resulted from weight training—specifically, full-body workouts done two or three times a week and consisting of three eight-repetition sets of each exercise at about 80 percent of your one-repetition maximum.

3. EAT RAISINS

Dried grapes are loaded with potassium and magnesium, two nutrients that help prevent the leaching of calcium from bones. In a recent Tufts University study, researchers found that those people who took in the least potassium and magnesium lost 4 to 5 percent more bone density than those consuming the most. "Think of what would happen if that loss occurred over a long period. In 20 years, you'd lose 25 percent of your skeleton," says Katherine Tucker, Ph.D., the study author.

How to stay rock solid: Fill up on potassium-rich foods, such as baked potatoes, tomato juice, and low-fat yogurt. As for magnesium, you can get some from oat bran muffins, almonds, and cashews, but you'll probably need a supplement, too. Look for one that contains magnesium gluconate; it's the form of the mineral that's least likely to give you the runs.

4. SAY "ESTROGEN"

We know it's a scary word, but estrogen tells our bodies to break down old bone and form new bone in its place. Of course, women are loaded with the stuff (until menopause, at least), but men have to rely on an enzyme to convert testosterone into the female hormone. As a result, a guy's bones run into trouble when his testosterone levels drop, whether due to age, stress, or diet. "Men who don't have enough testosterone end up with terrible bone loss," says Dr. Strewler.

How to stay rock solid: Snack on a handful of macadamia nuts every day. USDA researchers found that macadamias are one of the best sources of monounsaturated fat (17 grams per ounce), a nutrient that's believed to increase resting testosterone levels. And when you're not eating, you should be lifting; the more muscle you pack on, the more testosterone your body will produce.

5. WATCH THE STEROIDS

Rhinocort, Nasonex, Flonase—these widely prescribed nasal sprays may be sabotaging your skeleton. Each contains corticosteroids, powerful anti-inflammatory agents that, when used in asthma inhalers, have been shown to prevent new bone from forming and even to cause it to break down faster. "Research suggests that if you use these nasal sprays consistently, there is some risk that they'll also lower your bone mass," says Joan Lappe, Ph.D., a professor of medicine at Creighton University in Nebraska.

How to stay rock solid: "Use the lowest effective dose," says Lappe. For most corticosteroid nasal sprays, that's one spray in each nostril daily. Before you go higher than that, try complementing the spray with a noncorticosteroid remedy, such as Claritin-D.

Smile! This Won't Hurt a Bit

New high-tech tools at your dentist's command promise a perfect smile without the pain

By Christopher McDougall

Pain, noxious odors, and ugly stains: An entire multisensory alert system was going off in my mouth, warning that the situation inside was bad and approaching critical. Naturally, I took immediate evasive action: I began chewing on the other side of my mouth and kept my lips clamped tight when I smiled. As long as it kept the drills and needles at bay, I was willing to shut my trap and hope for a spontaneous self-cure.

I didn't realize that in the 4 years since my last checkup, new techniques and high-tech equipment had revolutionized modern dentistry. Thanks to soft-tissue lasers, digital and video imaging, high-propulsion jets, and new plastics-compounding agents, many of the procedures that once left me clawing at the arms of the dentist's chair are now performed in minutes—with no drills, no needles, and no pain.

Or so I was promised when I finally sought help from Mel Burchman, D.D.S., a suburban Philadelphia dentist who calls himself Doctor High Tech. Dr. Burchman is among a growing group nationwide specializing in laser care and digital diagnostics. He agreed to spelunk between my deteriorating jaws and do a complete oral overhaul. Right up front, I had to admit my apprehension; I've had bones set and once stitched a gash in my hip without much moaning, but I can't stand that whining dental drill and those unpredictable flashes of nerve pain.

"Believe me, there are kids I treat who have no *idea* that a dentist visit is supposed to be painful," says Dr. Burchman, a fit 52-year-old whose Mario Brothers mustache and muscular arms make him look like a trusty mechanic. "I will have a whole generation of patients who think going to the dentist is about as scary as getting a haircut."

A NEW WAY TO GET CLEAN

As the exam begins, I try to calm myself with these assurances. Dr. Burchman steers me toward a small booth for a panoramic x-ray. Instead of taking multiple conventional x-rays, a dentist can now use a single panoramic x-ray to quickly scan the entire jaw. I'm getting one because I haven't had a checkup in more than 3 years, and I may have bite problems and bone loss due to periodontal disease. As I stand in the booth, he fits me with a mouthpiece, then activates scanners that circle my head like a pair of rotating cafeteria trays. In less than 30 seconds, he's done a complete mock-up of my teeth and jaw.

Then it's into the treatment room, where the only standard equipment in view is the classic dental Barcalounger. Mounted on the ceiling are both a computer monitor and a TV screen. (Dr. Burchman gives patients control of the remote but bans Jerry Springer: "Makes patients too jumpy.") Once I'm seated, Dr. Burchman uses a matchbook-size sensor to take digital x-rays of my questionable teeth. "The digital negatives deliver a level of detail that the panoramic x-rays don't show," he notes. In seconds, the digitized images are downloaded from the office computer network and flash on the ceiling-mounted monitor, where they can be magnified and adjusted for contrast. "And if you ever change dentists," adds Dr. Burchman, "I can just e-mail him your entire file."

X-rays completed, I notice that Dr. Burchman is now holding an odd-looking wand with a fish-eye lens. "This is an intraoral camera," he says before carefully positioning the thing inside my mouth like a tongue depressor. Instantly, full-color close-ups of my teeth appear on the TV screen. "A broken tooth, cracked filling, or cavity doesn't always show on x-rays," says Dr. Burchman. Also, photos are a far more effective way to convince patients that work needs to be done: Early-stage gum disease is invisible on x-rays but dramatic in photos, and hidden cavities can be shown in detail and from various angles.

He discovers that I have four main problems: cavities (two), widespread staining (including a grayish cast from a childhood dose of the antibiotic tetracycline), a small but serious patch of gum disease, and three misaligned front teeth. The crooked teeth are more than a cosmetic concern, Dr. Burchman warns; besides looking a little too Austin Powers, they mean the impact of my bite isn't being evenly distributed, which could lead to hairline cracks and eventual jaw problems.

Dr. Burchman first goes after the surface stains and cementlike deposits of tartar. Ordinarily, that would mean intensive flossing and scraping with a steel scaling tool. But because my tartar buildup isn't too severe, he'll need to use only the Prophy-Jet, a bicarbonate spray that acts as a pressure washer for teeth. The sensation is surprisingly pleasant—it's cool and abrasively minty, like brushing with baking soda toothpaste, and the whooshing jet is much more tolerable than the sound of a rasping scaler.

The cleaning is done in less than 4 minutes. Dr. Burchman takes new photos with the intraoral camera, then flashes before-and-after images on the

SMILE FOR SALE

Here's the tab for a mouth makeover, and the odds your dentist has the training and the tools to do it.

Procedure	Average Cost	Typical Insurance Coverage	Availability
Intraoral photos	$10 to $15 each, $70 per series	100% if part of a checkup	About 20% of dental offices
Prophy-Jet cleaning	$50	100%, limited to two cleanings per year	Widespread
High-pressure cavity repair with surface particle-bond filling	$90 and up	80% to 100% after the deductible (usually $25 to $50)	Still limited
Periodontal laser surgery	$400 to $600 per diseased section	100% after the deductible	Still limited
Occlusal equilibration, a.k.a. reshaping of the teeth	$250 and up	100% after the deductible	Widespread
Acrylic laminate veneers	$400 to $500 per tooth	No coverage for cosmetic purposes, but 50% for reconstruction	Widespread

monitor. The difference is amazing, and embarrassing: Before, my smile was dingy with stains, and the backs of my front teeth were brown and mossy from coffee and missed food particles, providing ripe material for bad breath and future decay. Afterward, my teeth are brighter than I've ever seen them. Besides its speed, comfort, and power, Dr. Burchman says, the Prophy-Jet is more thorough than a rubber-cupped polisher and does less damage to tooth enamel than a scaler. "I'm blasting away more stains, and no metal instrument is scratching your teeth."

SPRAY AWAY THE DECAY

One week later, I return for the most serious work: my cavities and infected gums.

For the first cavity, Dr. Burchman briefly sprays a jet inside my mouth, tests the tooth with a thin instrument, then asks if I'm ready. "Okay?"

"Okay," I respond. "Go ahead."

"No," Dr. Burchman says. "I meant, 'Okay, that one's done.'"

It took about 90 seconds. When I thought Dr. Burchman was prepping the tooth, he was actually using an aluminum silicate spray, which blasts away decay with a hail of fine particles. Once the cavity was cleaned out, Dr. Burchman troweled a tooth-colored bonding adhesive into the gap, instead of the usual silver amalgam . . . and that was it. Not only is the new filling tinted to match my teeth, but it's also laced with fluoride to prevent future cavities.

Filling the next cavity goes just as quickly. Dr. Burchman seals both of them with a Pac-Lite, a blue-light wand that dries and hardens the adhesive at a speed of about 10 seconds each. The entire procedure for both teeth, including before-and-after photos, takes about 5 minutes. It involves no novocaine, no drilling, and no swelling. "This way, you can have a cavity filled on your lunch break and still have lunch," Dr. Burchman says. And the only drawback really isn't one: Compound fillings hold up for only 3 to 5 years—compared with 30-plus for silver fillings—but the ease of replacing them makes that a negligible concern.

On to my gums, a trickier proposition than the cavities. Because I'm a crummy flosser, bits of food lodged under my gums are being eaten by bacteria and excreted as flesh-corroding acid. Most dentists have to cut away the infected areas with a scalpel, requiring several painful novocaine shots directly into the sensitive hard palate. Afterward, the gum remains swollen and acutely tender for weeks.

A laser, however, is much gentler and requires far less anesthetic. "Patients used to schedule 3 days off from work for gum surgery, and would have to come back four times if they needed treatment on all four sides," says Dr. Burchman. "This way, I can do a side in an hour, and you'll be eating dinner tonight." There's also no need for antibiotics or gauze packing since the laser's high heat sterilizes the cut and instantly coagulates the blood.

Dr. Burchman gives me two shots of novocaine, both in the outer gum instead of in the more sensitive palate. With the area properly numbed, he sets to work. Occasionally, I feel a tiny pricking sensation, like being scratched by a pin, but mostly I'm watching CNN on the ceiling-mounted TV. Within 40 minutes, Dr. Burchman has cut away all of the infected flesh. He then uses the laser to recontour my gum so that it fits flush against the teeth, making it less likely to act as a storm gutter for food scraps.

I'm out of his office by 7 that evening. By 8, the novocaine has faded and I'm feeling a little sore, as if I'd been elbowed in a basketball game. By 9, however, I'm eating Chinese food and feeling only a little tenderness. When I wake up the next morning, it takes me a minute to remember I've just had surgery.

NOW, LET'S GET THIS STRAIGHT

Dr. Burchman's next challenge is to straighten my crooked front teeth. The best and most permanent solution, he stresses, would be braces. There are a number of jazzy new options, including transparent ceramic models and the invisible lingual type, which are positioned on the back of your teeth. But they all have the same downsides: They need frequent adjustment during the first few months, they require 2 to 3 years to "take," and a tooth or two may have to be extracted for optimal straightening.

In my case, because the alterations are small and I don't want a multi-year investment, Dr. Burchman recommends veneers—superhard plastic shields that are glued over teeth to help compensate for their misalignment. (Think of them as siding for your teeth.) Veneers require no anesthetic, and you can be chomping away as soon as you leave the chair. The catch? Some teeth (like mine) need to have protruding sections ground down with a high-speed, diamond-tipped burr before they can be fitted.

THE STATE THAT EARNED
THE BEST RATING FOR ITS
PREVENTIVE DENTAL CARE: SOUTH CAROLINA

THE STATES
RATED THE WORST: CALIFORNIA, ARIZONA, MISSISSIPPI, NEW JERSEY, NEW HAMPSHIRE

LICENSED TO ZAP

Dr. Burchman goes to work on my crooked canines. In a few minutes, he has ground the edges and given each misaligned tooth a nice, smooth shape. He evens them until they form a symmetrical row with the rest of my front teeth. I keep expecting pain, but I don't feel the slightest twinge because he's not hitting any nerves.

Satisfied with the basic tooth shape, Dr. Burchman applies a bonding adhesive. Next, he searches through a selection of veneers until he finds one that exactly matches my tooth color. After custom-shaping the veneers, he presses them onto the adhesive, dries it with a zap from the Pac-Lite, and then buzzes the plastic with a diamond polishing paste. Elapsed time: 1 hour.

I can't believe the result—it's like looking into someone else's mouth. My wolfman cuspids are gone, and that one jagged chopper is smoothed into conformity with the rest of the crew. For the first time in my life, my entire mouth looks clean, bright, and uniform.

Dr. Burchman's one remaining task is a full-scale whitening. The most advanced option is laser whitening, in which the teeth are pretreated with an acid gel so that a peroxide solution can penetrate the enamel. A laser is then used to activate the bleaching action. It can take multiple visits, however, and even then, knockout pearlies aren't guaranteed.

In my case, though, Dr. Burchman doesn't recommend it. Tetracycline staining is among the most stubborn of tooth discolorations, and he believes that no current technology will yield satisfactory results. In fact, he gives a discounted rate to tetracycline patients who insist on laser whitening, as a way of buffering their disappointment in advance. I could try home bleaching, but he doubts that the outcome will be worth the effort.

I'm a bit let down, but quickly perk up with my after-office-hours treat. No free toothbrush for me—instead, Dr. Burchman hands me a nice, frosty can. Toasting my gleaming new mouth, he says, "Here's another benefit of high-tech dentistry—you can crack an ice-cold beer a week after gum surgery."

KNOW THIS

Go over the Counter

It might not be that weekly game of basketball that's keeping your sprained ankle from healing. Researchers at the University of North Carolina at Chapel Hill found that a class of anti-inflammatory pain medications can actually slow down your body's natural healing process. The most common culprit: drugs called COX-2 inhibitors, which include the medications Celebrex and Vioxx. "These drugs are marketed as being gentler on your stomach than other pain medications, but if you can get by on aspirin or ibuprofen, you should. They're cheaper and less harmful to your body," says Laury Dahners, Ph.D., a coauthor of the study.

Conquer Congestion

Stuffed up? It might be acid reflux. Researchers at the University of South Florida analyzed the upper airways of 150 people, half with frequent heartburn and half without. They found that 60 percent of people with reflux disease also had chronic nasal congestion, compared with just 27 percent of people without reflux. Treating chronic heartburn (reflux) with Prilosec or Prevacid might help improve your breathing, says Dennis Ledford, M.D., the study author.

Better Vision in Sight

Throw away your reading glasses. The FDA has just approved conductive keratoplasty, a technique that improves farsightedness, including a person's ability to read things like fine print up close. To perform the procedure, doctors blast your eye with radio waves, which gently heat the surface of the cornea so that it can be reshaped to correct farsightedness.

More good news: If you're not ready to get your eyes blasted, at least you won't have to stick your fingers in your eyes so often. A new type of contact lens can be worn continuously for up to a month without damaging your eyes. "The lenses look and feel identical to existing contacts, but the material they're made from is fine enough to allow up to seven times more oxygen to reach your eyes," says H. Dwight Cavanagh, M.D., the project's lead researcher. The lenses received FDA approval last year and are now available from Bausch & Lomb at a cost of just a few dollars more than regular contacts.

Painkilling Plant

A Yale University study has confirmed that the anti-inflammatory herbal supplement feverfew—available at health food stores and pharmacies—does provide relief for men who suffer from chronic migraines.

Head Cold

Your job may not be the source of your headaches after all. According to research by the New England Center for Headache, more than 50 percent of migraines are caused by changes in the weather. In the study, 77 men and women recorded the dates and severity of their migraines. Researchers then tracked weather conditions and average temperatures and compared both sets of data. "We found that 25 percent of migraines occur during periods of low temperatures or low humidity levels," says Alan Rapoport, M.D., the study supervisor. Sufferers of frequent migraines should monitor the weather and take preventive medications at the onset of weather changes.

Wheezy Weather

Severe weather can wreak havoc on asthma sufferers as well. Researchers at the University of Sydney studied emergency room admission records of six Australian towns and found that asthma attacks were 15 times more common during thunderstorms than during calm weather. The reason is basic meteorology.

"Most thunderstorms push a wave of cool air ahead of them. That can lead to concentrations of ground pollen four to 12 times higher than normal," says Guy Marks, Ph.D., the study author.

NUMBER OF AMERICANS WHO SUFFER FROM MIGRAINES: 28 MILLION

NUMBER WHO SUFFER FROM BACK AND NECK PAIN: 27 MILLION

DOWN THE PIKE

Warning Sickness

Doctors may eventually be able to tell you when you're going to be sick, days before your symptoms develop. Researchers at the University of Maine recently discovered that levels of nitric oxide in your breath are 10 times higher when your body is trying to fight off an infection than they are when you feel fine. The body appears to produce nitric oxide to help it fight off viral infections. "Levels appear to be highest when you first come down with something," says Robert Lad, Ph.D., codirector of the project. Lad hopes to create a breath analysis device, based on the discovery, that could warn people when they're on the verge of getting sick.

Roma Therapy

Vaccinations with needles? That's so 20th century. In the future, protecting yourself from disease may be as simple as eating a raw tomato. Researchers at the Institute of Plant Biochemistry and Biotechnology in Germany have developed a genetically modified tomato capable of storing and replicating human vaccines. "Proteins from different vaccines can be inserted into the chloroplast of the tomato plant, where they will then multiply as the tomato grows and develops," says Ralph Bock, Ph.D., who developed the new plant. In addition to vaccines, the tomatoes—which so far lack FDA approval—could also be altered to carry some drugs and multivitamins.

Sight for Sore Eyes

Researchers at Vanderbilt University are working on an implantable contact lens that will give older people with cataracts virtually the same vision they had before the cataracts formed. The lens is made up of six overlapping plates that focus when muscles in the eye move. Clinical trials may begin within 2 years.

OF 605 LASIK PATIENTS WHO WERE SURVEYED, PERCENTAGE WHO COMPLAINED OF NIGHT-VISION PROBLEMS: 25

Breathe Easier

Only a small fraction of the medication in a traditional asthma inhaler reaches the lungs. That can make stopping an asthma attack tough. However, Dutch researchers are developing a new inhaler that uses much smaller drug particles, which can be inhaled more deeply, providing the patient with a more powerful form of treatment.

That's One Hip Joint

University of California engineers have devised an artificial tissue with the self-lubricating properties of real cartilage. Once implanted, the new artificial tissue might help repair injured or arthritic joints, restoring flexibility.

In related news, researchers at Case Western Reserve University are working on a new, longer-lasting type of artificial joint. Every year, nearly 1.5 million people get joint replacements. "Most of those joints wear out within 10 years, forcing people to undergo a second, corrective surgery," says Steve Kurtz, Ph.D., an engineer working on the project.

DOES IT WORK?

Bacteria Blasters

All those antibacterial products now in stores can make you think you're an extremely dirty person—and not in the good way. Our infectious disease experts found some debugging devices worth buying, and some not.

Deodorant

 Sweat doesn't have a bad odor until it mixes with bacteria. Cutting down on germs could make you smell better, says Schwab. Most antibacterial antiperspirants and deodorants contain natural germ fighters. **Buy it?** If you reek, give it a try.

Bar Soap

 The times you really need to wash with soap are after using the bathroom, before preparing or eating food, and when cleaning a cut. The everyday bacteria on your skin won't make you sick, but when they mix with sweat, you can start to smell. Triclosan—found in antibacterial soaps—could help with body odor, says Kellogg Schwab, Ph.D., an assistant professor of environmental microbiology at Johns Hopkins University. But repeated use can generate resistant bacteria, he warns. And besides, ordinary soap does a good job of removing bacteria.

Buy it? If odor is a problem, try a bar that contains triclosan.

Hand Soap

 Ordinary soap and water will kill germs as long as you wash for 30 to 60 seconds, says Gerba. If you don't, an antibacterial soap could make up the difference.

Buy it? Yes, if you always rush your hand washing.

Hand Sanitizer

 These little bottles are perfect when you can't get to soap and water, though the gel will turn dust and dirt into a muddy paste, says Gary Noskin, M.D., a specialist in infectious diseases at Northwestern University Medical School. For the dirty work, an antibacterial premoistened wipe is better.

Buy it? Yes. Toss a bottle and some wipes in your travel bag.

Bandages

 Dr. Noskin says bandages with germ-fighting pads reduce the need to reapply antibacterial ointment. Keeping a wound free from bacteria can help prevent infection and scarring.

Buy them? Sure—look for bandages that contain polymyxin and bacitracin.

Kitchen Sponge

 New antibacterial sponges won't kill germs in your kitchen, but they could smell fresher longer. Bacteria make regular sponges stink, Dr. Noskin says.

Buy it? No. Just run your regular one through the dishwasher.

WHAT'S THE DIFF?

Corn vs. Bunion

A corn is thick skin that forms on your foot from pressure. Wear a corn pad or have the corn removed. A bunion is a deformity of the joint between the foot and the big toe. There's a bump, and the big piggy points toward the little one. If it hurts, wear wider shoes or orthotics, or have surgery to remove it.

Ophthalmologist vs. Optometrist vs. Optician

An ophthalmologist is your one-stop eye care M.D., offering exams, prescriptions, and surgery. He's not the same as an optometrist, who does exams and writes prescriptions, and treats some eye diseases, but generally doesn't perform major surgery. And whatever you do, don't call him an optician, who's the guy at Walnut and Main who makes, sells, and fits the lenses that you hope will make you look smarter.

M.D. vs. D.O.

Medical doctors focus on conventional treatments based on symptoms, tests, and diagnoses. Doctors of osteopathy see the body as a whole, focusing on how one symptom can affect another. Both go to medical schools.

TAKE ACTION

Besides grape-flavored medicine and pitying girlfriends who pamper you, there aren't many perks to being sick. Well, here's your ticket out of the infirmary, friend. No matter what's got you down—anything from a cold to a headache to a kidney stone—these 10 tips will help you feel better fast, not to mention keep you from getting sick in the first place. So you can put those sick days to better use—like when you come down with a bad case of, uh, spring fever.

1. Take a hike, fight a cold. Scientists at Oklahoma State University tracked 79,000 people for a year and discovered that those who exercised just 20 minutes twice a week were significantly less likely to call in sick to work than nonexercisers. A brisk walk a couple of times a week can help keep you healthy, says Bert Jacobson, Ed.D., the study's lead author and a health professor at Oklahoma State University.

How does exercise defeat germs? Researchers at Texas Christian University, in a related study, measured immune system cells and found that people who exercised had significantly higher counts.

2. If you avoid that annual flu shot . . . Protect yourself the old-fashioned way: Become a compulsive hand washer. A recent Naval Health Research Center study found that when recruits washed their hands at least five times a day, they had 45 percent fewer respiratory illnesses, such as infection by the flu virus.

"Vaccination is the best preventive measure, but hand washing is a good alternative," says Carolyn Bridges, M.D., a medical epidemiologist with the Centers for Disease Control and Prevention.

3. Soothe a sore throat. If you go to your doctor, there's a 50/50 chance he'll accurately diagnose whether you have a viral or bacterial infection. Rather than take your chances with an antibiotic—which may or may not make you feel better—ask about a steroid called Decadron (dexamethasone). In a study of 118 patients with colds, flu, or other hard-to-swallow maladies, Mayo Clinic researchers found that this steroid is effective at relieving sore throats, and, unlike antibiotics, it works on both bacterial and viral infections. Plus,

PERCENTAGE OF PEOPLE WITH SORE THROATS WHO ARE GIVEN ANTIBIOTICS UNNECESSARILY: 62

Decadron provides longer-lasting relief—up to 24 hours per dose—says Julie Wei, M.D., the study author.

4. Know when to call in sick. When the inevitable strikes this winter, ask yourself these three questions to separate the sniffles from the serious stuff. And stay well away from us.

Did your temperature spike within 24 hours? A gradual temperature rise means it's most likely a cold. Flu knocks you out faster than a whiff of Homer Simpson's underwear—temp soars within a day to enable your immune system to work in its optimal climate.

Have you lost your appetite? If you're still hungry as a horse, it's a cold. With the flu your body warns you to eat less. The digestion process uses up vital energy resources that could be fuelling a D Day attack on the virus. Because colds are milder, less energy needs to be conserved.

Do you feel exhausted? If you just feel tired, it's a cold. Flu brings genuine, can't-get-out-of-bed exhaustion.

5. Try a new position. A bit of variety in the bedroom is good—even if it doesn't involve sex. According to a 2-year study at the University of California at San Francisco, regularly sleeping on the same side of your body makes you much more likely to develop kidney stones. Of 93 patients with recurring kidney stones, 75 percent developed them only in the kidney on the side they slept on. "Sleeping in the same position each night appears to alter bloodflow to that kidney, impairing the organ's ability to clear itself of stone-forming crystals and deposits," says Marshall Stoller, M.D., a UCSF professor of urology.

6. Cure contact lens woes. Contact lenses are like television—usually great, often annoying. Some ways to cope:

The problem: Dry eyes

The solution: Artificial tears, as often as needed. Buy preservative-free brands like Refresh since contacts absorb chemicals that further irritate your eyes. Left your rewetting drops at home? Close your eyes for 3 minutes for natural rehydration.

The problem: Itchy eyes

The solution: Take out your contacts and apply a cold compress to your closed eyes to reduce swelling. Use artificial tears to rinse out allergens.

The problem: Stranded overnight without case and contact solution

The solution: Sleep in your contacts. For one night, it's less risky than putting your contacts in tap or bottled water. Neither is sterile, so you'd be chancing infection.

The problem: Recurring protein buildup

The solution: Add a drop of a daily protein remover like Opti-Free Supra Clens onto each side of your lenses before storing in the multipurpose solution in your case, and allow it to clean overnight.

7. Cut? Call Dr. Pepper. Next time you nick yourself in the kitchen, reach for the black pepper. Run cold water over the wound to clean it, using soap if you were handling meat. Then sprinkle on the pepper and apply pressure. In no time, the bleeding will stop. Turns out black pepper has analgesic (that's painkilling), antibacterial, and antiseptic properties, according to Roberta Lee, M.D., medical director of the Beth Israel Center for Health and Healing in New York City. Pepper doesn't sting, either—but don't tell that to your audience.

8. Make your headache split. You may think you've pinpointed the cause of your headaches, but honestly, quitting your job in this economy isn't wise. Instead, try these new weapons.

Alka-Seltzer Morning Relief. Bayer's new effervescent hangover remedy packs 1,000 milligrams (mg) of aspirin and 130 mg of caffeine in each dose for pain relief and alertness.

Amitriptyline. Tiny doses of this antidepressant can be effective for migraines, says Lawrence Robbins, M.D., author of *Headache Help.*

Frova. Newly approved by the FDA, frovatriptan succinate is the longest-lasting of the migraine medicines called triptans.

Feverfew. If you suffer from migraines, ask your doctor if you can try this herbal supplement. As we mentioned in the "Know This" section, a Yale University study recently confirmed that feverfew effectively combats chronic migraines. Dr. Robbins says many of his patients get relief with two 325 mg capsules a day.

9. Survive the drive. If you get a headache every time you slide behind the wheel, the blame may fall on that hot new car you just financed, not on the stress of dealing with road wackos. According to an Australian study, that "new-car smell" everyone loves is often strong enough to trigger headaches, fatigue, nausea, and drowsiness. "It can take up to 6 months for the quantities of chemicals inside a new car to drop to safe, acceptable levels," says Stephen Brown, Ph.D., the study author. But don't sell your new wheels just yet. You can avoid "new car illnesses" by driving with your windows open at least a crack, keeping the fresh-air vent open, and leaving your windows down when you park, says Brown. Also, avoid parking your car in the sun; more toxins are released as the temperature rises inside the car.

10. Get the most out of your checkup. If you're going to have to put on one of those silly little paper gowns, you might as well make the humiliation worth your while. Here's how.

THE MOST COMMON REASON PEOPLE VISIT DOCTORS: COLDS

THE SECOND MOST COMMON REASON: PAIN

Practice e-medicine. A preparatory e-mail to your doctor can make your appointments more efficient, says Daniel Z. Sands, M.D., of Harvard Medical School. Just make sure beforehand that your doc welcomes e-mails—and checks his mailbox. E-mailing is especially good for follow-up questions.

Later is better. To get undivided attention, being the day's first appointment is ideal. But being the last isn't bad, either. "There's just not the same urgency as when he has 20 people in the waiting room," says Jon Pryor, M.D., chairman of urology at the University of Minnesota.

Finish your sentence. One study shows that doctors interrupt patients' descriptions of their ailments in more than 70 percent of cases, and the likelihood of returning to the patient's agenda is only 8 percent. So make a list of everything you want to discuss—and insist your doctor hear you out. Write down your exact symptoms, when they started, when they're worst, and what seems to trigger them, says David Pepper, M.D., of the University of California at San Francisco–Fresno. And don't forget to bring test results and any medications you're taking.

Try a female doctor. Male patients who have female physicians are the most satisfied with their care, a study published in the *Journal of General Internal Medicine* showed. After all, who do you want holding your *cojones* when you cough.

PERCENTAGE OF MEN WHO DON'T HAVE A REGULAR PHYSICIAN: 33

PERCENTAGE OF WOMEN WHO DON'T: 19

PERCENTAGE OF MEN WHO HAVEN'T MADE A DOCTOR'S VISIT IN THE PAST YEAR: 24

PERCENTAGE OF WOMEN WHO HAVEN'T: 8

ANY QUESTIONS?

Sapped by Spring

Every spring, I start out feeling really tired. Could it be allergies even though I never get sneezy and weepy-eyed?

—G. H., Austin, Texas

You bet. While excessive fatigue can be a symptom of lots of things—stress, depression, lack of exercise, poor diet, reading 8,000-word magazine profiles of Strom Thurmond—it's practically guaranteed with springtime allergies. Your body treats pollen as an infection and has no qualms about tapping all your energy to fight it off, says David Tanner, M.D., of the Atlanta Allergy and Asthma Clinic. To see if your fatigue is a pollen problem, try this simple allergy season precaution. Wash your hair before you go to bed. Outside, your head is just a big Swiffer for pollen. If you don't flush out the spores, they coat your pillow and you marinate in them through the night. Same goes for clothes, so change them as soon as you get home. Also, wash your sheets (in the hot cycle) once a week.

Halt-Rock Cafe

I never, ever want to get another kidney stone. So I drink plenty of water and avoid calcium, but what should I eat—or not eat?

—C. E., Atlanta

Poor man. Patients like you show up in doctors' offices all the time. All that squirming and wincing and groaning—as though someone slipped a Chris Kattan movie into the waiting room VCR. As for your diet, a recent study says one that's low in animal protein and salt is more effective at preventing a recurrence than a low-calcium diet, the old, traditional recommendation. Study participants consumed 4 ounces of protein per day, but only about a quarter of that came from meat.

Get most of your protein from whole grains, beans, vegetables, cereals, and dairy products, suggests Leslie Spry, M.D., a nephrologist in Lincoln, Nebraska, and spokesman for the National Kidney Foundation. Yes, calcium is fine. Just stick to about 1,000 milligrams—that's what you'd get from a cup of skim milk, 8 ounces of yogurt, and two slices of provolone. And keep drinking all that water; it's crucial for avoiding stones.

Sleep on It

Out of the slew of "therapeutic" mattresses on the market, once and for all, what's the best one for a bad back?

—P. H., Houston

The best back saver is a Tempur-Pedic mattress (you can order one at www.tempurpedic.com), says Jeffrey Bergin, D.C., the dean of clinics at the National University of Health Sciences in Lombard, Illinois. The Tempur-Pedic is made of a high-density, heat-sensitive type of foam that conforms to your body's exact topography. It's super-easy on your back and will lessen the strain on your wallet as well. Count on about $1,500 for a queen-size.

To get better back support from your existing mattress, top it off with one of those egg-crate pads, says Bergin. The pointy bits help by redistributing your weight equally—just like a bed of nails, but without the tetanus.

Comfy Commute

The seats in my new car adjust in about 12 different ways: up, down, lumbar support, backward, forward. What's the healthiest position to drive in? Does it really make a difference?

—K. K., Toronto, Ontario

Unlike your mother-in-law's, these buttons are well worth pushing. "Sitting for long periods with the spine misaligned is a major cause of back pain," says Edward Hanley, M.D., chairman of the orthopedic department at the Carolinas Medical Center in North Carolina. Here are three pointers to help you get properly seated.

I. Lower back: Supporting the lower back keeps the entire spine properly aligned. Adjust the seat so that the small of your back is against the seat back, with no space in between.

HOW MUCH LIKELIER SMOKERS ARE THAN NONSMOKERS TO DEVELOP LOWER-BACK PAIN: NEARLY TWO TIMES

2. Hips: With the vertical adjustment, make sure your hips are at the same level as your knees so your thighs are parallel to the floor.

3. Neck: Most men tend to overrecline seats. If you recline the seat so far back that you have to crane your neck to see in front of you, you're putting a dangerous strain on the lower neck. You should be able to see a full view of the road with your head against the headrest.

Drug Deadline

Should I toss out my OTC medications as soon as they reach their expiration dates?

—R. C., Cambridge, Massachusetts

No. If you've stored them properly—tightly capped and away from heat and humidity—they can be effective up to a year past the drop-dead date. "Those dates assume that a product has been stored in the worst possible conditions," says Steve Clement, president of the Illinois Pharmacist Association. "The date is the minimum time the drug is guaranteed to be effective."

Ironically, the worst place to store your stash is the bathroom medicine cabinet. Heat and humidity chemically break down tablets and negatively affect a drug's ingredients and materials. "It mimics what happens when you swallow a tablet and it goes to your hot and humid stomach," Clement says. He recommends storing medications in a bedroom dresser drawer, where it's dark and cool. Drugs that have narrow therapeutic uses and require very specific dosages, such as thyroid medications, are usually the first to lose their potency, Clement says. Drugs with hard shells, like coated aspirin, are the hardiest. A good rule of thumb: If it's been a couple of months since your drugs celebrated their 1-year anniversary, chuck 'em.

PERCENTAGE OF MEN WHO RATE THEIR PHYSICAL HEALTH AS GOOD OR EXCELLENT: 81

PERCENTAGE OF WOMEN WHO DO: 76

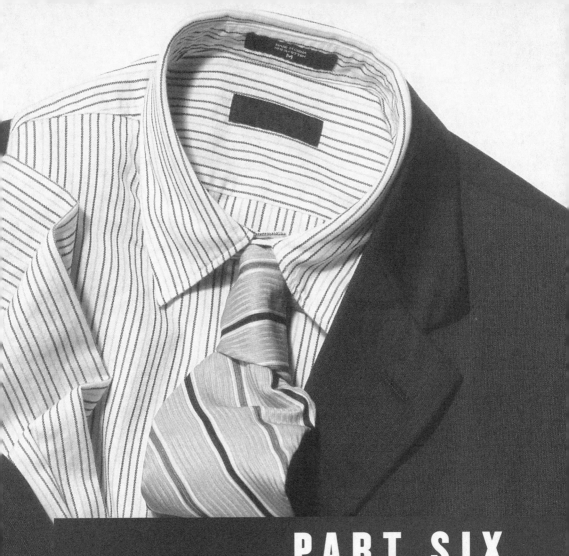

PART SIX
MAKE AN
IMPRESSION

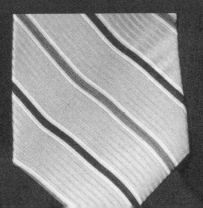

Who Will Get Hired First?
One of these hungry job hunters? Or you?

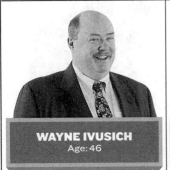

WAYNE IVUSICH
Age: 46

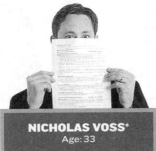

NICHOLAS VOSS*
Age: 33

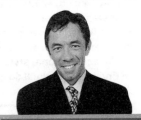

THADDEUS GRIMES-GRUCZKA
Age: 33

EDUCATION
- M.S., professional writing, Towson University
- B.A., general studies, Towson University

EXPERIENCE
- More than 20 years in various sales positions. Spent the past 11 as a sales manager.

INTERVIEW STYLE
- Articulate, casual, and humorous; confident in his ability.

ADVANTAGES
- Has strong communication skills, especially in writing. He's adept at breaking down complex issues into simple language, a valuable trait for a manager. He also has experience in public speaking; he regularly gives talks and runs seminars at trade shows.

DISADVANTAGES
- He is overweight and wears a suit that looks several years old.
- He's the oldest of the three candidates.

WAYNE'S PREDICTION
- "If the company wants sound experience, I will get the job. I won't make the mistakes a younger, less experienced person will."

EDUCATION
- M.B.A., University of Southern California
- B.S., business administration, Berkeley

EXPERIENCE
- Held managerial positions of increasing responsibility over a 9-year career.

INTERVIEW STYLE
- Personable and confident. He's passionate about his long-term goals and speaks highly of his current colleagues.

ADVANTAGES
- His M.B.A. could be a plus. And he has shown career growth, having been promoted four times in 7 years at his first employer and once by his current employer.
- Well-groomed and professional.

DISADVANTAGES
- Voss embellished a title on his résumé and exaggerated his length of employment at his first job. "Everyone pumps up a résumé," he explains.

NICHOLAS'S PREDICTION
- "I bring fresh ideas and enthusiasm wherever I go, and that will get me this job."

*Not his real name

EDUCATION
- M.A., English literature, University of Cambridge
- B.A. cum laude, philosophy and East Asian studies, Columbia University

EXPERIENCE
- Held vice-president positions in public relations and marketing in his past two jobs.

INTERVIEW STYLE
- Articulate and highly confident, bordering on cocky.
- He speaks poorly of his former employer, which is inappropriate in an interview.

ADVANTAGES
- He's fit and well-groomed, and he looks "executive" in his $700 suit.

DISADVANTAGES
- He has worked for three companies in the past 4 years. He was recently laid off, and he has never held a position for longer than 3 years. An employer could be wary of his job-hopping.

THADDEUS'S PREDICTION
- "Not to be snotty, but a younger, good-looking guy with an Ivy League education will always fare better in the job market."

And the Winner Is . . .
Thaddeus
Grimes-Gruczka

Carole Martin, an interview coach at Monster.com, helped us devise the test on the opposite page to determine who has the best combination of credentials, interview skills, and personal style. Take the test yourself to find out how you'll do in the job market.

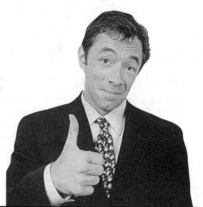

FINAL ANALYSIS

Without knowing the exact job description, all three contestants could qualify for the "management" position we advertised, but Grimes-Gruczka and Voss have the advantage over Ivusich in the personal-style category.

In a study, 472 members of the Society for Human Resource Management Association (SHRMA) viewed video résumés of four candidates and were asked to rate the applicants' employment prospects. The results showed a clear bias against overweight candidates. Other studies have shown that what we say accounts for little of an interviewer's first impression of us, while body language accounts for upwards of 55 percent, says Carole Martin, an interview coach at Monster.com

Though Voss has solid experience, Martin feels his résumé "embellishment" will likely be revealed by a background check. (If we caught it, human resources is bound to.) According to another SHRMA survey, 89 percent of hiring managers regularly check the references of prospective hires, investigating length of employment, titles, and salary history. "There are just too many good candidates out there right now for any company to hire someone with a possible character flaw," says Martin.

Also, although Voss's M.B.A. is an asset, it may not be enough. "The M.B.A. is most valuable when you're making a major career switch," says Jon Houseman, founder of *MBA Jungle* magazine. "But after years in the workforce, performance and experience are what counts."

Grimes-Gruczka has experience managing a large staff, which counts for a lot, says Martin. "Thaddeus was well-prepared for the interview, very confident—and he looked the part." All this could outweigh his spotty employment picture, according to Martin. "In today's economy, there has been a great deal of job instability."

Employment Figures

FACTOR	POINT VALUE	WAYNE	NICHOLAS	THADDEUS	YOU
RÉSUMÉ Your key to getting the interview.	Well-written, shows advancement? +1	+1	+1	+1	
	Typos, careless mistakes, no advancement? −1				
ADVANCED DEGREES Employers tend to look for postgraduate degrees in related fields when initially screening candidates.	Advanced degree related to field? +2		+2		
	Postgrad degree in unrelated field? +1	+1		+1	
EXPERIENCE The most important aspect in landing a job.	More than 3 years' managerial experience? +4	+4	+4	+4	
	Less than 3 years' managerial experience? +2				
	Less than 3 years' experience and no management background? 0				
APPEARANCE Research suggests that looking fit and well-groomed during the interview gives you an advantage over similarly qualified candidates who are less attractive or not as professional looking.	Well-groomed and -dressed, fit, and good-looking? +2		+2	+2	
	Average looks, well-groomed and -dressed? +1				
	Overweight or poorly groomed? −2	−2			
COMMUNICATION SKILLS Effectively articulating what you have to offer the company illustrates how well you'll communicate with your employees and management.	Excellent speaking and writing skills? +1	+1	+1		
	Poor communication skills or speak negatively? −1			−1	
DEVELOPING OTHERS A manager who forms a solid team and cares for his colleagues and employees is an asset to a company.	Hiring and team-building skills? +1		+1	+1	
	Little team-building experience? −1	−1			
INTEGRITY As many as 53 percent of applicants regularly or sometimes lie on their résumés. Getting caught may land you in the reject bin.	Truthful about qualifications (or not caught exaggerating)? +1	+1		+1	
	Caught lying about qualifications or achievements? −10		−10		
TOTALS		+5	+1	+9	

▶ **IF YOUR SCORE IS 6 OR MORE:** You're hired!

▶ **IF YOUR SCORE IS 3 TO 5:** We'll keep you on file.

▶ **IF YOUR SCORE IS 2 OR BELOW:** Don't call us. We'll call you.

MUST READS

Presidential Poise

Fifteen years ago, he was an undisciplined party boy, the floundering scion of a famous family. Today he is the man in charge during one of this nation's most hazardous passages

By Bill Minutaglio

What a miserable morning. It was the summer of 1986, and George W. Bush was deep into a getaway weekend with his wife and a handful of friends at the Broadmoor Hotel, a lavish 3,000-acre golf and tennis resort in Colorado Springs. He awoke that day, like so many days, with a piercing hangover—courtesy of a late night out hurling down drinks and being the life of the party. It was another of those dicey moments in what Bush would later ruefully call his "young and irresponsible" years.

That summer, as he celebrated his 40th birthday, one thing was clear—Bush's life was not exactly a raging success, particularly when compared with that of his accomplished father. Unlike his famous dad, W. was a failure at politics—he'd been whipped in his first and only run for office, a 1978 congressional race in Midland, Texas. (Bush won only three of 17 counties.) Nor had his business career amounted to much. While his father had made a fortune in the oil business, Bush's drilling company, Arbusto (the Spanish word for bush), lost so much money that his own friends had started mocking him. "Ar-BUST-o!" they dubbed the failing venture.

Then, of course, there were Bush's notorious run-ins with alcohol and the law. A disorderly conduct charge in college. A drunk driving arrest in Maine in the mid-1970s. As recently as the spring of 1986, Bush made a drunken ass of himself by verbally accosting journalists (and husband and wife) Al Hunt and Judy Woodruff in a Mexican restaurant in Dallas. As the couple ate dinner with their 4-year-old son, Bush stepped to their table and began a drunken, cursing harangue about an item Hunt had written for *The Washingtonian* magazine. As Bush walked away, Hunt had one thought: "This guy's got problems."

That summer morning in Colorado, the hungover Bush somehow slipped out the door for a jog. He was trying to muscle his mind and body into being whole again—as if he could command his inner army into action. It was what he had always done on mornings like this. But as he labored along, inhaling the thin mountain air, George W. Bush came to a disturbing realization: He wasn't able to simply press some internal button and unleash another endless blast of energy.

I thought of that moment in Bush's life—a low point for him, but also a turning point—as I watched our 43rd president stand before Congress and deliver a confident, defiant, rousing speech in the wake of the September 11 attacks. The contrast was stark: The Bush of 1986 was a wastrel, a prodigal son, a wise guy who had the essential physical package but seemed to be squandering it. The Bush of September 2001 was vigorous, muscular, and focused, a man who appeared ready, both mentally and physically, for his defining moment.

It's way too soon, of course, to know how history will judge Bush, his presidency, and his performance during the recent national crisis. But one thing is remarkable—the sheer willpower it took for Bush to remake his life and even reach that defining moment. It was a reinvention built on three key principles, and it offers lessons for any man about the importance of discipline.

ONE GOOD TURNAROUND

You can change your life, W. style, even if you don't want to be president. Here's how.

• **Make time to exercise,** and the rest of your life will follow (as George W. Bush discovered). Regular training not only makes you healthier physically but also provides "enduring resilience" to depression, anxiety, and stress, according to a recent British review of exercise studies. The result is more energy, discipline, and focus for everything else.

• Bush was inspired by baseball players, but there are role models everywhere. "There are many people in your life already who are worth emulating—just pay attention," says Mark Goulston, M.D., author of *Get Out of Your Own Way.* **Make a list of people you respect, and spend more time with them.** Then make another list of people who bring out your slacker side—drinking buddies, for instance—and lose their phone numbers. You won't miss them. A recent study found that these friends lead you to drink more and that the only thing you have in common is alcohol. Drop them, and you stand a better chance of dropping your bad habits.

• Bush doesn't call it meditation, but his daily ritual of reading Bible verses is just that. "Anytime that you **take on a routine to calm your mind,** it's meditation—and psychologically and physically beneficial," says Diane Reibel, Ph.D., of Thomas Jefferson University. Reibel found that meditating 20 minutes a day for 8 weeks slashed patients' anxiety, depression, and bodily pain symptoms by more than 25 percent.

TRAIN THE BODY

Ever since he was an unfettered puppy growing up on the flatlands of west Texas, Bush was irrepressible. Mr. Energy. The guy who couldn't sit still. The son who loved slamming across the links with his father in another rapid-fire game of "aerobic golf."

Which is why it hit him so hard that morning in Colorado when he realized he wasn't tapping into what had once been, for him, a bottomless well of energy. He suddenly understood that drinking was sapping his lifeblood. By the time he returned from his run, Bush had made an enormous decision, and he delivered a simple message to his wife and friends, a steady crew from deep in the west Texas oil patch: He was giving up drinking. Right now. Cold turkey. Years later Bush would say he didn't know whether he had a clinical problem with alcohol, but he knew that he was betraying his body.

By most accounts, Bush just walked away from booze and has never had another drink (when he ran for governor of Texas in 1994, wags noted he had quit drinking the "Republican" way, while his opponent, Ann Richards, had beaten her alcohol problem with a "Democratic" approach—group rehab). With his decision to quit, two things happened. First, the pure energy Bush had always relied on slowly but steadily began to creep back into his life. For a man like Bush, who'd played baseball, football, and basketball in prep school and who had always been such a physical creature, it was like rediscovering an old ally. Second, the success gave him the strength and inspiration to muscle his way through other physical changes—changes that would leave him today, in his mid-fifties, in better shape than in his mid-thirties.

One morning, for instance, Bush arrived at the Chevy Chase Club outside Washington, D.C., to play a round of golf with his old college roommate, Terry Johnson. Bush announced he had quit smoking. Johnson asked when. "This morning," cracked Bush. "I told Laura I'm not going to smoke anymore."

The pair teed off. By the ninth hole, Johnson could see that Bush was actually starting to shudder and shake. Johnson suggested they retreat to the clubhouse and take a breather, but Bush waved him off and insisted they finish the round.

In time, Bush found a rhythm, and a new addiction, that lingers to this day. Though he'd always been a jogger, he became more dedicated than ever to his daily workout. Today he runs whenever he can, trying to get in at least 3 miles and trying to finish each mile in less than 8 minutes. In 1992, he entered a marathon in Houston and finished in 3 hours and 44 minutes. Not long after, he compared politics to running. "It's a stamina race," he told a neighbor.

PERCENTAGE OF PEOPLE WHO SAY THEY RESPECT A PERSON LESS IF HE SMOKES: 21

INSPIRE THE MIND

When he was a kid, Bush's heroes (aside from his father) were baseball players. He pitched for the Yale freshman team. He idolized Willie Mays. He mailed baseball cards to the game's best players and asked for autographs. Today he has a treasured collection of 250 autographed baseballs that he takes to every new office he settles into.

In early 1989, Bush borrowed $600,000 from friends and bought himself 1.8 percent of the Texas Rangers. The result was not only the first real business success Bush ever had (he eventually sold his interest for nearly $15 million) but also an environment in which he thrived personally. Suddenly, he was surrounded by men who inspired him—men who, it's worth noting, knew better than most the value of perfecting the body and the mind–body connection.

During that period, Bush grew especially close to someone he would simply identify as a hero—Rangers pitcher Nolan Ryan. Baseball's all-time strikeout king was one of the most disciplined men ever to play the game, and he was famous for pushing himself to extremes in the gym—and for defying old, stale notions of what the body can do as it ages. If Bush needed somebody to serve as a role model, Ryan was it. Well into middle age, Ryan could still throw as hard as a teenager, and that fact rubbed off on the people around him. Consciously or unconsciously, Bush had gravitated toward someone whose example could keep him motivated and working hard.

"Nolan and I often exercised together," Bush once said. "I would run on the warning track or on the streets around the ballpark, and then go to the clubhouse to lift weights. He was almost always there. I marveled at Nolan's work ethic and intensity. I watched him prepare for games, then come back to the clubhouse to work out again after a game. God gave him the talent to be a good player; his hard work and drive made him great."

As the public face of the Rangers, Bush thrived in a way he never had thrived before. Friends said he seemed happier than ever, and the job gave him the profile and credibility he needed to make a successful run for governor of Texas in 1994.

FEED THE SOUL

Bush is much better at impulse than introspection. One day, when a veteran Texas writer came to interview him for an in-depth piece, Bush stared across his cluttered desk. "You're not going to write some goddamned psychobabble, are you?"

But as he searched for more discipline in his life, Bush attended to mental and spiritual sharpness as well. He cleared his mind and restocked his soul. He grew especially close to Donald Evans, now secretary of commerce and perhaps Bush's best friend in life. Evans was a jogging partner, but also someone who taught Bush to focus, relieve stress, and take time to replenish his mind and body. Bush and Evans co-owned a boat in Texas, and Evans encouraged his friend to use it often.

Bush also began to pay more attention to his spiritual side. There's little evidence that he was overtly religious before the mid-1980s. He had grown up Episcopalian, but converted to Methodism when he got married in 1977 (though he once told a reporter he was unclear what the exact doctrinal differences were). But around the time he quit drinking, Bush began talking to the evangelist Billy Graham, a longtime friend and advisor to the Bush family. In the aftermath came an apparent religious awakening that continues to this day. Did his public embrace of religion help Bush politically? You bet. Christian conservatives have been key to his electoral success. But discovering his spiritual side truly seems to have helped the impulsive Bush stay focused. Every morning, according to one friend, he takes a quick-hit read from a book

LOOK COMMANDING, CHIEF

Just like his predecessor, George W. Bush likes to run. But instead of topping off his 30-minute jog with a Big Mac, Bush hits the weights.

"He wants to make sure he looks good in a suit," says Jeff Madden, strength and conditioning coach at the University of Texas, where Bush worked out when he was governor of Texas. So he tries to run 4 days a week to stay lean, and follows with an intense upper-body workout twice weekly to build a powerful-looking chest and chiseled shoulders and arms.

But the workout is for more than just vanity's sake. "His goal is to project a strong image to the country and the world," says Madden. And that helps Americans feel more secure, which in turn makes his job more secure. "Having a strong physical appearance helps reassure people the guy in charge is on top of his game," says Lee Sigelman, Ph.D., Columbian Professor of Political Science at George Washington University.

Try the President's workout, courtesy of the White House. It'll keep you looking strong and fit, which benefits you even if people don't preface your job title with the word "mister."

The Cardiovascular Workout

Run for 30 minutes 4 days a week at an intensity that allows you to talk only in short spurts. President Bush manages 3 to 5 miles each workout, keeping at least an 8-minute-per-mile pace.

The Resistance Workout

The President's weight workout usually consists of upper-body exercises only, with the focus on his chest, shoulders, and arms.

The Exercises:

- Arm curl—three sets of 10 repetitions
- Incline bench press—one to three sets of 10 repetitions
- Chest fly—one to three sets of 10 repetitions
- Bench press—one to three sets of 10 repetitions
- Lat pulldown—one set of 30 repetitions

For exercise descriptions, go to www.menshealth.com.

of easy-to-digest Bible verses called *One Minute Bible*. For him, it's a simple way of feeding his mind and soul.

TAKE COMMAND

Bush's presidential honeymoon seemed to expire quickly; by the time August 2001 rolled around, even some members of his own party had doubts. That month, he ducked out of Washington and headed to his ranch to chop trees and run miles through the withering, smothering Texas heat.

For some people, just walking from an air-conditioned SUV to the front door of the mall is grinding when temperatures are well above 100°F. But Bush stuck to his plan. He kept jogging. He cut down more cedars. He broke a sweat. And he made time to nourish his mind, listening to the rhythm of the water and watching the arc of his fishing line.

Through it all he didn't seem disturbed by the critics who were railing about his being away from work too long—that he was out there getting in shape while there was "real" work to be done.

And then, of course, came September 11—among the most brutal days any president, or this nation, has endured.

The people, reeling and wounded, waited to study Bush's language. Not just the words coming out of his mouth but the physical language, the way he delivered the words, the way he carried himself. And he impressed nearly everyone. In the days, weeks, and months that followed, even his fiercest critics (including the ones who still want to debate him on his policies) began to concede that at least he was walking tall, looking in charge.

These days, President Bush is clearly resolute. He goes to work at 7 A.M., but he still takes time to hit the weights and put in the miles on the treadmill (or the trails around Camp David). He knows the steps that have brought him this far, and he's determined to stick with them as he—and the rest of us—wage the fight of our lives in this war against terrorism.

Know Your Power Hours

Want to make your day more productive? Start watching your body clock

By Francine Parnes

Think of the things in your life that don't run on time—trains, planes, the cable guy. Now think of the things that actually stick to their prearranged schedules—ball games, bowling leagues, happy hour.

Common theme: Where there's chaos, there's stress. Where there's order, there's beer.

So why should we tolerate workdays that feel as chaotic as January at O'Hare? Because, between meetings, phone calls, and surprise Gorilla Grams, it's almost impossible to stick to your well-intended plan. But if you can follow these simple guidelines throughout the day, the payoff will be huge: less stress and more energy, which means bigger raises and earlier quitting times.

No, we can't tell you how to do your job better. But your body can.

BEST TIME TO DO THE HARDEST THING YOU'LL DO ALL DAY

Early morning. Your personal periscope isn't the only thing to rise a couple of hours before you wake up. The stress hormone cortisol does, too. And this change increases your blood sugar level, giving you the energy and momentum to manage difficult situations effectively, says Norbert Myslinski, Ph.D., an associate professor of neuroscience at the University of Maryland. While too much cortisol can make you feel overwhelmed, it's also what contributes to the "fight-or-flight" ability to finish that project that's hanging over your head—or to storm in and ask for a raise. Bonus: The morning is also the time when you're least likely to activate ulcers.

BEST TIME TO MAKE A PRESENTATION

10 A.M. Morning is the time of day when your voice is most rested. And by 9 or 10, you've had a chance to drink some water; a good dose of hydration will help eliminate early-morning raspiness. Avoid milk, though. For some people, dairy products can increase mucus production, says Clark A. Rosen, M.D., director of the University of Pittsburgh voice center. Phlegm impresses first graders, not the chairmen of the board.

BEST TIMES TO STRETCH

10:30 A.M., 2:30 P.M., 4:30 P.M. Stretch every few hours to avoid back and shoulder tightness that comes from hunching over a keyboard, says Keith Cinea, C.S.C.S., of the National Strength and Conditioning Association. Clasp your hands behind your back and lift them straight up; hold for 10 seconds. This will open your chest and relax your shoulders and back. To stretch your glued-to-the-chair glutes, cross your left leg over your right, resting your left ankle on your right knee. Bend forward at the waist and hold the stretch for 10 seconds. Then switch legs and repeat. Don't forget to close the door first.

BEST TIME TO MAKE MAJOR STRATEGIC DECISIONS

Late morning. This is when your body temperature is rising, your alertness is up, and your brain's ability to process information is at its best, says Timothy Monk, Ph.D., a psychiatry professor at the University of Pittsburgh's sleep and chronobiology center. Most people also find they're best at problem solving around now. Scientists think your rise in temperature may be what keeps your mind more aroused. And why we keep asking for a transfer to Curacao.

BEST TIME TO MAKE YOUR MOVE ON THE NEW TALENT DOWN THE HALL

11:55 A.M. Lusting after a coworker? Ask her out just before lunch—when her mood is likely to be best, says James Sniechowski, Ph.D., coauthor of *The New Intimacy*. "People are usually more receptive right before they leave for lunch because their minds aren't cluttered with what they have to do that day or what they're planning to do when they get home," Sniechowski says. Even if she responds with "Cou—(loser)—gh," it won't bother you. Depression tends to peak early in the day.

BEST TIME TO READ TEDIOUS REPORTS WITH LOTS OF NUMBERS IN THEM

Early afternoon. Your vision is often a bit blurry in the early morning and sharpens over a few hours, says Thomas Friberg, M.D., chief of retina services at the University of Pittsburgh medical center.

BEST TIME TO SNACK

2 P.M. Eat a handful of nuts. The protein will increase your energy, and the fat will keep you full until dinner. "You wouldn't drive your car to the office with the 'empty' light flashing at you," says Jackie Berning, Ph.D., R.D., a spokeswoman for the American Dietetic Association. "But that's basically what you're doing to your body if you don't have a couple of snacks throughout the day."

BEST TIME TO FIRE SOMEBODY

Midafternoon. Even if you have to ruin your employees' day, you don't have to ruin their lives. Heart attacks are more likely to hit in the first 3 hours after you wake up than at any other time, says Richard Stein, M.D., a spokesman for the American Heart Association. So avoid doing dirty work before 10 A.M.—when stress can trigger a coronary.

PERCENTAGE OF MEN WHO SCRIBBLE NOTES ON SCRAPS OF PAPER TO REMIND THEM OF APPOINTMENTS: 53

PERCENTAGE WHO KEEP THEM IN THEIR HEAD: 55

PERCENTAGE WHO SCROLL THEM ON THEIR HANDS: 16

BEST TIME TO DRINK COFFEE OR TAKE A WALK

3 P.M. While other people rely on the caffeine method to jump-start their central nervous systems in the morning, you can use it to get you through the afternoon slump. Drink 8 ounces of a caffeinated drink about 30 minutes before a meeting, and you'll feel more alert. Sworn off the stuff? Take a brisk 15-minute walk around the halls. It'll help restimulate the hormones associated with alertness, says David Pearson, Ph.D., an exercise scientist at Ball State University.

BEST TIME TO MAKE OR RETURN CALLS

3:30 P.M. Waiting for that caffeine to kick in? Do mindless tasks (ones that won't get you fired). Some person-to-person stimulation—even over the phone—can help revive you enough so you can finish the day strong, says Martin Moore-Ede, M.D., Ph.D., president of Circadian Technologies in Lexington, Massachusetts.

BEST TIME TO TEE OFF WITH CLIENTS

4:50 P.M. Typically, hand–eye coordination reaches optimal levels in the late afternoon, says Lynne Lamberg, coauthor of *The Body Clock Guide to Better Health*. So put it to good use by squeezing in nine holes, answering e-mail, or shattering your record in Quake III.

The *Men's Health* Charm School

Sure, brains and brawn come in handy. But they're nothing compared with the fine art of smooth

By Hugh O'Neill

Men are suspicious of charm. The word is freighted with suggestions of superficiality, of a guy who only talks a good game. Charm evokes images of oily 18th-century French guys in wigs, usually played by John Malkovich. Or even worse, for those of us with gender anxiety, charm seems female. Jackie Onassis and Pamela Harriman were charming, dynamos in the drawing room. Men don't do drawing rooms. We aspire to be strong, skilled, and steady in a storm. But charm isn't always high on the male ambition list.

NUMBER OF TIES THE AVERAGE GUY OWNS: **20**

NUMBER OF PAIRS OF UNDERWEAR HE OWNS: **15**

Big mistake. Though charm is no substitute for competence or character, for any of the traits with *cojones*, it's a keen extra arrow for your quiver. Genuine American male charm makes colleagues more cooperative, rivals less determined, clerks less rude, and women more willing to take off their clothes and rub up against you.

Note the modifying adjectives: *American* and *male*. The charm we covet is no Euro polish, and no mere liturgy of fork selection. Yes, a man should be able to dine at the palace without an international silverware incident. But we're stalking bigger game here. We're after a graciousness of spirit that makes etiquette seem silly, one that springs, when rightly summoned, from some kink of the Y chromosome.

Forget all those charm *tricks*, like parroting a person's name every 6 seconds or imitating his pattern of speech. The charm we seek isn't studied or deliberate; it grows from the inside out, nourished by fundamental male energies. Once you have a charming heart, you won't need no stinking rules for 163 different occasions. The right moves will just come to you, the way they come to Jordan once he's airborne in the lane.

Start by accepting the beguiling ideas below. Then you'd better brace yourself, boy, because your life is about to be filled to the brim. You're about to get much of what you've wished for.

CHARM PAYS ATTENTION

The most oft-cited feature of charm is the ability to focus on the person you're interacting with. Over and over, people describe charmers with some version of "He makes you feel as though you're the only person in the world." Former top kick Clinton is famous for his ability to make every housewife in Hot Springs believe he felt her particular pain. By my lights, Bubba abused the blessing, but it's tough to argue with his career arc. And anyway, the principle trumps politics. The best gift we can bestow is our attention. It makes people feel valuable.

A brief aside: Occasionally throughout what follows, I may suggest that treating people with respect is the backbeat of male charm. If you, like most of our staff members, are sickened by that idea, keep this in mind. The goal remains as self-serving as it gets. In return for a little fake respect, you'll be able to charm the pants off anybody you'd like to see with no pants.

Some so-called experts say lots of eye contact is the key to paying attention. Wrong. In my view, this intense eye contact stuff is creepy. To women, the term "stalker" is rarely a charming word association. And to men . . . well, let's just say that when guys lock onto me with their lamps, I find myself vibing, "Hey, look somewhere else, Svengali, or I'll clean your clock for you." Sure, now and then it's important to look into folks' eyes. It's even a pleasure to witness the plain humanity in faces. But skip the psychohypnotist Death Stare routine. Instead, try this broader attentiveness head game.

Every time you interact—be it an early-morning driveway exchange with a neighbor or a meeting of a dozen heroic editors dedicated to enriching the lives of men everywhere—imagine that you're a chosen few, the knights of some round table. You're in a bubble together; the rest of the world doesn't exist. No matter how modest the exchange, feel that everything that really matters is happening right here and right now.

CHARM IS MISCHIEVOUS

Don't let life's routine put out the gleam. To wit, it's 1965 and a father is driving along the Garden State Parkway with all nine of his clan jammed into the family Ford. Right after greeting the toll taker as though he's actually happy to see him, our man extends a dollar, saying, "Take out for the guy behind me, too."

On the far side of the tollbooth, there is much headlight flashing and horn honking, kids waving in solidarity from backseats. And as the stranger sweeps by, two American fathers at full throttle salute each other. This is among the most charming dimes ever spent. The gesture had an impish quality. It said there are surprises out there yet. We need not be hobbled by habit. We're free to resist, in little ways, the soft shackles that subdue us.

You know that woman you're married to? Try something just a little different tonight when you get home from work. Hug her softly from behind and kiss her head tenderly. Leave her an affectionate note because she deserves an affectionate note and because it jumps the tracks of till-death-do-us-part familiarity. This shouldn't happen often—just now and then. Charm is just a little playful, polishes up common days.

A note on language: Clichés scream routine, send the message that we're just hamsters on this wheel. Consider the Grand Canyon of charm between the hackneyed "Nice to see you" and the very similar but far more charming "It does me good to see you." (Hit the "you" just a touch.) The first bromide sucks the air out of a room; the second twist actually suggests that a person's mere presence is tonic for your weary soul. The charming man creates something brand new for your ears. You're much too special for off-the-rack language; you get the custom-made.

CHARM SMILES—SORT OF

Technique-oriented charm mavens often recommend deploying a smile. I'm skeptical. To be sure, the full-wattage smile of an exuberant male is currency. But only if it's the good goods. For my money, deliberate smiles tend to look just that—deliberate.

Real men are quick to laughter, but they don't slap on a grin for a purpose. They're what Roald Dahl called eye smilers. Their eyes twinkle, betraying a readiness for the game. By me, constant smiles are weak, even silly. But a glint in the eye is strong. It suggests that you're more than momentarily

CHARMS AND THE MAN

Making an Escape

The party is cooking, and you're trapped talking with Paul, who is telling you all about these mysterious structures in Egypt. ("They're called pyramids!")

First, don't feel guilty. You're entitled to enjoy life. Second, don't slip away subtly. Charming men don't disappear from conversations. They check out of them—often reluctantly, always politely.

Tell Paul you're fascinated ("What did you say they were called? Pyramids?") and you've enjoyed talking to him, but you need to catch a colleague before he splits. Then, as you turn to leave, ask Paul for his business card—as though he's a guy you definitely want to stay in touch with.

Here's Looking at You, Kid

We like a fellow who has a low-key respect for occasions, whether they happen in a baptismal or a barroom. A man who can propose a toast, stand and deliver just a few simple words to exalt the assembled, is much to be cherished.

Most common mistake: Men clink their glasses to show off—either their cleverness or their baritone. Keep in mind (1) brief, (2) sincere, and (3) big picture. A proper toast chooses a small detail about our man—a trademark phrase, a characteristic gesture, a favorite point of view—and uses it as a window into his greatness. Yeah, that's right, greatness. A toast doesn't use such words, but it finds heroism in all the daily things we do. Remember, the target of a toast is actually everybody in the room. We're all enriched just by knowing the toastee.

Democratic Spirit

Men with charm treat both the doorman and the duke with the deference a child of God deserves. They're interested in the human flame, not accidents of biography.

Chauffeuring a Sot

Your ex-roomie is drunk again, headed for his Cutlass. Don't open with the old hurl-his-keys-into-the-reservoir trick. Your first move shouldn't even mention his condition. Shaming intoxicated men in public is only a good plan if you want a police car on the scene. Sidle up to him, with your own keys clearly jangling in your hand, and say, "Take a quick ride with me, old buddy. . . ." Your tone suggests you've got something you need to talk to him about—and only he will do. Then add, "I need 10 minutes with you, my man . . ." and finish your thought with either "to pick your brain about how I'm going to salvage what's left of my career" or "to tell you an unbelievable story about the new redhead in accounting."

As you steer him toward your car, sweep him up in your enthusiasm about talking to him. Guide him into the passenger seat, and end up driving him home.

Death-Defying Style

Men are important at mourning moments. In part, just because we're big and strong. Women and kids look to us for hope when the boats hit the rocks. Going to funerals is charming. It's a sign of respect.

Along with your dark suit, remember to pack a reminiscence or two of the deceased. Best are brief, simple, and specific memories that savor one of the deceased's distinctive traits—her kindness, her laugh, her fanatical devotion to the Mets. If you've got recollections her kids haven't heard before, great. But originality doesn't count here. Familiar stories unite tribes, too. Sharing them is tribute.

And remember to reach out. A man's hands are powerful tools, too rarely deployed. They break the shell between us with a pat on the forearm, a squeeze of the upper arm, a momentary touch on a shoulder or back. In moments of pain, pass love and reassurance through your hands into others' hearts.

amused, but rather constantly delighted by the whole, ever-loving human comedy. Charm is a pilot light of possibility, not an open flame.

CHARM THINKS YOU'RE GREAT

According to an almost surely false legend, someone once asked Queen Victoria, who ruled for 64 years back when the throne had influence over something other than tabs, if she preferred the company of Benjamin Disraeli or the other dazzling prime minister of her day, William Gladstone. She replied that when she dined with Mr. Gladstone, she left the meal thinking he was the most interesting person in all of England, but that when she ate with Disraeli, she felt *she* was the most interesting person in all the realm.

That's about as good a definition of charm as you'll find. Our man makes others feel proud of themselves. I've heard F. Scott Fitzgerald get credit for the line that the greatest gift you can give anyone is to see them exactly as they wish to be seen. If he didn't say it, I hereby claim it.

Unfortunately, sometimes this element of charm is blindsided by our Hemingway gene—also known as our stupid all-American male compulsion to tell it like it is. *Hey, man,* whispers the gene, *we haven't got time for this bullshit or that charade.* Plain truth: Seeing through people is big-time boring. It takes no ingenuity to catalog the myriad ways in which people are limited or preposterous or clumsy or vain. Fish in a barrel, my brother. The intrigue lies in digging the thousands of small ways in which many of us are splendid. Charm spotlights our gifts and is uninterested in our limitations.

Charm allows your brother the harmless belief that he's got vertical game. People don't have much to cling to in the storm. Make somebody feel like the most interesting person in all of England.

CHARM APPRECIATES

Frequent, low-key acknowledgment of our links is a hallmark of charm. Remember Mom's wisdom: Say thank you to the nice man. Be grateful for even small considerations.

Get epistolary. No, this doesn't mean "Buy a handgun." It's just a fancy phrase I've been trying to trot out ever since I learned it in college. It means "Write letters." In our rat-a-tat-tat, e-mail, download world, letter writing is a potent weapon. Actually, letters are too much work. Try notes. Master the art of the high-minded seven-word note.

Buy the following charm equipment: (1) Some cream-colored personalized stationery. (I like initials centered up top, but I'm not rigid.) (2) A foun-

PROPORTION OF MEN WHO HAVE THROWN OUT A PIECE OF CLOTHING BECAUSE IT WAS MISSING A BUTTON: 1 IN 4

tain pen. Yup, a fountain pen. Just do it. (3) A book of stamps. Stash the supplies in your desk. And every now and then, whip off a brief note of thanks to whomever—a business associate for a meal, your mother for teaching you how to swim, your buddy for lying to the cops.

The language should be simple and straightforward. It should feel like a fragment, just a yelp of much obliged. It's best if you have dashing penmanship, but your crabbed scrawl will do. Phone calls of thanks are okay; e-mails, too. But both are dwarfed by a handwritten huzzah delivered through the U.S. Postal Service. The moment of opening a letter is truly intimate. The sender had you in his heart as his sentiments passed through pen to paper.

CHARM REMEMBERS

Who among us hasn't met (or been) the following perfect example of not charming? Prince Charmless takes the new guy out for lunch—not his idea, the boss's. Over burgers, Fresh Meat mentions that this past summer he climbed Everest and earned that jagged scar across his face in a close encounter with an ice cave. Four days later, Mr. Clueless asks New Man if he's ever done any serious hiking.

We're often so swamped and/or self-centered—that would be a critique from a woman, but it's a secret password from me—that information about others bounces off our brains. It's not that we forget what folks tell us, but that we never actually bother to download the info in the first place.

When you first meet somebody, or when an acquaintance reveals some new little wrinkle, make a mental note of a few key details. ("Andy has a side business raising hamsters.") If you've got a lousy memory, buy a little book and jot things down. These notes, recorded right after my first meeting with some of the *Men's Health* editorial crew, helped convince them I was paying attention when they spoke.

"Joe Kita: grown man obsessed with the fact that he didn't make his high school basketball team."

"Dave Zinczenko: appears to believe he was once the best high school wrestler in Pennsylvania."

"Tom McGrath: insists the evidence was planted."

Nobody likes feeling that he's wasted his breath telling his epic story. You should have seen McGrath's face light up during our second meeting when I used the phrase "unlawful search and seizure." His passion had found a spot in my hard drive.

CHARM IS CONTRARIAN

Just as gems are valuable in proportion to their rarity, so too with some parts of the charm equation. Since we live in times that are informal and smart-assed, he who would stand out should swim against the tide—be a little bit formal and even, dare I say, sincere.

Speak with just a trace of courtliness. "Forsooth" is not required. But in our "Yo, bro" age, old-fashioned phrases like *I beg your pardon* and *I hope I haven't disturbed you*, mark you as a . . . what's that word? Oh, yeah . . . a gentleman. Through the talk radio spew, politeness actually makes a distinctive noise.

So, too, with being plainspoken. In our sarcastic society, men have lost the male power of plainness. We've traded Gary Cooper for David Spade. We've been diminished by the need to be clever, to make a joke out of everything. A charming man says what he thinks. Straight up, like whiskey. No smirks. No winks. It's no snap to go through an entire day saying exactly what you mean—without teasing, without any irony in your voice. Because we live in compulsively clever times, plain often becomes quite charming.

CHARM SINGS

Perhaps the most common male obstacle to charm is a little grouch who lives inside lots of men's heads. This grouch is suspicious of enthusiasm, of exuberance. Most of our fathers, not to mention most icons of male strength, are understated, strong silent types. We often confuse strength with severity. And we're just the slightest bit reluctant to risk being shamelessly upbeat.

Ten minutes ago, I overheard one of my colleagues shout out to another, "You make my job fun." He said it in a straight-ahead tone, joyful in his gratitude, unashamed by the simplicity of the sentiment. Charming. Strong. "I hate a song that makes you feel you're no good," said the troubadour Woody Guthrie. "I'm out to fight those songs to my very last breath of air and my last drop of blood." Charm has the confidence to sing praises.

CHARM IS ON A MISSION

Most of the charming men I've known are dashing, with a trace of the military officer about them. This doesn't mean they'll ask you to drop and give them 50, but just that they emanate a sense of shared purpose. We're in this together, sergeant. My father somehow managed to make you feel as though you and he were on a mission together—a mission to enjoy each other and to be mindful of everything you had. He made you feel as though he were a commissioned officer, charged with an obligation to shine up the small corners of every day.

CHARM LOVES WOMEN

A charming man makes women of all ages feel like beautiful young things. This is not accomplished by remarks like "Hey, Marie, your ass looks great in that skirt!" nor the more popular "Nice rack, Flo!" No, it's achieved by vibing an enthusiasm at a physical level.

Sure, maybe it's not going to happen because I'm married or I'm gay or I'm old enough to be your father or young enough to be your son. But the charming man somehow suggests—respectfully, of course—that if the two of us had met in another time and place, if the tumblers of fate had but put us together under different circumstances, I would have made a big-time run at you.

A woman should feel in the back of her mind that you've noticed her—as a sexual creature—and that her allures have you slightly pixilated. Of course, it all has to be conveyed with subtlety, grace, even a gentlemanly respect. But make no mistake, the most charming thing a man can be by a woman is dazzled.

OF THE MUSIC MAN AND GUYS LIKE YOU

The final truth about male charm is in *The Music Man,* the Meredith Wilson musical featuring our irresistible American rogue, Professor Harold Hill. Our man sells the parents of River City, Iowa, on the idea that the town needs a boys' band. Further, he peddles the Think System of musical instruction. Pay me now, goes his spiel, and the instruments will arrive next week, and, presto, 76 trombones in the morning sun.

The moms and dads want to believe that their kids are special and that there's beauty somewhere out there. When the charlatan Hill is revealed and he's hightailing it out of town ahead of a mob equipped with tar and feathers, he runs into Winthrop, the little boy who has fallen under his spell and is crushed by the thought that his hero is a shill. When the kid indicts him for pretending there was a band, Hill pauses for a moment and replies, as though just realizing something about himself, "I always think there's a band, kid."

Our man, the ultimate charmer, has fooled himself. He, too, wants to believe. He's determined in his soul to make the air sweeter. Finally, charm is no trick. It's not superficial at all. It's as deep as love. Charm is a generous con, a willingness of the heart. Charm hears the music, and wants to help you hear it, too.

My Quest for Cool

How a middle-age man discovered his inner James Dean

By Colin McEnroe

If it weren't for the Argentinian erotic aerialist performance artists, I would not have embarked on a project to see how cool I could become.

On the evening of February 24, 2000, I was at something called *Villa Villa,* which has been running for a long time in New York City, down at Union Square, and which involves young, attractive people, many of them Argentinian, swooping around on ropes while mist and rain pour down from the ceiling and wild carnival music plays. Occasionally the aerialists land and

DUMB THINGS GUYS OVER 40 DO TO LOOK COOL

- Get an earring
- Grow a ponytail
- Wear baggy jeans
- Buy "dude" cowboy boots
- Be the old guy at the young bar
- Buy a Harley (and it's your first bike)
- Get into rap music

- Say "Keep it real"
- Start tanning again
- Buy a shiny sports car
- Wear jeans shorts
- Take up snowboarding
- Get tattooed

dance semi-lewdly on the sopping floor with the audience and, in some cases, interact with the audience in a fully lewd manner. In the presence of untamed Third World carnality, it's hard not to feel frumpy, especially if you're 45 and escorting children, which I was. Even without children at my side, I was a poor candidate for flinging myself heedlessly into the happy madness, and if I did, would any of the cool, young people want me there?

I went home thinking there was nothing to be done, except to mark time until death, which I was already doing. I would simply live out my days, becoming gradually less cool. Eventually I would be so dull and out of touch that cool people would not be able to see me. I would be a poltergeist of unhipness, knocking over Palm Pilots to demonstrate my existence to pierced and scarred people listening to Chilean art rock.

But then I decided not to.

I thought of Fitzgerald's Nick Carraway and his "thinning briefcase of enthusiasms," of Prufrock measuring out his life in coffee spoons, and of Thoreau's claim that "the mass of men lead lives of quiet desperation." The greatest writers of Western civilization were telling me: Be cool or die. Okay, Thoreau would not have been down with the money I wound up spending at Urban Outfitters, but, hey, did I tell him what kind of beans to grow?

Why be cool?

Why not? Why not crackle with a little electricity when you walk through the produce department? Why not go through life being asked, "Where'd you get that shirt/haircut/CD/dog/wallet/entourage/grail/scar/Tibetan gong?"

The only real question is: How cool can you get?

Down the hall from my office is Athreb's Kinky Kinks, a creative hair salon catering to persons of color. Everybody who walks out of Athreb's Kinky Kinks looks cool. And when the stylists have nothing better to do, they work on themselves, which is how I happened to get on the elevator with a stunning young African-American woman whose hair was somehow braided and gathered into little neolithic spearheads.

"Wow," I said, adding, "I suppose there's not much you can do with boring middle-age White-guy hair."

"This is the year 2000," she shot back. "There's nothing we can do with our hair that we can't do with yours."

Somehow, this became a statement about something larger than just my hair. It's the 21st century. We have Prozac for dogs, and onions genetically modified to score in the 400s on the SATs. We have smart toilet paper and Ginkgo biloba Fizzies and Rick Lazio, the first android politician. Surely we have ways to make me cool.

I got off the elevator and walked back into my office. I looked out the window at the city spread out below me. Okay, so it was only Hartford; I have to live *somewhere*. I placed my hand on the dictionary and vowed, "By the ghost of Bobby Darin, I shall be cool again."

I didn't do much about it for several weeks.

"Won't everybody know what you're doing?" asked Tim Helmecki, one of the producers on my radio show. Helmecki is 27 and pulls off a sort of low-budget geek cool surprisingly well. "You go away for a day or two and come back with a new haircut and new clothes and stuff—how cool is that going to be?"

He had a point.

I decided I would start with something very simple. I would get cool shoes.

LA DOLCE FEETA

Where I live, there is a store, Strada, that sells nothing but capricious European shoes with names like Mephisto. I decided that the longest journey to cool would begin with a single step in these shoes.

The owner greeted me and showed me around.

"Have you ever owned shoes that address your feet?" he asked.

"I don't think so," I said. Maybe my shoes have always been addressing my feet, but both parties always seemed to be doing their best to ignore each other, under the circumstances.

I bought some Ecco shoes. It sounds Italian, but they seem to be made in Slovakia. When they began addressing my feet, what they said was "Get out! Or we will pinch the insides of your heels!" They were angry Slovakian shoes, still brooding about the forced Magyarizations of 1918. I was about $150 in the hole and had blown my shoe budget for the next 2 years, and I was not noticeably cool.

Cool people, however, do not worry about money.

AMOUNT OF MONEY THE AVERAGE MAN SPENDS ANNUALLY ON CLOTHES: 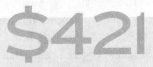 **$421**

AMOUNT THE AVERAGE WOMAN SPENDS: $584

THE APPLE

With nothing but the chump threads on my back, I went to New York City.

I had arranged to meet with Amanda Freeman, a "cool-hunter" with a firm called Youth Intelligence, based in a little brownstone in the West Village. They make money by figuring out what people in Gen X and Gen Y are going to want and then selling that information to Corporate America.

In me, a person too depressed to work backward through the alphabet and figure out whether he was Gen U or V, they faced a special challenge.

"You have to be true to yourself," said Freeman. "You could dress up in 18-year-olds' clothes, but you would look like you were trying too hard, and that wouldn't be cool."

If you want to have a "meeting" at YI, you sit down on an unoccupied couch, and other cool-hunters, as they drift around, plop down, and join the discussion if they feel like it. This resulted in several terrifying moments of cool-hunter frenzy, in which the YI people all began shouting (at me) the names of, say, wristwatches or eyeglass frames or, for all I knew, neurologists.

They were also willing to talk about the complexities of cool. Barbara Coulon observed that, as cool-hunters, they were regularly in touch with trendsetters who, by definition, were cool in ways that were not evident to the people around them.

"They tend to have something that nobody else has yet," she said.

"Does a fungus count?" I asked.

It was hard pinning them down to any specific program for me because if I did anything just because they told me to, instead of because I wanted to, it wouldn't be cool.

We finally agreed on a few things.

OVER-40 COOL

You know what's really cool? Being an adult. True cool rules when you've reached 40. Until then, the best you can do is be precool.

Consider these cool cats, and how you didn't hear a meow that mattered from them until they hit 40: Christopher Walken, Iggy Pop, Fred Rogers, Dennis Hopper, B. B. King, Humphrey Bogart, Charlton Heston, John Malkovich, Norman Schwarzkopf, Lou Reed.

These guys came close to cool but passed 40 and missed it forever: Sting, Charles Grodin, Bill Clinton, O. J. Simpson, Jackson Browne.

These yutzes will never be cool, unless they live to be 100 and die in bed surrounded by naked nurses: Al Gore, Brent Mussberger, David Spade, Ted Turner.

And the few, the proud, the drop-dead cool guys: Jimi Hendrix, Steve McQueen, Lee Marvin, William Holden.

- I would get my hair cut at the Astor Place salon, which is very cheap but, in a weird way, has become a hipper joint than many of the tony hair salons.
- I would get some different shoes, possibly at a place nearby on Broadway that nobody could remember the name of, except that the last word was "Shoes."
- I would come up with a look that was "simple, not crazy," possibly involving "a clean-looking outfit: a T-shirt with a simple design and plain-looking pants but in a different fabric" (one with a sheen or one that made noise when you crinkled it).
- I would try to layer, instead of wearing a sport jacket. "A sport jacket is something that will say you're 45," observed one of the trend spotters, who is so cool that her boyfriend was forced to become Cuban just to be cool enough for her, even though he is, technically, from suburban Connecticut.
- I would, at some point, get funky eyeglass frames. I've been stalling about getting bifocals, so much so that I actually have to remove my glasses and touch a menu to my cornea to read it. It seemed to me that buying really cool frames might cancel out the AARP ennui of that bifocal moment.
- I would pluck a lily growing between the feet of a giant and stain it with blood from the heart of a hummingbird. I made that one up, but there was kind of a fairy-tale-task quality to all of this.
- If I were caught or captured in my current chump condition, I would deny all knowledge of Youth Intelligence.
- The most important thing, said Amanda, was to remember that it is not necessary to be cool in every way. Most cool people are cool because they are passionate about one or two things.

"Actually, I think you're cool already," said Barbara Coulon.

Everybody nodded uneasily. The unspoken understanding was "You are cooler than you will be if you try to become faux cool and turn into some kind of a-hole."

FEAR ITSELF

Back out on the street, I walked a few blocks toward Broadway and was seized by a panicky desire to run back to YI and pound on their little door and beg them to come with me. Cool suddenly seemed too big for me to tackle alone. I had become codependent with my cool-hunters.

I made myself keep walking toward the shoe place, which turns out to be called No Difference Shoes, unless it's called something else. The last word is definitely "Shoes."

There were all kinds of fabulous shoes, but I really fell in love with a shoe by Camper, which is made in Spain and has soft, pliant leather uppers and thick rubber soles. They look kind of like bowling shoes, and each one is the weight of a good-size pork roast, and everybody cool in New York is wearing them.

I had to have them. They cost $150, which meant that I would have spent as much for shoes, in a week's time, as I had the rest of my adult life. I did not care.

I put them on and walked over to Astor Place. There were pictures of customers ranging from Judd Nelson to Jeff from 98 Degrees.

"Can you make me look cool?" I asked Luigi, my haircutter.

"I make you cool," he said.

After an interval of snipping, he said, "I got to ask you. There's cool, but, you know, I don't know how old you are. I mean, we get rid of this professor thing, but you don't want to look . . ." Here he struggled for a genteel version of "like an a-hole."

"Luigi," I told him, "I trust you. Do what you think is right."

He proceeded to give me a terrific haircut. I looked a little bit like the father of a guy from 98 Degrees, but in a good way.

I could feel layers of frumpiness being stripped away.

I was now cool enough to buy a bulky but funky wallet at Triple 5 Soul, virtually the only purchase in the store that did not require being a tautly muscled, rail-thin 22-year-old.

SHERBET

I had arranged to meet, the next day, with John Seabrook, author of *Nobrow: The Culture of Marketing—The Marketing of Culture.*

Seabrook, who writes for the *New Yorker,* specializes in the study of buzz and how buzz kind of trumps the old class-and-power structure.

It seemed to me that I should present myself as a newly minted cool person. I was waiting at the doors when Urban Outfitters opened. I bought a Ben Sherman shirt, shiny blue with a sort of motherboard print and notched short sleeves. I went to a street fair and bought some simple T-shirts.

I was running out of time before my appointment, but I was swept by a wave of revulsion for my pants. The pants I had worn to the city, plain chinos, had been plenty good enough for me until now. Now I could not face the prospect of meeting John Seabrook in SoHo in loser pants.

In a formal ceremony in the apartment, I repudiated my pants. "By the power of Helmut Lang, I renounce you!" I shouted at them. Then I put them back on because I still had to go shopping.

I began racing around the East Village, clutching my huge and compli-

NUMBER OF MEN WHO LET THEIR WIVES OR GIRLFRIENDS DO THE CLOTHING SHOPPING: 2 IN 3

THINGS TO DO AT 40 THAT, SURPRISINGLY, WILL MAKE YOU COOL

- Lose some weight
- Vote for someone who will cut taxes
- Yell at "those neighbor kids"
- Cut your hair short; pluck anything coming out of your ears and nose
- Don't make excuses

- Appreciate alcohol instead of gulping it
- Appreciate women rather than gulping them
- Say "I don't know" when you don't
- Scare your daughter's boyfriend because you can

cated Triple 5 Soul wallet and looking for those plain pants in a "different fabric," but I couldn't find anything that wouldn't look ridiculous on a middle-age mesomorph. I was in trouser hell.

In panic, I grabbed a pair of lightweight, artificially distressed, karate-style pants in an infected-snot color called moss. Back in the apartment, I combined them with the shiny blue Ben Sherman shirt and, trying to layer, put on a kind of raspberry-colored T-shirt underneath.

And then, in my thuddingly heavy pork roast shoes, I ran to meet Seabrook in SoHo. He showed up in a Chemical Brothers T-shirt and normal Banana Republic pants.

"I've never dressed like this in my life," I blurted, and then, in my shiny blue shirt, raspberry tee, and moss karate pants, I wailed, "I look like sherbet!"

"You're a little on the sherbety side," Seabrook agreed calmly.

He took one step back and said, "It doesn't all quite come together."

Without really linking this remark to my absurd outfit, Seabrook observed, "There is sort of a cool way of dressing that is not ostentatiously cool. If you want to look cool and it does not come from long years of looking cool, you have to do stealth cool."

Right before showing me places in SoHo where one could easily spend $1,200 and wind up looking like a slightly shinier version of the old Unabomber police sketch, he assured me that cool does not have to cost a lot of money.

Sometimes, said Seabrook, being able to tell a story of getting something cool for $3 is the coolest possible statement.

ALL COOL ON THE WESTERN FRONT

"Why are you wearing bowling shoes?" Helmecki demanded, looking at my Campers.

"These are not bowling shoes. These are Campers. They're incredibly cool. You can't even buy them around here. I bought them at that place at Broadway and 12th. I forget the name, but the last part is 'Shoes,'" I said.

"Never heard of it," he said. "They look like bowling shoes to me."

This was so unfair. I had the coolest shoes in Hartford, was the only person for miles around who had seen *The Virgin Suicides*, had the only ex-professor–98 Degrees–Astor Place haircut in my county. I was incredibly cool, and nobody knew it but me.

By experimenting, I discovered that to be recognized as cool these days, you have to dance right up to the line of nerd. One day I wore a Hawaiian shirt, khaki shorts, socks, and my dark brown Campers. I looked way cool, but an argument could also be mounted that I looked geeky and impaired.

I also discovered that if I did not make nearly constant efforts to reload my coolness clip, I would slide back into frumpiness.

One day, aware that I had not been noticeably cool for half a week, I begged Natosha, the stylish young Black woman at the front desk of the health club, to give me something cool to say.

"I want to say something that white people aren't saying yet."

She laughed.

"It's all good," she offered.

"Really?"

"It's all good," she said again.

I started saying it. Everybody says it now, but—you have to trust me—if I died tomorrow, my obit would include "He was probably the first White person in Hartford to say, 'It's all good.'"

I got better at layering. On a riverboat cruise, I had layered an old khaki shirt over a dark-gray T-shirt, which I wore with my infected-snot distressed karate pants and my ever-present Campers.

"I like your outfit," said a pert blonde woman not of my acquaintance.

"I'm trying to look cool, but I have no sense of clothes," I apologized.

"Yes, you do! Did you pick out that outfit?"

"Well, yes. Sort of." It seemed impossible to tell her that I had, as my pit crew, a high-priced New York cool-hunting firm and a best-selling author on trends.

"Well, then, you do understand clothes."

"It's all good," I told her.

NUMBER OF MEN WHO DESCRIBE THEMSELVES AS "EXCELLENT DRESSERS": 1 IN 2

KNOW THIS

Schmooze On Up

So you're notorious for wandering down the hall to sample the hazelnut blend in the marketing department's kitchenette. It's not goofing off; it's networking—and it can help your career. Researchers at the University of Cincinnati and Penn State found that office workers who take the time to venture out of their departments for a chat are likely to receive better evaluations from their bosses. The researchers say these cross-pollinators are able to bring fresh ideas to their departments and know how to act on them. Plus, they know where the best doughnuts are.

Pull the Plug

Hair plugs look fake, but there's a better reason to avoid getting them: You could easily end up with an infection. In a study published in the journal *Infectious Diseases in Clinical Practice*, researchers described the case of one man whose hair plugs got so badly infected that his body went into septic shock—a deadly condition in which bacteria spread through his entire body. "About one out of every thousand guys who get hair plugs ends up with an infection," says Bruce Hirsch, M.D., the study author. Fortunately, most hair plug infections aren't serious and can be treated with antibiotics. Your ugly new hair will persist, however.

Hair's the Answer

Here are three more newsflashes on the hair front.

- Harvard researchers have discovered that a protein called VEGF improves bloodflow to hair follicles, producing thicker hair. Drugs to increase VEGF production are in development.
- Clogged hair follicles and excess scalp oil cause a reversible form of balding called hair shedding. The dandruff shampoo Nizoral, however, appears to fight both symptoms and prevent thinning hair.

• Men taking Propecia have 280 more scalp hairs per square inch than men using placebos, according to a new 5-year study.

Zit Zapper

A new prescription gel combining two existing acne treatments (clindamycin and benzoyl peroxide) may be the most powerful topical treatment yet for the prevention of pimples. In clinical trials, the gel BenzaClin reduced the average number of acne-causing bacteria on patients' faces by 99.7 percent—within just 1 week of treatment. "Before BenzaClin, the best treatments reduced bacteria levels by only 30 to 60 percent," says James J. Leyden, M.D., a professor of dermatology at the University of Pennsylvania. The most common side effect of BenzaClin is dry skin.

Smelly Up to the Bar

Polyester was once known as the wonder textile. As in *I wonder why anyone would wear this.* Now the fab fabric of the 1960s and 1970s is making a stylish comeback. And it turns out that polyester is the material of choice for going to bars—it absorbs far less smoke than natural fibers. A physician and chemist in San Francisco, Rudolf Noble, M.D., Ph.D., found that polyester soaks up 30 times less smoke than wool, cotton, linen, or even rayon. Silk finished a respectable second to polyester.

DOWN THE PIKE

Regrow Your Mop

GlaxoSmithKline has developed a new hair-loss drug called dutasteride. In early clinical trials, men taking the drug experienced dramatic regrowth of hair. The company is awaiting FDA approval to sell the drug.

DOES IT WORK?

Wrinkle Remover

 We picked up a bottle of Downy Wrinkle Releaser ($4) and gave it a try. While it's no replacement for ironing, spraying it on a cotton dress shirt allowed us to smooth out even heavily creased areas with just one pass.

An iron-free trick for travelers: De-wrinkling your suit jacket in a steamy bathroom actually works. Except when the steamy bathroom is in a cheap motel with wire hangers, which are death to jackets. Or in a nice but distrustful hotel that locks . . . the damn . . . hangers . . . to the . . . closet rod! So pack the Lexon Passenger Folding Hanger ($25), with its wide shoulder supports. It even folds into a lint brush. Look for it at www.lexondirect.com.

Invisible Teeth Aligners

Do they work as well as braces? Yes, but only for minor crowding or gaps between teeth. If you have an Austin Powers–esque overbite, brace yourself—or, rather, have an orthodontist do it. The see-through technology, called Invisalign, is ideal mainly for cosmetic enhancements, says Normand Boucher, D.D.S., a clinical professor of orthodontics at the University of Pennsylvania. The dentist will take a mold of your surly whites and create a series of 12 to 40 nearly invisible plastic aligners. Each aligner is worn for approximately 2 weeks, incrementally straightening your chops in 6 to 18 months (the same time required for braces). Twenty-five percent of those in the market for straighter teeth are good candidates for Invisalign, says Dr. Boucher.

Under 21? Sorry, metal mouth. The precision of the Invisalign mold doesn't allow for still-maturing jawlines.

NUMBER OF TIMES THE AVERAGE GUY WILL
WEAR A PAIR OF JEANS BEFORE WASHING THEM: 12

WHAT'S THE DIFF?

Chinos vs. Khakis

Chinos are boring medium-weight cotton pants. Khaki is the boring tan color of those boring cotton pants. Khakis are boring tan chinos.

Pants vs. Slacks vs. Trousers

You wear pants, your dad wears slacks, Brits wear trousers. They mean the same thing—over here. The Brits, however, call underwear *pants*. Which is why, when visiting London, we avoid the whole subject. There was this misunderstanding, see . . .

Your Excuse vs. Your Explanation

Your excuse: "I forgot about dinner with your parents tonight because I was preoccupied." Your explanation: "I forgot about dinner with your parents tonight because I was preoccupied with thoughts of homeless puppies and trying to find a cure for cancer—while watching the NHL draft." Your better explanation: "I wasn't listening because I was too distracted by how darn beautiful you are."

Reluctant vs. Reticent

The first usually refers to an aversion—you're reluctant to go down on her. The second is about speech—you're reticent about asking her to go down on you.

TAKE ACTION

Hey, man, we know you work hard to bring home the bacon. So do we. And it's our job to make *yours* easier. That's why we've put together this top-notch list of strategies that will help you get ahead at work—without having to suck up to or sleep with your boss. (Note: If your boss looks like Halle Berry, skip this list and turn back to part two of this book, Turbocharge Your Sex Life.)

1. Give your boss an earful. Here's an easy trick to make your boss think you're bright: Speak loudly and quickly. A psychologist taped high school kids answering tough questions, and listeners were asked to rate the speakers' intelligence. Kids who spoke loudly and avoided *ums* and *uhs* were perceived as smarter. And it was easier to judge IQ accurately when listening without looking. So for job interviews and sales pitches, "phone contact first may help," says the psychologist Robert Gifford, Ph.D., of the University of Victoria in British Columbia. Same for a blind date.

2. Give 'em the business. Back when a cup of coffee cost a dime and a movie cost a nickel, the mass of men made their livings with their muscles. They built the Hoover Dam, erected the Empire State Building, and turned millions of damp basements into paneled palaces. Nowadays few of us wrestle with I beams, and far more make a living by tricking people into giving us money. The venue? The business meeting. Here are a few pointers for prevailing in style.

Stand tall. Before you walk into a room, stand sideways in front of a mirror. Your ears, shoulders, and hips should be in alignment; if anything slouches, suck it up.

Shake on it. The handshake may be old, but it's tried and true. Single pump. Go with firm but brief. Deal maker trick: You want the webbing between your thumb and index finger to touch the webbing between his.

Keep it small. A meeting should have three or four people. Fewer is a staring contest; more feels like an Expos game. The best ideas and deals come from three or four.

PERCENTAGE OF WORKERS WHO
WOULD SLEEP WITH THEIR BOSS FOR A RAISE: 9

WHO WOULD GO ON A DATE WITH THE BOSS'S KID: 5

WHO WOULD PICK UP THEIR BOSS'S DRY CLEANING: 2

Put your best foot forward. When you sit, sit back in the seat, but don't rest your back against the backrest, which can encourage slouching. Put one foot slightly in front of the other, which forces your hips forward and makes you look involved. If you have to cross your legs, go for ankle on knee. Avoid that slithery thigh-over-thigh look at all costs.

Toss them a slow pitch. Speak simply, and just a tad slower than you normally do. Use your natural voice; to find the perfect, grown-up tone, hum a few bars. The pitch at which you hum is the natural pitch of your voice. No squeaking, no barking.

Avoid coming on too strong. Don't suggest either (1) that you're convinced or (2) that you're trying to pressure him. He'll sign on when he sees the great opportunity you represent.

Show enthusiasm. Not the bubbly cheerleader kind, but the male energy that comes out of a man who knows his business and, more to the point, believes it matters.

Dole out the orders. Every meeting should end with a plan of action, and every attendee should have an assignment. Dan pulls the numbers from manufacturing. Judy drafts a preliminary letter of agreement. Fred works the shredder. Marching orders are vital—or you'll have the same meeting next week.

3. Tell 'em to "buzz off." Distractions at work waste your time. Here's how to banish them instantly.

E-mail alarms. Ring, squeak, buzz. Ah, new e-mail. You've got to see who it's from. *No, you don't.* Disable the e-mail announcement feature in Outlook by clicking on Tools/Options/E-mail Options/Advanced E-mail Options. Keep ads from popping up during your Web research by downloading NoAds, a free program at www.southbaypc.com/NoAds.

The great flood of office visitors. Close the door and tape a "Please do not disturb" note on it, asking coworkers to use e-mail instead. Route calls to voice mail.

The meeting staller. If a side conversation drains the mojo from your presentation, go silent. Soon you'll have everyone's attention, says Ginny Pulos, CEO of Ginny Pulos Communications, which coaches executives in leadership skills.

The office mouth. When a chatty coworker comes into your office, stand up or meet him at the door. This says, "I'm here but I'm busy," says Paul Radde, Ph.D., an organizational consultant in Austin, Texas. It's your time—defend it.

**IN A STUDY OF 1,400 MANAGERS,
THE PERCENTAGE OF MANAGERS WHO PREFER
E-MAIL OVER OTHER CHANNELS OF COMMUNICATION: 41**

The poorly timed phone call. Take control of the conversation to get the caller to cut to the chase. State your time limit, but frame it with encouragement: "I'm glad you called, Jim. I only have a minute. How can I help you?"

The noisy open office. If your cube is next to the watercooler, pick up Sony's MDR-NC5 Noise Canceling Headphones ($100; www.sonystyle.com). Designed to block out engine noise on a jet or train, they'll also filter out office chatter.

4. Lead by example. Whether you're the boss or an underling, it's best to keep cool when the heat is on. Boston chef Eric Brennan has handled dinner rushes at high-end restaurants for 25 years. Have a late project going up in smoke? Try his recipe for staying focused amid chaos.

Plan ahead and prioritize. "I'll look at the reservation list, and if I see that we're going to get creamed at 8 P.M., I'll shuffle guys around to a needed area, even ask for help from the in-front managers."

Fake calm. "I can't show any panic if I want my staff to remain focused. When it gets busy and I need them to step up the intensity, I'll change the tone of my voice and get rid of all outside influences in the kitchen. That lets them know that it's time to concentrate."

Never whine. "I never tell my staff how busy I am. They don't want to hear it. If they can physically see me working hard, that can be motivating. But just telling them of my busy life shows insecurity."

Don't scream at the staff. "I might not be consistently nice when it's tight, but afterward, I let them know it's not personal."

5. Recover gracefully from a screwup. Dave Righetti, the former Yankee pitcher, tells us that when he gave up a big hit, he'd keep his head up and trust his ability. That's good advice you can use at work. Here's more you can employ when you bungle things at the office.

'Fess up. Figure out who was affected, then quickly explain to your supervisor what happened, says Paul R. Timm, Ph.D., a management professor at Brigham Young University. Just the hint of a cover-up is a career crippler.

Offer solutions. Have strategies ready that will fix things—like landing another client or apologizing—says Audrey Lavine, who advises companies on efficiency.

Seek advice. Here's a trick. Ask your boss how he would have handled a similar situation. Suddenly you're showing good character, a desire to improve, and respect for his opinion.

Fix what's broke. Fix the system to prevent further mistakes, and present it in a written plan to your boss.

Take it seriously. Don't joke about the mistake; rationalize it; broadcast it; or blame others, says Bill Coleman, a senior VP at Salary.com.

Kick butt on your next project. If it's well-received, gracefully point it out to your superior, but don't brag, says Lona O'Connor, author of *Top Ten Dumb Career Mistakes and How to Avoid Them.*

6. Look the part. While wearing a clean, ironed shirt will certainly score you some points, the shirt has to fit, too. "Men tend to buy shirts that don't fit because they don't try them on before heading to the register," says David Stewart, a manager of men's wear for Kenneth Cole. Pick out your size shirt, pull it on, and drop your hands to your sides; the sleeves should end exactly $1/2$ inch below your wrist bone. A little long? Ask for a free alteration.

7. Go barber shopping. You're in Atlanta and need a trim before the big meeting. How do you avoid looking like Wile E. Coyote after the dynamite? Take a chair, pal. No waiting.

Talk to the man. "The biggest mistake a guy makes is getting a haircut that's wrong for him," says Peppe Baldo, who's been cutting rich and powerful hair at the Plaza Hotel in New York City since 1969. Barbers are trained to cut to the shape of your face—full or thin, square jaw or no jaw—so a good one will take a good, long look. Point out what matters to you: the thin spot on top, the annoying neck hair, that odd growth.

Never say "short." Drastic instructions lead to drastic actions, says Curtis Baker, owner of the Florida Barber Academy in Deerfield Beach. If all you want is a little trim, say you want a little trim. He'll know you mean haircut.

Share your history. Barbers know that hair grows $1/4$ to $1/2$ inch a month. So if it's been 6 weeks since your last cut, he'll know how short you like it by how much it's grown.

Show, don't tell. Indicate how long you want your 'burns. You want the hair on the sides of your head to fall above the ear? Put your finger on it. Don't like where he put the part in your hair? Draw one for him.

Keep talking. A good barber always asks how he's doing, says Baldo. Like it so far? Short enough? If he doesn't ask, tell him anyway.

8. Come out smelling like roses. What do you do when your deodorant deserts you, the Certs is long gone, or you've picked up an errant odor? We've assembled three common stinkin' scenarios and fumigated each one.

• Your breath is about to screw up a job interview.

The instant deodorizer: a packet of salt. Stir the salt into a cup of warm water and swish it around your mouth for about 30 seconds. "Odor-causing bacteria feed on an acidic environment," says Eric Shapira, D.D.S., a spokesman for the Academy of General Dentistry. "The salt solution helps neutralize the acidity by raising the pH level." No salt? Swish with plain water; it'll still help lower the bacteria.

THE MOST COMMON FASHION MISTAKE THE AVERAGE GUY MAKES: HIS SHIRTSLEEVES ARE TOO LONG

Sidestep the stink. Don't just swish your mouthwash; gargle, too. "The back of the tongue is the only place where the bacteria that cause bad breath grow in substantial quantities," says Jon L. Richter, D.M.D., Ph.D., of the Richter Center for Diagnosis and Treatment of Breath Disorders. Brush your tongue, and then gargle for 10 seconds with an antibacterial mouthwash, he recommends.

- You're giving off nervous premeeting B.O.

The instant deodorizer: the men's room. Grab two paper towels; put a small shot of hand soap on each, but wet just one. Now head into a stall, scrub your pits with the wet, soapy towel, and then wipe your skin with the drier, soap-only towel. According to John Romano, M.D., a professor of dermatology at Cornell Medical Center in New York City, this process will kill the offending bacteria while leaving behind just enough scent to pull you through the meeting.

Sidestep the stink. Wash with an antibacterial soap and dam the sweat flood with Certain Dri, a powerful antiperspirant. "It contains aluminum chloride, which forms little plugs in the sweat glands," says Dr. Romano.

- Your flatulence is going to kill the carpool.

The instant deodorizer: fresh air. Quick! Crack both front windows. The low-pressure zone outside the windows will suck out the gas. Key note: Keep the back windows closed. "When all the windows are open, inside air doesn't exit but is forced into the back," says Lou Bloomfield, Ph.D., a professor of physics at the University of Virginia.

Sidestep the stink. Eat less of whatever food triggered your spontaneous eruptions, and add more yogurt to your diet. "The active cultures will displace the bacteria that make the gas smell," says Mary Ellen Camire, Ph.D., a professor of food science and human nutrition at the University of Maine.

ANY QUESTIONS?

Parched at the Podium

Whenever I give a speech, my mouth gets so dry I almost choke. What can I do?
—G. B., Arlington, Texas

You could lip-synch, but you'd be screwed during the Q & A. Instead, try this. Just before taking the podium, eat a Granny Smith apple. It's the tartest of the apple bunch; the acidity stimulates saliva production, which will help keep your talk crisp and fluid. If things still feel gummy, try a chaser of olive oil. Swish a spoonful in your mouth and spit it out; it will keep your lips from sticking to your teeth, eliminating that annoying lip smack when you're behind a microphone, says Dan Zitt, a Random House executive who coaches authors who will be recording audio books.

If your talk goes into extra innings, keep a glass of water with a wedge of lemon handy. The water keeps you hydrated, and like the apple, lemon's acidity sparks saliva production. Just skip the coffee (caffeine can dry your mouth) and stay away from milk, yogurt, and ice cream; dairy products turn saliva thick as soup.

Don't Stretch the Youth

My bosses keep getting younger. Should I be dressing younger to keep up?
—J. I., New York City

Never. If you're in your thirties, say, and you start wearing young, trendy styles like Phat Farm, B.C. Ethic, and Stussy, you're going to look as if you're trying too hard to be hip. "Focus on dressing well, not younger; good taste and classic style are timeless," says Brian Boyé, *Men's Health* fashion director, who offers these guidelines.

Dress up: Stick to single-breasted, two- or three-button suits. They'll never be out of style.

Dress down: Go classic: A dark-colored three-button blazer and striped button-down shirt with khaki pants and black dress shoes.

PERCENTAGE OF PEOPLE WHO SAY THEY FEAR PUBLIC SPEAKING: 40

Casual: Don't take this word too literally. Sport a short-waisted solid-color jacket (breast pockets and zipper closure okay), long-sleeved button-down shirt, chinos, and brown leather shoes that tie.

On-the-Cuff Remarks

When I buy pants, I'm always wondering how much cuff should be riding on my shoes. What's the right place for a pant leg to break?
—K.Y., Olympia, Washington

To avoid bunching, a classic 1½-inch cuff should have a ¼-inch to a ½-inch break, says Richard Bowes, vice president and fashion director at Bergdorf Goodman in New York City. We didn't know what this meant either, but Bowes was nice enough to explain that when you're standing straight and still, the bottom ½ inch of the cuff should lie on the shoe. If your pants have slightly narrower cuffs—say, 1¼ inches—you should still keep an inch off the shoe so that just ¼ inch rests on it.

Fashionable at 40

I'm 40 and just got divorced. What should I wear when I go out so I won't look as if I'm trying to be 18 again?
—J.S., San Francisco

Besides Charlize Theron on your arm, your best tactic is to keep it simple, says Boyé. By now you probably have more money, experience, and taste than 18-year-olds (at least ones who aren't NBA lottery picks), so put that advantage in the form of a leather jacket or sport coat, a crisp white shirt, and a good pair of jeans. The message: You have style, cash, and, in the ladies' eyes, lots of potential. We like DKNY's leather jackets and Lucky jeans. And if you don't already have a classic white shirt, go find one at www.brooksbrothers.com.

The Name Game

Why do I sometimes blank on names of people I know? Any tricks for remembering and not looking like an idiot?
—G.L., Reno, Nevada

Think of your brain as an overworked phone system, says David Masur, Ph.D., director of neuropsychology at Montefiore Medical Center in New York City. Your cortex is the receiver, and its neurons are a web of phone wires that patch through information. You see hot lady X slinking toward you, and you know you know her. The switchboard lights up, neurons spark your long-term memory, but all you get is static. And here's the kicker. When you get static, you naturally think harder, mentally pummeling your brain for the information. "All that does is activate more neurons, which only increases the interference," says Masur. Blanking on names is a natural phenomenon that everyone experiences. Unfortunately, forgetting names becomes more frequent as we age and can start as early as 30, adds Masur.

Here's how to get total recall. If you need her name now, don't focus on the word itself. "That may bring up similar-sounding words you use more often, totally blocking the word you really want," says Daniel Schacter, Ph.D., a professor of psychology at Harvard University. Instead, try to remember where you met her—the supermarket, a buddy's party, the dressing room at Victoria's Secret. "Remembering the context of the meeting can spark the retrieval clues necessary for remembering her name," says Schacter. Bra . . . panties . . . belly. . . . "Hi, Ellie!"

The Future's in Plastics

I spent a lot of cash on a bottle of wine for a dinner party, and it turned out to have a plastic cork. Did I get ripped off?
—E. S., Washington, D.C.

Don't judge a wine by its stopper, says Jamal Rayyis, author of *Food & Wine magazine's Wine Guide 2002*. First ask yourself this question: Did your party enjoy the wine? If the answer's yes, you weren't ripped off. Odds are that your plastic-corked wine was actually in better condition than one with a natural cork, he says. More than 5 percent of wines sealed with cork are contaminated by a harmless but pungent compound called TCA (trichloroanisole). "It infuses the wine with the taste of wet cardboard," says Rayyis. Synthetic corks—made from plastic composites—are nearly immune to infection and are now used in about 10 percent of domestically produced wines. European vintners have been slower to go synthetic, but with the gradual decline of cork forests in Spain and Portugal, natural corks are becoming more porous, and more vulnerable to bacteria, says Rayyis. Expect to see even some of the world's premier wines sporting plastic tops in the coming years.

NUMBER OF MEN WHO, IN AN EMERGENCY, WOULD SECRETLY USE ANOTHER PERSON'S TOOTHBRUSH: 1 IN 8

NUMBER WHO WOULD EVENTUALLY CONFESS: 1 IN 4

Index

Underscored page references indicate boxed text. **Boldface** references indicate illustrations.